Study Guide
Cooper & Gosnell

Foundations and Adult Health Nursing

Eighth Edition

Candice Kumagai

Formerly Instructor in Clinical Nursing
University of Texas at Austin
Austin, Texas

ELSEVIER

ELSEVIER
3251 Riverport Lane
St. Louis, Missouri 63043

STUDY GUIDE FOR FOUNDATIONS AND
ADULT HEALTH NURSING, Eighth edition

ISBN: 978-0-323-52459-9

Notices

Knowledge and best practice in this field are constantly changing. As new research and
experience broaden our understanding, changes in research methods, professional practices, or
medical treatment may become necessary.

Practitioners and researchers must always rely on their own experience and knowledge in
evaluating and using any information, methods, compounds, or experiments described herein.
In using such information or methods they should be mindful of their own safety and the
safety of others, including parties for whom they have a professional responsibility.

With respect to any drug or pharmaceutical products identified, readers are advised to check
the most current information provided (i) on procedures featured or (ii) by the manufacturer
of each product to be administered, to verify the recommended dose or formula, the method
and duration of administration, and contraindications. It is the responsibility of practitioners,
relying on their own experience and knowledge of their patients, to make diagnoses,
to determine dosages and the best treatment for each individual patient, and to take all
appropriate safety precautions.

To the fullest extent of the law, neither the Publisher nor the authors, contributors, or editors,
assume any liability for any injury and/or damage to persons or property as a matter of
products liability, negligence or otherwise, or from any use or operation of any methods,
products, instructions, or ideas contained in the material herein.

Content Strategist: Nancy O'Brien
Senior Content Development Specialist: Diane Chatman
Publishing Services Manager: Jeff Patterson
Project Manager: Carol O'Connell
Design Direction: Renee Duenow

Printed in the United States of America

Last digit is the print number: 9 8 7 6 5 4 3

Working together
to grow libraries in
developing countries

www.elsevier.com • www.bookaid.org

To the Student

Understanding fundamental concepts and principles of nursing will prepare you for patient care experiences. By mastering the content of your *Foundations and Adult Health Nursing* textbook, you will have the necessary knowledge and skills for nursing practice. This Study Guide was created to help you achieve the objectives of each chapter in the textbook, establish a solid base of knowledge in the fundamentals of nursing, and evaluate your understanding of this critical information.

Each Study Guide chapter is organized into sections, each with its own topic and related objectives from the textbook. Different types of learning activities, including short answer, multiple choice, table activities, matching, figure labeling, and critical thinking activities assist you in meeting these content objectives. To maximize the benefits of this Study Guide and prepare for the learning activities:

1. Carefully read the chapter in the textbook and highlight, note, or outline important information.
2. Review the Key Points, access the Additional Learning Resources, and complete the Review Questions for the NCLEX® Examination at the end of each textbook chapter.
3. Complete the Study Guide exercises to the best of your ability.
4. Time and pace yourself during the completion of each exercise. You should spend approximately 1 minute for each multiple choice and matching question, and approximately 2 minutes for completion activities or short answer questions.
5. After completing an exercise, refer to the textbook page references as needed. You can then repeat any exercises for additional practice and review. A complete Answer Key is provided on the Evolve Resources website.

ADDITIONAL LEARNING RESOURCES

Additional Learning Resources are available on the Evolve website at http://evolve.elsevier.com/Cooper/foundationsadult/.

Evolve

- Review Questions for the NCLEX® Examination (for each chapter)
- Calculators
- Fluids and Electrolytes Tutorial
- Immunization Schedule
- Spanish/English Glossary
- Additional Animations
- Additional Audio Clips
- Additional Video Clips
- Skills Performance Checklists
- Body Spectrum Electronic Anatomy Coloring Book

STUDY HINTS FOR ALL STUDENTS

- *Ask questions!* There are no bad questions. If you do not know something or are not sure, you need to find out. Other people may be wondering the same thing but may be too shy to ask. The answer could mean life or death to your patient, which certainly is more important than feeling embarrassed about asking a question.
- *Make use of chapter objectives.* At the beginning of each chapter in the textbook are objectives that you should have mastered when you finished studying that chapter. Write these objectives in your notebook, leaving a blank space after each. Fill in the answers as you find them while reading the chapter. Review to make sure your answers are correct and complete, and use these answers when you study for tests. This should also be done for separate course objectives that your instructor has listed in your class syllabus.

- *Locate and understand key terms.* At the beginning of each chapter in the textbook are key terms that you will encounter as you read the chapter. Page numbers are provided for easy reference and review, and the key terms are in bold, blue font the first time they appear in the chapter. Phonetic pronunciations are provided for terms that might be difficult to pronounce.
- *Review Key Points.* Use the Key Points at the end of each chapter in the textbook to help you review for exams.
- *Get the most from your textbook.* When reading each chapter in the textbook, look at the subject headings to learn what each section is about. Read first for the general meaning, then reread parts you did not understand. It may help to read those parts aloud. Carefully read the information given in each table and study each figure and its caption.
- *Follow up on difficult concepts.* While studying, put difficult concepts into your own words to see if you understand them. Check this understanding with another student or the instructor. Write these in your notebook.
- *Take useful notes.* When taking lecture notes in class, leave a large margin on the left side of each notebook page and write only on right-hand pages, leaving all left-hand pages blank. Look over your lecture notes soon after each class, while your memory is fresh. Fill in missing words, complete sentences and ideas, and underline key phrases, definitions, and concepts. At the top of each page, write the topic of that page. In the left margin, write the key word for that part of your notes. On the opposite left-hand page, write a summary or outline that combines material from both the textbook and the lecture. These can be your study notes for review.
- *Join or form a study group.* Form a study group with some other students so you can help one another. Practice speaking and reading aloud, ask questions about material you are not sure about, and work together to find answers.
- *Improve your study skills.* Good study skills are essential for achieving your goals in nursing. Time management, efficient use of study time, and a consistent approach to studying are all beneficial. There are various study methods for reading a textbook and for taking class notes. Some methods that have proven helpful can be found in *Saunders Student Nurse Planner: A Guide to Success in Nursing School* by Susan C. deWit. This book contains helpful information on test-taking and preparing for clinical experiences. It includes an example of a "time map" for planning study time and a blank form that you can use to formulate a personal time map.

ADDITIONAL STUDY HINTS FOR STUDENTS WHO USE ENGLISH AS A SECOND LANGUAGE (ESL)

- *Find a first-language buddy.* ESL students should find a first-language buddy—another student who is a native speaker of English and is willing to answer questions about word meanings, pronunciations, and culture. Maybe your buddy would like to learn about your language and culture. This could help in his or her nursing experience as well.
- *Expand your vocabulary.* If you find a nontechnical word you do not know (e.g., *drowsy*), try to guess its meaning from the sentence (e.g., *With electrolyte imbalance, the patient may feel fatigued and drowsy*). If you are not sure of the meaning, or if it seems particularly important, look it up in the dictionary.
- *Keep a vocabulary notebook.* Keep a small alphabetized notebook or address book in which you can write down new nontechnical words you read or hear along with their meanings and pronunciations. Write each word under its initial letter so you can find it easily, as in a dictionary. For words you do not know or for words that have a different meaning in nursing, write down how they are used and sound. Look up their meanings in a dictionary or ask your instructor or first-language buddy. Then write the different meanings or usages that you have found in your book, including the nursing meaning. Continue to add new words as you discover them. For example:

  - *Primary*—Of most importance; main (e.g., *the primary problem or disease*); The first one; elementary (e.g., *primary school*)
  - *Secondary*—Of less importance; resulting from another problem or disease (e.g., *a secondary symptom*); The second one (e.g., *secondary school* ["high school" in the United States])

Illustration Credits

Chapter 5
P. 26: Maslow A: *Motivation and personality*, ed 2, New York, 1970, Harper & Row.

Chapter 11
P. 63: Maslow A: *Motivation and personality*, ed 2, New York, 1970, Harper & Row.

Chapter 16
P. 92: Modified from Sheehy SB & Lombardi J: *Manual of emergency care*, ed 4, St. Louis, 1995, Mosby.

Chapter 17
P. 107: Clayton BD & Willihnganz M: *Basic pharmacology for nurses*, ed 17, St. Louis, 2017, Elsevier.

Chapter 23
P. 144: Elkin MK, Perry AG, Potter PA: Nursing interventions and clinical skills, ed 4, St. Louis, 2008, Mosby.

Chapter 31
P. 194: Hockenberry MJ, Wilson D: *Wong's essentials of pediatric nursing*, ed 8, St. Louis, 2009, Mosby.

Chapter 32
P. 203: Hockenberry MJ, Wilson D: *Wong's essentials of pediatric nursing*, ed 9, St. Louis, 2013, Mosby.

Chapter 41
P. 256: Harkreader H, Hogan MA, & Thobaben M: *Fundamentals of nursing: Caring and clinical judgment*, ed 3, St. Louis, 2007, Saunders.

Chapter 43
P. 270: Patton KT & Thibodeau GA: *The human body in health and disease*, ed 7, St. Louis, 2018, Elsevier.

Chapter 44
P. 275: Patton KT & Thibodeau GA: *The human body in health and disease*, ed 7, St. Louis, 2018, Elsevier.

Chapter 45
P. 281: Thibodeau GA & Patton KT: *Anatomy and physiology*, ed 10, St. Louis, 2019, Mosby.

Chapter 48
P. 301: Canobbio M: *Mosby's clinical nursing series: Cardiovascular disorders*, St. Louis, 1990, Mosby.

Chapter 51
P. 328: Patton KT & Thibodeau GA: *Anatomy and physiology*, ed 8, St. Louis, 2013, Mosby.

Chapter 52
P. 335: Thibodeau GA & Patton KT: *Structure and function of the body*, ed 14, St. Louis, 2012, Mosby.
P. 337: Seidel HM, Ball JW, Dains JE, et al.: *Mosby's guide to physical examination*, ed 7, St. Louis, 2011, Mosby.

Chapter 53
P. 343: Patton KT & Thibodeau GA: *Anatomy and physiology*, ed 10, St. Louis, 2019, Elsevier.
P. 344: Patton KT & Thibodeau GA: *The human body in health and disease*, ed 7, St. Louis, 2018, Elsevier.

Chapter 54
P. 351: Patton KT & Thibodeau GA: *The human body in health and disease*, ed 7, St. Louis, 2018, Elsevier.
P. 352: Ignatavicius DD, Workman ML, Blair M, et al: *Medical-surgical nursing: Patient-centered collaborative care*, ed 8, St. Louis, 2016, Elsevier.

Chapter 55
P. 359: Grimes D: *Infectious diseases*, St. Louis, 1991, Mosby.

The Evolution of Nursing

MATCHING

Directions: Match the nurse on the left with the contribution to nursing on the right. (4)

Nurse	Contribution to Nursing
_____ 1. Dorothea Dix (1802-1887)	a. Credited with the development of our present-day documentation system
_____ 2. Clara Barton (1821-1912)	b. Pioneer crusader for elevation of standards of care for the mentally ill
_____ 3. Mary Ann Ball (1817-1901)	c. Worked for acceptance of African-Americans in the nursing profession
_____ 4. Linda Richards (1841-1930)	d. Developed the American Red Cross in 1881
_____ 5. Isabel Hampton Robb (1860-1910)	e. Championed the rights and comforts of soldiers; organized diet kitchens, laundries, and ambulance service
_____ 6. Lavinia Dock (1858-1956)	f. Organized the first graded system of theory and practice in schools of nursing
_____ 7. Mary Eliza Mahoney (1845-1926)	g. Responsible for the development of public health nursing in the United States through the founding of the Henry Street Settlement in New York City
_____ 8. Lillian D. Wald (1867-1940)	h. Responsible, with Robb, for the organization of the American Society of Superintendents of Training Schools, which evolved into the National League for Nursing Education
_____ 9. Mary Adelaide Nutting (1858-1947)	i. Pioneer in nurse-midwifery
_____ 10. Mary Breckenridge (1881-1965)	j. Developed curriculum concepts and guidelines for student nurses

SHORT ANSWER

Directions: Using your own words, answer each question in the space provided.

11. Identify the role of the National League for Nursing (NLN) in nursing education. *(10)*_____

_____

_____

12. List the purposes of the National Association for Practical Nurse Education and Service (NAPNES) and the National Federation of Licensed Practical Nurses (NFLPN). *(10)*

_____

_____

_____

_____

13. Discuss the roles and responsibilities of the practical or vocational nurse in today's health care system. *(18, 19)*

_____

_____

_____

_____

MULTIPLE CHOICE
Directions: Select the best answer(s) for each of the following questions.

14. Which nursing actions are appropriate to the roles/responsibilities of the LPN/LVN? **Select all that apply.** *(19)*
    1. Uses active listening techniques when interacting with a depressed patient
    2. Reports changes in vital signs to the health care provider in a timely fashion
    3. Takes initiative to create a comprehensive care plan for a newly admitted patient
    4. Ensures that the correct medication is given to the correct patient at the correct time
    5. Collects data from the patient, the family, and previous medical records

15. Which statement by a male nursing student is **most** likely to represent a factor associated with the high attrition rate of male students from nursing education programs? *(8)*
    1. "The course of study is too prolonged and difficult."
    2. "I can make more money if I become a doctor."
    3. "The nursing instructors claim that I am not caring."
    4. "It's difficult for men to advance in the nursing profession."

16. A patient suddenly becomes unresponsive; therefore, he is unable to make decisions about health care options. What is the health care team **most** likely to do to determine the patient's wishes? *(6)*
    1. Contact the patient's closest adult relative.
    2. Determine if the patient has a personal attorney.
    3. Seek opinions from the patient's primary care provider.
    4. Review the patient's advance directives.

17. One of the major problems of hospitals of the early nineteenth century has been addressed by which measure in contemporary health care? *(2)*
    1. Focusing on women's health issues, such as heart disease
    2. Using Standard Precautions and improving hygienic practices
    3. Encouraging men to enter the nursing profession
    4. Reducing the nursing shortage during wartime

18. Which patient typifies the demographic changes of the population in the twenty-first century and represents an increased need for nursing care? *(8)*
    1. A 3-month-old infant with developmental disabilities
    2. A 15-year-old homeless adolescent
    3. A 45-year-old man with diabetes
    4. A 78-year-old woman with chronic illness

19. Which nursing action reflects Florence Nightingale's vision of how to improve patient care? *(3)*
    1. Includes the family in the patient education sessions
    2. Considers the patient's cultural and ethnic background
    3. Attends an in-service to learn about a new infusion pump
    4. Safeguards patient's privacy by maintaining confidentiality

20. Which situation includes the four major concepts that are the basis for nursing theories and models? *(17)*
    1. The home health nurse assesses the patient's health and the home setting.
    2. The nurse studies nursing theory in an advanced-practice nursing curriculum.
    3. Nursing programs draw from several psychosocial and nursing theories.
    4. The patient is treated for hypertension, diabetes, and obesity.

21. Which patient is **most** at risk for being one of the "medically underserved" in the United States? *(9)*
    1. A 30-year-old woman with newly diagnosed breast cancer
    2. An 86-year-old man who resides in a long-term care facility
    3. A 3-year-old whose parents recently emigrated for work
    4. A 65-year-old Vietnam veteran who lives on the street

22. Using Maslow's hierarchy of needs, the nurse gives **priority** to which problem? *(12)*
    1. Loneliness due to being away from family during hospitalization
    2. Inability to eat because of difficulty chewing and swallowing
    3. Anxiety due to recent diagnosis of cancer with poor prognosis
    4. Safety related to difficulty with balance during position change

23. A mother tells the nurse that her 17-year-old son, who is wheelchair-bound for 1 year following an accident, has been depressed because basketball season is starting and he was a star player for his high school team. Using Maslow's hierarchy of needs, which intervention would address the adolescent's **priority** need? *(12, 13)*
    1. Advise the mother to check the wheelchair access ramps for safe access to the gym.
    2. Explore other interests and activities that would increase his self-esteem.
    3. Initiate a review of body systems to identify the cause of depression.
    4. Suggest the mother and son seek out a wheelchair basketball team.

24. The nurse has identified that a 56-year-old woman has an increased risk for heart problems because of family history. Which modifiable factor(s) should be included in the teaching plan to promote health and self-help practices for wellness for this patient? **Select all that apply.** *(15)*
    1. Smoking cessation and stress reduction
    2. Use of advanced technology and new medications
    3. Weight reduction and decreased alcohol consumption
    4. Cost of health insurance and specialist care
    5. Control over decision-making that affects the patient's own body and health

25. Which set of tasks should be assigned to an unlicensed assistive personnel who has been cross-trained as a unit secretary? *(15)*
    1. Direct visitors and give out patient information.
    2. Take vital signs and restock medications.
    3. Validate transcriptions and interpret vital signs.
    4. Ambulate patients and order unit supplies.

26. Which action **best** demonstrates the nurse's consistent effort to contribute to cost-containment? *(26)*
    1. Obtains malpractice insurance
    2. Uses time and materials economically
    3. Questions excessive diagnostic testing
    4. Refers patients with no insurance to a sliding-scale clinic

27. The nurse is caring for a patient with immobility related to a chronic musculoskeletal disorder. Using Orem's theory of nursing, what would the nurse do? *(18)*
    1. Monitor for self-care deficits.
    2. Arrange pillows to provide joint protection.
    3. Support existing coping mechanisms.
    4. Encourage ambulation down the hallway.

28. The nurse is caring for several patients on the medical-surgical unit. Which action(s) indicate(s) that the nurse is providing care that adheres to the American Hospital Association's Patient Care Partnership? **Select all that apply.** *(6)*
    1. Ensures that the housekeeping staff empties the trash receptacles in a timely fashion
    2. Assists a patient to make a list of questions to ask about a surgical procedure
    3. Identifies a problem with a broken side rail and contacts the maintenance department
    4. Keeps up to date with the latest information on medications and side effects
    5. Ensures that every patient gets a private room with a window and private bathroom
    6. Contacts the hospital's financial counselor if a patient has questions about the bill

29. An intoxicated patient comes to the walk-in clinic and verbally threatens a nurse with bodily harm. The nurse refuses to care for the patient and informs the supervisor about the threats. Which document/concept supports the nurse's right to refuse to care for this patient? *(16)*
    1. Patient Care Partnership
    2. Position Paper of the American Nurses Association
    3. Health Care Providers' Rights
    4. Resident's Bill of Rights

30. Which action is outside the scope of practice for the LPN/LVN? *(19)*
    1. Offers suggestions to improve the patient's fluid intake
    2. Collects data on the patient while giving medication
    3. Makes independent decision about altering the care plan
    4. Uses therapeutic communication with a patient's family

CRITICAL THINKING ACTIVITIES

31. The nurse is interviewing a 65-year-old woman who has hypertension, which is well-controlled by blood pressure medication. She is retired, but recently started volunteering at her church. She describes herself as having some problems, but is happily coping and looking forward to spending time with her grandchildren. Describe this woman's state of health by placing an X on the Wellness-Illness continuum and give a rationale for the placement of the X. *(12)*

Wellness ⟷ Illness

Highest level of optimal health   Diminished or impaired state of health

_____

_____

_____

32. a. Compare and contrast the historical significance of the white pleated cap and the apron that were originally part of the nurse's uniform with contemporary mandatory dress codes for nursing students and nurses. *(7)*

_____

_____

_____

_____

b. Compare and contrast your personal point of view about uniforms with patients' and families' points of view. *(7)*

_____

_____

_____

_____

_____

33. The patient is admitted to the medical-surgical unit for exacerbation of a chronic respiratory disease. While in the hospital, he requires medication, oxygen therapy, and diagnostic testing. In addition, the nurse notes that he smokes. He is overweight and making very poor food choices for between-meal snacks. He is unsteady when he ambulates and requires some assistance for activities that require bending and lifting, such as tying his shoelaces or picking up his suitcase. On further assessment, the nurse finds out that the patient lives by himself in a second-story apartment and his primary source of income is from a small pension.

a. Identify all of the participants in the health care delivery system who will be involved in this patient's care and briefly describe their roles and responsibilities. *(13, 14)*

_____

_____

_____

_____

_____

b. How could the nurse apply the concepts of health promotion and illness prevention to assist this patient? *(13)*

_____

_____

_____

_____

_____

Legal and Ethical Aspects of Nursing

chapter

2

MATCHING

Directions: Match the terms on the left to the correct definition on the right.

		Terms			**Definitions**
_____	1.	malpractice *(24)*		a.	Defines acts whose performance is required, permitted, or prohibited
_____	2.	accountability *(25)*		b.	Legal responsibility
_____	3.	standards of care *(26)*		c.	Professional negligence
_____	4.	liability *(25)*		d.	Process of self-evaluation that helps gain insight into personal values
_____	5.	value clarification *(14)*		e.	Being responsible for one's own actions

MULTIPLE CHOICE

Directions: Select the best answer(s) for each of the following questions.

6. The nursing student needs to obtain patient information to prepare for the clinical experience and decides to stop and say hello to the patient. While they are talking, the patient suddenly stops breathing and becomes unresponsive. What should the student do **first**? *(24)*
   1. Call the nursing instructor and write an incident report.
   2. Call the primary nurse and apply oxygen.
   3. Call the Rapid Response Team and get the crash cart.
   4. Call for help and initiate cardiopulmonary resuscitation.

7. In which case is the nurse **most** likely to be charged with malpractice? *(24)*
   1. The nurse explains the restraint policy to the family and later the older adult patient climbs over the side rail and sustains a hip fracture.
   2. The patient becomes very angry when the nurse refuses to give an additional dose of pain medication before the prescribed time.
   3. The family wants the provider called at 3:00 AM because "something is wrong;" the nurse waits until 7:00 AM, but the patient is unharmed.
   4. The patient is very demanding and unpleasant so the nurse ignores the call bell; the patient sustains tissue injury at the IV site.

8. The patient asked the unlicensed assistive personnel (UAP) to apply a heating pad to her back, despite the fact that the home health nurse had instructed both the patient and UAP to avoid using the device. The patient sustained a burn and decided to sue the UAP and the nurse. Which documents are likely to be used in this case? **Select all that apply.** *(24)*
   1. Policies and procedures
   2. Standards of care
   3. Equipment maintenance records
   4. Patient's medical records
   5. UAP's personal health records
   6. Personnel files for UAP and nurse

9. The nurse recognizes that in today's health care climate, there is an increased likelihood of being involved in litigation. What action could the nurse take to improve the overall situation in the work setting? *(25)*
   1. Agree to care for a limited number of high-acuity patients.
   2. Work on a committee to improve discharge teaching.
   3. Work at a facility that covers nurses with malpractice insurance.
   4. Ensure that others are accountable for their own actions.

10. A new UAP is assigned to do a task that was reviewed and demonstrated in orientation and practiced on a mannikin. The UAP tells the nurse that she does not know how to do the task. What should the nurse do **first**? *(24)*
    1. Ask the UAP to recite the steps of the task and assess readiness to perform.
    2. Go with the UAP and perform the task while the UAP observes.
    3. Instruct the UAP to try to perform the task to the best of her ability.
    4. Pull the UAP's orientation file and see if competency was established.

11. The LPN/LVN is instructed by a provider to start a unit of blood on a patient, but the institution's policy indicates that LPN/LVNs can monitor blood transfusions, but RNs must initiate blood transfusions. What should the LPN/LVN do? *(31)*
    1. Start the blood transfusion as ordered, because the provider is supervising.
    2. Locate the RN in charge so that he/she can start the blood transfusion.
    3. Tell the provider that hospital policy prohibits blood transfusion by LPN/LVNs.
    4. Obtain the unit of blood and assist the provider as he/she initiates the transfusion.

12. A nursing student must write a clinical report about the care that was given to a patient in the hospital. What should the student do to prevent a Health Insurance Portability and Accountability Act (HIPAA) violation? **Select all that apply.** *(29)*
    1. Do not use the patient's name in any section of the paper.
    2. If laboratory data are used, make sure no identification numbers are included.
    3. Avoid including the provider's name in the report.
    4. Do not refer to the room number or the specific unit.
    5. Do not include the patient's vital signs.
    6. Avoid using details about the patient's medical condition.

13. Which unaccompanied minor requires parental consent prior to treatment? *(29)*
    1. A 17-year-old who wants a prescription for insulin
    2. An 18-year-old who needs sutures for a laceration of the hand
    3. A 14-year-old who was sexually assaulted by a family member
    4. A 16-year-old who is independent and self-supporting and wants birth control

14. The nurse is working on the medical-surgical unit and answers the telephone. The caller wants to know, "How is Mr. Smith doing?" What is the **most** important factor that affects the nurse's response? *(30)*
    1. The identity of the caller
    2. The stability of Mr. Smith's condition
    3. The hospital's policy for releasing information
    4. HIPAA

15. A mother brings her 8-year-old son to the clinic for a broken arm. There are no other apparent injuries and the child and mother appear to have a supportive relationship; however, review of the chart indicates that this child has frequently been treated for other fractures and injuries. What should the nurse do **first**? *(31)*
    1. Ask the social worker to consult for possible child abuse.
    2. Call child protective services and make a report.
    3. Point out the history of injuries to the provider.
    4. Take the child aside and assess his true feelings.

16. The nurse stops at a traffic accident and offers aid to victims. In which circumstance are Good Samaritan laws **less** likely to provide the nurse immunity from liability? *(31)*
    1. The nurse initiates cardiopulmonary resuscitation after cardiac arrest occurs.
    2. The nurse directs bystanders to move a victim and a spinal cord injury occurs.
    3. The nurse uses the victim's coat and applies pressure to a bleeding wound.
    4. The nurse pauses to call 911 before assessing or assisting victims in distress.

17. Which action by the nurse is the **best** to avoid a lawsuit? *(31)*
    1. Remain current on practice developments.
    2. Know the legal definition of terms such as *negligence.*
    3. Obtain professional malpractice insurance.
    4. Validate nursing actions with a supervisor.

18. The nurse performs a dressing change on a surgical wound. The procedure is routine and there are no signs of infection or excessive drainage. What should the nurse do about documentation? *(32)*
    1. If using charting by exception, "dressing changed" is adequate.
    2. Document appearance of wound site and type of dressing used.
    3. There is no need to document because there are no problems with the wound.
    4. Read the previous entry about the wound and document "unchanged as above."

19. The nurse has to go before the state board of nursing because there is a question about her nursing license. Which type of insurance will provide a qualified attorney to represent the nurse? *(32)*
    1. Claims-made policy
    2. Occurrence basis policy
    3. "Tail" agreement for extended coverage
    4. Disciplinary defense insurance

20. A newly graduated nurse has completed orientation and is assigned to take care of a patient who has a tracheostomy. The nurse has never done tracheostomy care. What should the nurse do **first**? *(26)*
    1. Ask to be reassigned to a different patient.
    2. Review the procedure using a textbook or the Internet.
    3. Report that orientation did not include tracheostomy care.
    4. Seek instruction and supervision for any unfamiliar procedures.

21. An older adult patient begins to cry during review of the advance directive information and refuses to sign. What should the nurse do **first**? *(33)*
    1. Encourage the patient to express his feelings about the advance directive.
    2. Reassure the patient that his wishes will be respected above all else.
    3. Alert the family to support the patient in the decision.
    4. Document in the patient's record that the information was given and declined.

22. A patient is in very critical condition and unable to make decisions about ongoing treatment. There is conflict among family members on what should be done. Which source, if followed, is the **most** likely to protect the health care team from liability? *(33)*
    1. Agency's policy and procedure manual
    2. Patient's living will
    3. Patient Self-Determination Act
    4. Accreditation criteria of the Joint Commission

23. A mother and her pregnant 13-year-old daughter are arguing; the mother wants her to keep the baby and the girl wants to have an abortion. The nurse feels very angry toward the mother and very protective toward the girl. What should the nurse do **first**? *(35)*
    1. Take the girl aside and assess her feelings and wishes regarding the pregnancy.
    2. Ask another nurse to assess the mother's rationale for opposing her daughter.
    3. Seek advice from a supervisor about who can legally make decisions about the pregnancy.
    4. Reflect on his or her own feelings and ability to be supportive and caring toward this family.

24. Which actions indicate that the nurse is practicing within the code of ethics developed by the National Federation of Licensed Practical Nurses (NFLPN)? **Select all that apply.** *(36)*
    1. Collects data about the patient's skin and reports it to the RN
    2. Gives change-of-shift report to the oncoming nurse and the nursing student
    3. Wears professional attire and adheres to the facility's dress code
    4. Observes another nurse being rude and demeaning toward a patient
    5. Cares for a patient with an infectious disease and follows isolation precautions
    6. Uses a cell phone to text messages about another nurse's behavior toward coworkers

25. Nurse A knows that Nurse B is stealing small items from older residents in the long-term care facility, but Nurse A hesitates to report Nurse B because they are friends and Nurse B gives good care to the residents. Whom should Nurse A talk to **first**? *(36)*
    1. Ask the residents if they have any complaints about Nurse B.
    2. Speak to the families of residents to see if the thefts can be substantiated.
    3. Speak to the supervisor and give facts; do not offer suspicions.
    4. Talk to an objective third party about personal values clarification.

26. Nursing Student Apple posts a detailed description of caring for an older patient on social media. Nursing Student Orange sees the Facebook post. What should Nursing Student Orange do **first**? *(29, 30)*
    1. Review the post to see if any patient identifiers are included.
    2. Give positive feedback to Student Apple for sharing the experience.
    3. Tell Student Apple that the nursing instructor should be informed.
    4. Do nothing; no harm is done if just a few people see the post.

27. Which nurse is appropriately incorporating cultural considerations while providing nursing care? *(34)*
    1. Nurse A expects the patient to make better food choices to lose weight and thereby control his diabetes.
    2. Nurse B assumes that the patient understands English because the family is speaking English.
    3. Nurse C treats all patients the same, regardless of ethnicity or cultural background.
    4. Nurse D listens while a patient expresses feelings and thoughts related to a situation.

28. Which nursing action incorporates the ethical principle of nonmaleficence? *(36)*
    1. Provides high-quality care to a homeless man who has no health insurance
    2. Advocates the need for better pain control for a patient who has cancer
    3. Encourages the patient to ask questions and make an informed choice
    4. Calls the provider about a medication prescription because the dose seems too high

CRITICAL THINKING ACTIVITIES

29. A new nurse has just started his first job after graduating from nursing school. The nurse receives a surgeon's order to "get surgical consent form." The nurse is unsure what the order means, so he calls the surgeon for clarification. The surgeon is a little terse on the phone and says, "Just get the consent form signed." The nurse is unsure what to do, so he consults the charge nurse, who says, "Oh, the doctors here are too lazy to get their own consent forms signed, so we always do it for them." *(27, 29)*

    a. Discuss the nurse's responsibilities when obtaining an informed consent from a patient before a procedure.

    _____

    _____

    _____

    _____

    b. The nurse is new to the city and this is his first job, so he has limited experience, but he clearly remembers what was taught in school about informed consent. What should he do?

    _____

    _____

    _____

    _____

30. Nurse A is assigned to care for a patient with AIDS, but asks Nurse B to switch patients. Nurse B readily agrees because Nurse A always helps other nurses and members of the health care team. Together, they inform the charge nurse, who gives the okay for the switch of assignments. At the end of the day, Nurse A thanks Nurse B for taking the patient with AIDS because "those kinds of people really bother me." Nurse B feels a little confused by the comment, but shrugs it off. *(35, 36)*

    a. Discuss the behavior of Nurse A and Nurse B, as related to the NFLPN code of ethics.

    _____

    _____

    _____

    _____

    b. Nurse B goes home and thinks about the day and about Nurse A's comment. Nurse B realizes that the situation has created some uncomfortable feelings and a potential problem if Nurse A makes a future request to change patient assignments or makes additional comments. What should Nurse B do?

    _____

    _____

    _____

    _____

31. The nurse is caring for a patient who has been quadriplegic for 3 years following a diving accident. One morning, the nurse notes that the patient has redness on the sacral area and informs the patient that there is a risk for a pressure injury and that very careful turning and scheduled assessment will need to be started. The patient politely thanks the nurse, but informs her that he intends to refuse any treatment for pressure injuries and is likely to start refusing other nursing measures as well. The nurse is stunned and upset because the patient has always been cooperative and generally very satisfied with the care. *(37)*

    a. What should the nurse do? _____

    _____

    _____

    _____

    _____

    b. How can the nurse continue to interact with this patient if he continues to refuse therapies? _____

    _____

    _____

    _____

    _____

    c. How would you feel if a patient refused to allow you to meet basic needs such as food, hygiene, or preventive care like turning or receiving immunizations?

    _____

    _____

    _____

    _____

32. The nurse has been working for several years in the hospital. The patient assignments are always very heavy and there has been a continuous nursing shortage. Two patients have died within the past year and although there have been no legal actions taken against the hospital or the staff, the general feeling among the nursing staff is that working conditions are going to result in more harm to the patients. The nurse has talked to her supervisor about her concerns for the patients' safety and the morale of the staff. The supervisor has assured her that everything that can be done has been done. Discuss the legal and ethical implications of these working conditions and the actions that the nurse could take. *(36)*

_____

_____

_____

_____

_____

Documentation

MATCHING

Directions: Match the abbreviations on the left to the correct terminology on the right.

Abbreviation	Terminology
_____ 1. CBE *(48)*	a. Plan, intervention, evaluation
_____ 2. DRGs *(41)*	b. Data, action, response, education
_____ 3. EHR *(42)*	c. Situation, background, assessment, recommendation, read back
_____ 4. HIPAA *(56)*	d. Charting by exception
_____ 5. MDS *(55)*	e. Subjective, objective, assessment, plan, evaluation
_____ 6. POC *(42)*	f. Electronic health record
_____ 7. DARE *(47)*	g. Minimum data sets
_____ 8. SBARR *(43)*	h. Point of care
_____ 9. PIE *(48)*	i. Diagnosis-related groups
_____ 10. SOAPE *(46)*	j. Health Insurance Portability and Accountability Act

SHORT ANSWER

Directions: Using your own words, answer each question in the space provided.

11. The nurse does not have time to document a procedure after it was completed. Discuss how the nurse would handle a "late entry." *(44)*

   _____

   _____

12. Compare and contrast focused charting, charting by exception, and narrative charting. *(45, 47, 48)*

   _____

   _____

   _____

13. Briefly identify how long-term care and home health care documentation are different from acute care (hospital) documentation. *(55)*

   _____

   _____

TABLE ACTIVITY

14. In the right-hand column of the table, indicate all of the potential places where the examples of documentation could be recorded. *(41)*

Nursing Process	Where to Document
Assessment	
Alert and oriented to person, place, and time.	
Ambulates independently to bathroom.	
Family assessed for knowledge of wound care.	
Diagnosis or problem	
Risk for infection of surgical wound	
Needs review of wound care at home	
Outcomes Identification/Planning	
Patient will participate in wound care prior to discharge.	
Family will demonstrate ability to perform wound irrigation.	
Implementation	
Wound care procedure demonstrated to patient and family.	
List of supplies and how to obtain reviewed with family.	
Referral made to home health agency.	
Evaluation	
Patient and family participated in wound care. They had questions about asepsis in the home setting; principles of hand hygiene and asepsis were reviewed. They acknowledged understanding of written and verbal information and agreed to follow up with the home health nurse.	

MULTIPLE CHOICE

Directions: Select the best answer(s) for each of the following questions.

15. Which actions by members of the health care team reflect the basic purposes of accurate and complete patient records? **Select all that apply.** *(41)*
    1. Risk manager uses patient's records to investigate accusations of staff abuse of patient.
    2. Nursing instructor directs the students to look at nurses' notes written by expert nurses.
    3. Medicare auditor reviews patient records to observe for evidence of minimum data sets.
    4. Nursing student reads the patient's flow sheets to observe for trends in the vital signs.
    5. Nurse discusses the provider's documentation with the patient to clarify medical diagnosis.

16. Which nurse is **most** likely to expect a peer review? *(41)*
    1. Nurse A submits a research article to a nursing journal.
    2. Nurse B queries a provider's medication prescription.
    3. Nurse C fills out an incident report for a patient fall.
    4. Nurse D completes an admission assessment and history.

17. In using the hospital's computer information system, where is the nurse **most** likely to find documentation about the patient's response to the last dose of pain medication? *(42)*
    1. Individualized care plan
    2. Medication administration record (MAR)
    3. Automated Kardex form
    4. Narrative notes

18. An auditor is randomly reviewing the nurses' charts and the nurse manager has agreed that the auditor can ask questions and give feedback as necessary. Which example of documentation is the auditor **most** likely to query? *(54)*
    1. Ambulated independently with steady gait to bathroom
    2. Instructed on method of clean midstream urine collection
    3. Discharged to home accompanied by spouse
    4. Placed side rails up x3 with call bell in place

19. The nurse is working on a medical-surgical unit in a large hospital and observes an unfamiliar person looking at a patient's chart. What should the nurse do **first**? *(56)*
    1. Call hospital security and report the person's behavior and description.
    2. Ask for identification and determine if the person can look at the chart.
    3. Allow the person to continue unless there is suspicious behavior.
    4. Request that the chart be returned and contact the charge nurse.

20. The nursing student attempts to document AM hygiene care, but several computers are broken and the remaining functional computers are being used. What should the student do? *(44)*
    1. Make a note to self of time and relevant details and document at the end of the shift.
    2. Report to the instructor and ask for advice about what to do.
    3. Document the care on a hardcopy form and add it to the patient's chart.
    4. Jot down the time that care was given and document when a computer is available.

21. It is 10:00 AM, and the nurse needs to give a patient a blood pressure medication but would like to know what the morning vital signs were before administering the medication. The nurse looks at the flow sheet, but the vital signs are not there. Which action should the nurse take **first**? *(44)*
    1. Give the blood pressure medication now and then check the blood pressure in 30 minutes.
    2. Find the unlicensed assistive personnel (UAP) and ask why the morning vital signs have not been documented.
    3. Check the blood pressure, give the medication as appropriate, and then document both.
    4. Check in the nurses' notes to see if the vital signs were documented there.

22. The nurse phones the provider to report a change in the patient's condition using the SBARR (situation, background, assessment, recommendation, read back) method of communication; however, the provider declines to listen to the "read back" and then hangs up. What should the LPN/LVN do **first**? *(43)*
    1. Call the provider back and insist on "read back."
    2. Carry out the orders if they are clear.
    3. Consult a supervisor about the incident.
    4. Document the provider's exact words in the patient's chart.

23. The LPN/LVN is reading the documentation that was written by a newly graduated RN. There are numerous spelling mistakes and the grammar is terrible. What should the nurse do? *(43)*
    1. Do nothing; an RN is not accountable to an LPN/LVN.
    2. Offer to teach the new nurse how to document.
    3. Ask the charge nurse to review the documentation.
    4. Correct the spelling errors and initial the changes.

24. The student nurse sees that it is time to give medication to a patient, but the patient is currently in radiology. The student is aware that there is a 30-minute time window to administer the medication, otherwise it will be considered late. What should the student do? *(45)*
    1. Document that the medication was given at the correct time and then give it as soon as the patient returns from radiology.
    2. Call the pharmacy and inquire if a delay in administering the medication or holding it until the next dose is harmful to the patient.
    3. Document that the patient is in radiology, advise the charge nurse, and administer the medication when the patient returns to the unit.
    4. Hold the medication and fill out an incident report that explains the circumstances and details of why the medication was not administered.

25. A patient is admitted to the hospital for a total hip replacement. Care and documentation are performed according to the facility's clinical (critical) pathway for this condition. What information is likely to appear in this documentation tool? *(54)*
    1. Level of activity on a day-to-day basis following surgery
    2. Unusual events that have a potential for injury
    3. Nursing care plan with diagnosis and detailed interventions
    4. The LPN/LVN's role in monitoring the patient's progress

26. A patient comes to the nurses' station and demands to have his chart because he has decided to leave the hospital and seek care from a different facility. What is the **best** response? *(42)*
    1. "Sir, all of the patient records are the property of the hospital."
    2. "Sir, let me contact your provider so you can talk to him before leaving."
    3. "Sir, please wait and I will call the nurse manager right now."
    4. "Sir, please return to your room and I will make a copy of the chart."

27. The nursing student leaves a copy of a patient's Kardex on a bedside table. A visitor finds the copy and reads it. What should the student do? *(56)*
    1. Take the Kardex out of the patient's room and immediately shred it.
    2. Apologize to the visitor and patient and explain the information on the Kardex.
    3. Obtain the copy of the Kardex and check for patient identifiers.
    4. Retrieve the Kardex, contact instructor, and complete an incident report.

28. The nurse is documenting with a black pen on the hardcopy nurses' notes about a patient's response to pain medication. The nurse suddenly realizes that she is writing the note in the wrong chart. What is the **best** action to take? *(45)*
    1. Draw a line through the error and initial it.
    2. Report the error to the charge nurse.
    3. Use white correction fluid to cover the error.
    4. Discard the page that contains the error.

29. An auditor is advising a nurse about possible inadequate or inappropriate documentation that could be involved in a malpractice suit. What types of documentation are likely to cause problems in malpractice cases? **Select all that apply.** *(44, 45)*
    1. Failed to document latex allergy
    2. Documented patient's complaint about care by using patient's remarks in quotes
    3. Charted medication that the patient claims he did not receive
    4. Documented amount of IV fluid, but no assessment of IV site
    5. Clustered information obtained from physical assessment
    6. Recorded verbal prescription using brand-name medication

30. Which nursing action/behavior would be considered a potential Health Insurance Portability and Accountability Act (HIPAA) violation? *(56)*
    1. Faxes a patient's medical records to a consulting specialist
    2. Leaves the computer monitor display open for easy access
    3. Discusses a patient's problem during handover with oncoming staff
    4. Shares a copy of an incident report with the risk manager

31. The nurse sees a medication prescription for a patient who has acute postsurgical pain. The prescription reads "3 mg oral MS as needed for pain." What should the nurse do **first**? *(44)*
    1. Report the prescribing provider for using an inappropriate abbreviation.
    2. Correct the prescription to read "3 mg oral morphine sulfate as needed for pain."
    3. Call the prescribing provider and ask for clarification of the abbreviation "MS."
    4. Ask the pharmacist to deliver the medication to the unit as soon as possible.

32. The nurse inadvertently gives the patient's 7:00 PM medication at 7:00 AM. What should the nurse do **first**? *(49)*
    1. Call the pharmacist and ask if there are specific side effects related to the time of day the medication was administered.
    2. Observe for adverse effects, notify the prescribing provider, and fill out an incident report.
    3. Notify the charge nurse and inform the patient about the medication error.
    4. Document the time and dose given and tell the evening shift not to give the PM dose.

33. The LPN/LVN arrives for her shift and is assigned to care for a patient who will soon return from surgery: acuity level 1. What should the nurse do **first**? *(49)*
    1. Ask the offgoing nurse to give a comprehensive hand-off report about the patient.
    2. Prioritize the care of other assigned patients to accommodate the arrival of the postoperative patient.
    3. Check the patient's medical records to find out about the patient's condition and type of surgery.
    4. Consult with the charge nurse about the appropriateness of the patient assignment.

34. Which nursing students have violated the guidelines for safe computer documentation during their clinical rotation? **Select all that apply.** *(56, 57)*
    1. Shares password so that a classmate can collect preclinical information
    2. Logs on and leaves computer terminal to respond to a call light
    3. Records information on the wrong chart; reports to the charge nurse
    4. Positions the monitor display so that it is visible to patient and visitors
    5. Prints and takes a hardcopy of patient data to complete case study assignment

CRITICAL THINKING ACTIVITIES

35. Review the documentation samples below and then refer to Box 3.2, Basic Rules for Documentation, and Table 3.2, Legal Guidelines for Documentation to identify errors and examples of poor documentation. *(44, 45)*

Sample #1

Sept, 2014 Patient had a good night. Status was escendially unchanged. Family in to visit and asked about storage of patient's belongings. Reassured that diamond ring and gold watch were in the bedside table. Patient went with family to cafeteria. S. Smith, LPN.

_____

_____

_____

_____

Sample #2

Sept. 24, 2014 2100 J. Jones RN gave a 500-mL SSE; patient assisted to CC for a return of 600 mL with brown formed stool noted. Procedure well tolerated. J. Jones said that patient had relief of adominal distencion and discomfort. S. Smith, LPN

_____

_____

_____

_____

Sample #3

Sept 24, 2014 Patient reported pain. Noted in chart that physician made an error and ordered MS. Consulted charge nurse who advised to give the dose morphine sulfate according to the written prescription. Patient was angry because he didn't get the pain medication as soon as he asked for it; called me a "stupid lazy fool." Pain medication given later in the shift.

_____

_____

_____

_____

36. Interview nurses during your clinical assignment and then compare and contrast electronic health record (EHR) systems to hardcopy (paper) record systems. *(42, 44, 45)*

_____

_____

_____

_____

37. Discuss how Medicare, Medicaid, and other types of insurance affect the documentation for home health patients. *(55)*

_____

_____

Communication

MULTIPLE CHOICE

Directions: Select the best answer(s) for each of the following questions.

1. In which circumstance would it be **most** appropriate to incorporate the phrase "nursing diagnosis" into the verbal communication? *(61)*
   1. The nurse tells the provider about a change in the patient's respiratory status.
   2. The nursing student and the nursing instructor discuss the patient's care plan.
   3. The home health nurse reviews the goals of rehabilitation with the patient and family.
   4. The offgoing nurse gives hand-off report about several patients to the oncoming nurse.

2. What type of eye contact would be **best** to use if the nurse is trying to involve the patient in a discussion about sexuality without being threatening or intimidating? *(61)*
   1. Lean slightly forward and maintain extended eye contact.
   2. Look downward if the patient uses slang terms related to sex.
   3. Maintain eye contact for 2 to 6 seconds during the discussion.
   4. Observe the patient and mimic the patient's eye contact.

3. A nursing student goes to an instructor's office to discuss an uncomfortable interaction that occurred with a patient during the last clinical experience. Which behaviors suggest that the student does not have the instructor's full attention? **Select all that apply.** *(65)*
   1. Instructor welcomes the student and offers 40 minutes for discussion.
   2. Instructor smiles and waves at others who walk past the office.
   3. Instructor offers advice before the student explains the details of the incident.
   4. Instructor appears relaxed and asks open-ended questions.
   5. Instructor frequently handles her cell phone.
   6. Instructor shuffles and rearranges papers on the desk.

4. The nurse is trying to interview a patient who is very hard of hearing. What strategy should the nurse try **first**? *(73)*
   1. Talk to the patient's spouse.
   2. Shout loudly into the patient's good ear.
   3. Use simple language and avoid medical terminology.
   4. Use normal volume and lower tone of voice.

5. The patient says, "I trust you, so I am going to tell you a secret. I am going to end it all by going for a long swim in the ocean." What should the nurse do **first**? (64)
   1. Tell the patient that intent to harm self must be reported to the provider.
   2. Ask the patient to elaborate on the meaning of "end it all" and "long swim."
   3. Thank the patient for the trust and promise to keep the secret confidential.
   4. Stay with patient and wait for him to express his thoughts and feelings.

6. The night nurse is giving report during shift change. A visitor passing by is an unintended receiver of the nurse's communication. What is the **best** method to prevent this type of occurrence? (71)
   1. Ask visitors to leave the unit during shift change.
   2. Give report in a private room with the door closed.
   3. Eliminate negative connotations during report.
   4. Make written notes that are passed only to staff members.

7. The nurse is attempting to elicit the patient's state of mind about an upcoming surgery. Which approach is likely to be **most** effective? (67)
   1. "Are you afraid of having the procedure?"
   2. "Let me give you information about the procedure."
   3. "Look at this series of pictures about the procedure."
   4. "What do you understand about the procedure?"

8. A patient is grimacing while trying to change his position in bed. He tells the nurse that he is feeling great and is ready to get up and go home. Which response **best** indicates that the nurse recognizes that the patient's communication is incongruent? (63)
   1. "Going home is the goal, but let me help you get up and you can walk around for a while."
   2. "Let me help you sit up and then you can get dressed and pack up your belongings."
   3. "Would you like a dose of pain medication before you go home?"
   4. "That sounds great! I'll call your provider and inform her that you are ready to go home."

9. The nurse is about to begin teaching a small group of adolescents about healthy eating habits. Which nonverbal behavior **best** indicates potential interest in listening to the nurse? (63)
   1. Talking on a cell phone and smiling at the nurse
   2. Staring at the blackboard with a bored expression
   3. Using the Internet to search for topics of interest
   4. Removing a notebook and pen from a backpack

10. The patient tells the nurse, "I'm supposed to check my blood sugar at least three times each day, but I can't always find the test sticks and they're very expensive." Which response by the nurse is the **best** example of effective clarification? (69)
    1. "When did you last check your blood sugar?"
    2. "I'll speak with the nurse practitioner about your situation."
    3. "I see that you know how important it is to check your blood sugar."
    4. "Let me make sure I understand what your concern is with the blood sugar testing."

11. The patient states, "I'm worried and don't know what to expect after my biopsy." Which question **best** encourages the patient to explain the problem to the nurse? (68)
    1. "Would you like to talk to your surgeon before the procedure?"
    2. "Are you feeling anxious about the results of your biopsy?"
    3. "What are you worried about?"
    4. "How can I make you feel better?"

12. The nurse is trying to take a patient's history, but the patient makes frequent references to her aunt's health, a neighbor's illness, and events that happened many years ago to him or others. Which therapeutic communication technique is the nurse **most** likely to use with this patient? (67)
    1. Clarifying
    2. Paraphrasing
    3. Restating
    4. Closed questioning

13. When communicating with a patient who has expressive aphasia, which communication strategy is the nurse **most** likely to use? (76)
    1. Encourage the patient to speak as much as possible.
    2. Use eye blinks, one for "yes" and two for "no."
    3. Ask family members for information.
    4. Speak loudly and slowly with good enunciation.

14. When communicating with a patient of an unfamiliar culture, what would the nurse do? **Select all that apply.** (72)
    1. Use formal names until preference is assessed.
    2. Realize that interpretation of social time versus clock time can differ.
    3. Be aware that touch varies according to gender and relationship.
    4. Assume that smiling and handshake are universal greetings.
    5. Use tone of voice that is soft and deferential.
    6. Understand that eye contact has different meaning among cultures.

15. When communicating with an older adult, what should the nurse do? (72)
    1. Speak loudly and at a very slow pace.
    2. Allow time for processing information.
    3. Provide a dark, quiet environment.
    4. Discourage anecdotal or tangential replies.

16. Which nurse behavior/response **best** indicates to the patient that the nurse is actively listening to what he or she is trying to say? (69)
    1. Says "Uh-huh"
    2. Smiles and nods at patient
    3. Says "So in other words, you are…"
    4. Looks at patient and leans forward

17. The patient will be discharged from the hospital tomorrow. During the discharge teaching, the patient states, "I don't know how I will be able to care for myself after I leave the hospital." What is the **most** therapeutic response? (69)
    1. "You don't know how you will take care of yourself when you leave the hospital?"
    2. "It sounds like you have some concerns. What do you think is going to happen?"
    3. "Would you like me to review the instructions so the information is clear?"
    4. "Could you get someone to stay with you until you are feeling better?"

18. The nurse is working with a patient from a different culture. Which action by the nurse is **most** likely to cause offense if patient's sense of intimate space differs from the nurse's? (70)
    1. Assists the patient to transfer from bed to chair
    2. Sits in a chair and speaks with the patient
    3. Speaks to the family in the presence of the patient
    4. Hangs the patient's clothes in the closet

19. The nurse is completing the patient's history. Which question encourages the patient to provide a specific answer with relevant detail? (67)
    1. "What type of surgeries have you had in the past?"
    2. "What kinds of problems do you have?"
    3. "Are you having any pain?"
    4. "How do you feel about your current health status?"

20. The patient tells the nurse that the unlicensed assistive personnel (UAP) is always making jokes. What is the **best** response? (70)
    1. "Laughter is the best medicine."
    2. "What do you think about the UAP's jokes?"
    3. "Yes, the UAP really is a funny person."
    4. "Would you tell me a joke?"

21. The nurse is explaining a change in a patient's condition to a provider. The provider rudely and sarcastically replies, "Well, what do you want me to do about that?" What is the **best** response? (63)
    1. "Well, mostly I just wanted you to know about the situation."
    2. "That's really your decision. I'm merely reporting the patient's condition."
    3. "Please come and examine the patient, because the condition has changed."
    4. "Sorry to bother you. I'll just keep monitoring the patient's condition."

22. The patient has just died. The wife and daughter are holding each other and crying at the bedside, while the little boy is standing apart staring out the window. Which communication approach would be the **best** to support everyone in the family? (62, 65)
    1. Talk to the little boy about what he is feeling and what he sees out the window.
    2. Stand beside the wife and daughter and direct the little boy to join the group.
    3. Use therapeutic touch with the wife and daughter and allow the little boy to have his space.
    4. Stand beside the little boy and keep an open body position toward the mother and daughter.

23. The nurse is present when the obstetrician informs a 17-year-old that she is pregnant. The adolescent shrugs, appears bored and says, "That's no big deal to me." The nurse, who has been trying to get pregnant for several years, feels angry and hostile toward the patient. What should the nurse do **first**? *(64)*
    1. Care for the patient and talk about the situation later with a friend.
    2. Perform a self-assessment of ability to convey acceptance.
    3. Be honest with the patient and express concern about her attitude.
    4. Ask another nurse to take over care of the patient.

24. An experienced UAP gives excellent care and is well-liked by all of the residents in the long-term care facility. She calls the female residents "Sweetie" and the male residents "Honey-bunch." The nurse is newly graduated but recognizes that the UAP is using "elderspeak." What should the nurse do? *(72)*
    1. Let a good thing continue because everyone seems happy and the care is good.
    2. Gain more experience and mimic the UAP's behavior and communication style.
    3. Report to the RN in charge about concerns for the UAP's disrespect of residents.
    4. Praise the UAP for giving excellent care and role-model use of "Mr.," "Mrs.," or "Ms."

25. Social isolation is one of the identified problems on the care plan for a resident with a hearing impairment in a long-term care facility. The nurse goes to the patient's room and finds that he is cheerful, conversant, and happy to engage. What should the nurse do **first**? *(73)*
    1. Suggest to the RN that social isolation does not seem to belong on the problem list.
    2. Assess the patient to determine his social skills and the extent of his social network.
    3. Spend more time with the patient because trust and rapport are established.
    4. Suggest that the patient go into the common room and talk with other residents.

CRITICAL THINKING ACTIVITIES

26. A 58-year-old man is admitted to the medical-surgical unit with a diagnosis of left-sided stroke. During the admission process, the nurse observes that the patient's speech is unclear and his words are slurred. The nurse also observes that when the patient is asked a question that can be answered with a "yes" or "no" response, he answers the question by moving his head to indicate "yes" or "no." Apply the nursing process to the given situation. *(76, 77)*

    a. Identify communication problems observed by the nurse during the admission process. _____

    b. Write a realistic goal that addresses the patient's verbal communication. _____

    c. Identify at least five nursing actions that can be implemented. _____

    d. Write a statement that reflects evaluation of the outcome. _____

e. What would the nurse do if the goal is not being met? _____

_____

_____

_____

27. The nurse is having a very rough day. Another nurse called in sick; a physician's assistant was very rude; several patients have extremely complex care needs; and Mrs. M., who is an older adult widow, has repeatedly used the call bell all morning. The nurse goes to Mrs. M.'s room and stands in the doorway with her arms across her chest, saying nothing, but looking directly at the patient. Mrs. M. says, "I'm sorry to bother you dear, but I thought I heard my husband in the hallway. Could you check and see if he is here?" The nurse shakes her head and walks out. Analyze this situation and the factors that are influencing the communication between the nurse and the patient. *(62, 70, 73)*

_____

_____

_____

_____

_____

_____

28. Recall a conversation you recently had with a family member, friend, coworker, instructor, or patient in which you used responses that blocked communication. Such responses include false reassurance, giving advice, making false assumptions, giving approval or disapproval, automatic responses, defensive responses, arguing, asking for explanation, or changing the subject. (See Table 4.4 for examples.) Record two or three responses that you used and describe how the other person responded to you. *(75)*

_____

_____

_____

_____

_____

_____

Rephrase your responses listed above so communication remains open. _____

_____

_____

_____

_____

_____

_____

_____

Nursing Process and Critical Thinking

SHORT ANSWER

Directions: Using your own words, answer each question in the space provided.

1. When identifying patient problems, what factors should be considered? *(83)*

    a. _____

    b. _____

    c. _____

2. Identify six elements that are included in well-written patient-centered goals. *(85)*

    a. _____

    b. _____

    c. _____

    d. _____

    e. _____

    f. _____

3. Identify three elements that are included in a correctly written nursing intervention. *(87)*

    a. _____

    b. _____

    c. _____

4. Identify four sources of evidence that are used to support evidence-based practice. *(89)*

    a. _____

    b. _____

    c. _____

    d. _____

5. List four or five advantages of using the standardized language from systems such as North American Nursing Diagnosis Association International (NANDA-I), Nursing Interventions Classification (NIC), and Nursing Outcomes Classification (NOC). *(90)*

_____

_____

_____

_____

FIGURE LABELING

6. Directions: On the figure below, use a-f to indicate where the following patient problems would be according to Maslow's Hierarchy. *(13, 86)*

a. Acute pain
b. Insufficient cardiac output
c. Situational low self-esteem

d. Potential for injury
e. Ineffective relationship
f. Hopelessness

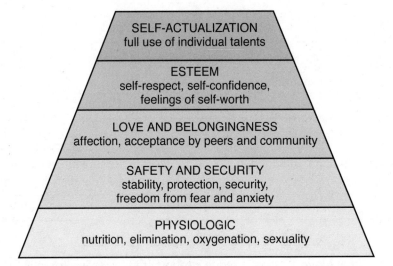

TABLE ACTIVITY

7. Directions: On the table below, list the conclusions that you would make based on the analysis of significant cues. The first block has been completed for you. *(83)*

Determination of Significant Cues

Patient Values	Normal Range	Conclusion
10-month-old child not babbling	Babbling usually starts at 9 months	Babbling delayed
38-year-old patient with potassium 6 mEq/L	3.5 to 5.0 mEq/L	
45-year-old patient with Glasgow Coma score of 15	15 is normal; score of less than 8 is severe brain injury	
22-year-old patient with blood pressure 120/76 mm Hg	<120/80 mm Hg is normal	
Adult male patient with sodium of 130 mEq/L	135 to 145 mEq/L	
Adult female patient with hemoglobin of 12 g/dL	12 to 16 g/dL	
65-year-old patient with 4+ pitting edema of lower legs	1+ is barely perceptible; 4+ is severe	
28-year-old female patient with pulse of 55 beats/min	60 to 100 beats/min	

MULTIPLE CHOICE

Directions: Select the best answer(s) for each of the following questions.

8. The nurse is caring for a patient who is 1 day postoperative for abdominal surgery. The patient reports that the abdominal pain is unrelieved by medication and seems to be getting worse. He also reports feeling dizzy, lightheaded, and slightly nauseated. What objective data should the nurse collect **first**? *(82)*
   1. Assess the dressing and observe for blood or drainage.
   2. Look at the most recent blood pressure and pulse.
   3. Check the last hematocrit and hemoglobin results.
   4. Assess the abdomen for distention and rigidity.

9. The nurse hears in report that the patient has a medical diagnosis of chronic obstructive pulmonary disease. Which data cluster does the nurse expect to find when assessing this patient? *(92)*
   1. Low oxygen level, chronic cough, dyspnea with exertion
   2. Low blood pressure, ascites, shortness of breath
   3. Decreased range of motion in extremities, orthopnea, stridor
   4. Low carbon dioxide level; shallow, rapid respirations; pallor

10. Which patient problem would be considered a collaborative problem? *(85)*
    1. The patient has sundown syndrome and the family is unsure what to do.
    2. The patient is reluctant to ambulate because of fear of falling.
    3. The patient has early Alzheimer's disease and shows early symptoms of dementia.
    4. The patient needs anticipatory guidance for transfer to long-term care.

11. Which intervention would be considered a prescribed nursing intervention? *(87)*
    1. Obtain and report peak and trough levels
    for vancomycin x3 days.
    2. Administer IV 5% dextrose and half nor-
    mal saline at 125 mL/hour for 8 hours.
    3. Make a referral to physical therapy to teach
    the patient to transfer from bed to wheel-
    chair.
    4. Encourage independence in hygiene by
    supervising while the patient washes face
    and hands.

12. The health care team is using a standardized
clinical pathway in the care of patients who require cataract surgery and follow-up care. The
nurse notes a "repetition of variances." What
is the **best** rationale for the nurse to report this
observation to the team leader? *(91)*
    1. The clinical pathway is not consistent with
    patients' medical diagnosis.
    2. Team should review the clinical pathway
    and possibly make revisions.
    3. Some team members are not reliable about
    documentation and followup.
    4. The team is not consistently interpreting or
    applying the clinical pathway.

13. Place the nursing actions in correct order according to the six phases of the nursing process. *(81)*
    _____ 1. Identifies outcome of "patient
    will demonstrate respiratory rate
    of 12-20 breaths/min after being
    positioned in high Fowler's."
    _____ 2. Assists RN to develop a plan of
    care that will improve the pa-
    tient's ability to breathe and ex-
    pand lungs.
    _____ 3. Collaborates with RN to make
    diagnosis of Ineffective breathing
    pattern related to positioning that
    prevents lung expansion.
    _____ 4. Observes position and respira-
    tory effort, counts rate, and aus-
    cultates lung fields.
    _____ 5. Assists to high Fowler's position
    or assists to sit in the bedside
    chair.
    _____ 6. Checks oxygen saturation and
    asks patient about subjective feel-
    ings of relief after being reposi-
    tioned.

14. The nurse is performing the assessment phase
of the nursing process. Which nursing action
would be done during this phase? *(81)*
    1. Observe a patient's ability to independent-
    ly perform AM hygienic care.
    2. Adjust a standardized care plan to meet
    the needs of the individual patient.
    3. Take blood pressure 30 minutes after giv-
    ing an antihypertensive medication.
    4. Assist the patient to make a list of ques-
    tions to ask the provider.

15. The nurse observes that the patient is pale;
diaphoretic; slightly hunched over; and demonstrates deep, rapid breathing. Based on this
objective data, which question will the nurse
use to elicit the **most** relevant subjective data?
(82)
    1. "Do you feel chilled or feverish?"
    2. "Do you need some help to sit up?"
    3. "Are you having any pain?"
    4. "When did you start feeling like this?"

16. The nurse has identified six relevant nursing
diagnoses that would apply to the patient's
care. Which nursing action is the **most** important? *(86)*
    1. Determine how the nursing diagnoses re-
    late to the medical diagnoses.
    2. Plan interventions that will address the six
    problems that were identified.
    3. Prioritize the nursing diagnoses from most
    urgent to least urgent.
    4. Ask the patient if the identified problems
    are consistent with his/her view.

17. The nurse is caring for a patient who is newly
diagnosed with asthma. On the care plan, there
is the patient problem of ineffective breathing
related to narrowing of airways, with an intervention of "use inhaler as needed (PRN) for
asthma attacks." How does the nurse implement this intervention? *(82, 83)*
    1. Consult the charge nurse to clarify the spe-
    cific parameters of the nursing order.
    2. Ask the patient how often he has asthma
    attacks and what triggers them.
    3. Keep the inhaler at the bedside and tell the
    patient to use it whenever he needs it.
    4. Observe baseline respiratory effort, fre-
    quently reassess and instruct the patient to
    call for help.

18. Which data would be included in a cluster relevant to the patient problem of constipation? **Select all that apply.** *(82)*
    1. Abdomen firm and nontender to touch
    2. Decreased bowel sounds
    3. Flat, brown, 1-cm lesion noted near umbilicus
    4. Takes opioid pain medications as needed
    5. Passed a small, hard stool yesterday
    6. Prefers to eat meat and potatoes, but lacks appetite

19. The nurse will perform a focused assessment on which patients? **Select all that apply.** *(81)*
    1. Newly admitted to a long-term care facility
    2. Has a head injury that was sustained during a fall
    3. Reports sore throat and a low-grade fever
    4. Comes to the clinic for a physical examination for a job
    5. Reports pain in the left leg that worsens with walking
    6. Reports back pain, painful urination, and low-grade fever

20. What is the **best** rationale for collecting a patient's biographic data such as age, weight, and place of employment? *(82)*
    1. Creates a complete and comprehensive legal document about the patient
    2. Is required by insurance companies and other third parties for reimbursement
    3. Helps the health care team identify potential risk factors for health problems
    4. Allows the patient to participate more fully and have a say in his/her own care

21. What is the **major** advantage of using the nursing process to identify nursing diagnoses? *(83)*
    1. Helps nurses identify a disease or illness that creates problems for the patient
    2. Allows nurses to use clinical judgment about actual or potential health problems
    3. Permits nurses to use standardized care plans for common patient problems
    4. Limits the type of problems that nurses are responsible for treating

22. The nurse has completed the assessment and reviewed the patient's record. The patient has potential for impaired skin integrity. Which datum supports this problem? *(84)*
    1. A deep pressure injury is noted over the sacral area.
    2. Documentation includes descriptions of many skin lesions.
    3. The patient reports a painful, open sore on the left ankle.
    4. The patient is underweight and has trouble changing position.

23. What would be an example of a *collaborative problem*? *(85)*
    1. Edema
    2. Anxiety
    3. Coping
    4. Social isolation

24. The home health nurse needs the patient's complete medication history, but the patient tells the nurse that many changes were made in the hospital and at discharge, so he is not sure what to tell her. What would be the **best** secondary source of this information? *(82)*
    1. Patient's family
    2. Discharging provider
    3. Medication reconciliation form
    4. Local pharmacist

25. The postsurgical patient reports that he is having lower abdominal pain. What would the nurse include in the focused physical assessment? *(81)*
    1. Check peripheral pulses and sensation.
    2. Check for rigidity and rebound tenderness.
    3. Assess the patient's mental status.
    4. Auscultate the lung sounds.

26. The caregiver of a patient with Alzheimer's disease reports that the patient is unsteady and easily loses his balance, leaves the house, and needs coaching to accomplish tasks. Which nursing diagnoses will apply to this patient? **Select all that apply.** *(83)*
    1. Acute confusion
    2. Self-care deficit for activities of daily living
    3. Wandering
    4. Potential for caregiver role strain
    5. Potential for falls

27. An older adult patient is wetting the bed because he is unable to independently get up and go to the bathroom. For this particular patient, which phase of the nursing process is **most** critical to address the patient's needs? *(86)*
    1. Assessment
    2. Diagnosis
    3. Planning
    4. Evaluation

28. The home health nurse has been visiting a patient for several months. One of the patient's problems is that she is reluctant to leave the house. The goal of "patient will attend a social function two times per month" has not been met. What should the nurse do **first**? *(89)*
    1. Document the results obtained 89 interventions have been performed.
    2. Rewrite the goal and replace "two times per month" with "one time per month."
    3. Agree to visit the patient more frequently to decrease sense of isolation.
    4. Evaluate the factors that are affecting or interfering with the patient's response.

29. Which nursing action **best** demonstrates that the nurse believes that evidence-based practice is important for quality patient care? *(89)*
    1. Routinely reads research articles and applies research to patient care
    2. Works on a committee to update policy and procedure manuals
    3. Looks on the Internet to find clinically relevant data
    4. Asks a clinical nurse specialist to validate nursing care decisions

30. A patient comes to the clinic for a broken toe. The nurse checks the patient's pulse and then attaches him to the cardiac monitor, which reveals an irregular heart rhythm. What is the **best** rationale for the nurse's action? *(92)*
    1. The nurse saw that the patient had obvious risk factors for cardiac problems.
    2. Standard of care is a complete evaluation when patients first seek health care.
    3. A head-to-toe assessment is implemented when the patient is not distressed.
    4. Palpation of the pulse revealed irregularities, so the nurse considered pathophysiology.

31. The nursing student has diligently read all assignments, attended all lectures and skills practice sessions, but lacks clinical experience to improve critical thinking skills. What should the student do to improve critical thinking as it applies to patient care? **Select all that apply.** *(92)*
    1. Mentally rehearse clinical scenarios: "What would I do if…"
    2. Develop the habit of formulating relevant questions when listening or reading.
    3. Ask the instructor or nurse preceptor to "think out loud."
    4. Discuss with classmates how they reached a certain decision.
    5. Advocate for more clinical time with patients.
    6. Scan for nursing information from a wide variety of sources.

CRITICAL THINKING ACTIVITIES

32. Ms. M., aged 48 years, is admitted to the medical-surgical unit after an abdominal hysterectomy. Her vital signs are stable. The IV in her left forearm is patent, without swelling or tenderness. The dressings are dry and intact. Ms. M. has an indwelling urinary catheter in place that is draining clear, yellow urine. She was just transferred from the surgical recovery unit and is expressing severe pain. Select the priority problem for this patient and write a nursing care plan that addresses the problem. *(88)*

_____

_____

_____

_____

33. a.   Discuss the LPN/LVN's role in the nursing process. *(91)* _____

_____

_____

_____

_____

_____

b.   If the LPN/LVN disagrees with the RN about the choice or priority of a nursing diagnosis/patient problem statement, what should the LPN/LVN do? *(91)*

_____

_____

_____

_____

34. The nurse is working on a busy medical-surgical unit, and today has been particularly hectic. Upon entering a patient's room, the nurse notes that the patient seems upset. The patient's body language suggests that she would like to talk to the nurse. Discuss how the nurse would use critical thinking in the decision to stay (or not) and sit with the patient to talk. *(92)*

_____

_____

_____

_____

_____

Cultural and Ethnic Considerations

chapter

6

CROSSWORD PUZZLE

1. Directions: Use the clues to complete the crossword puzzle.

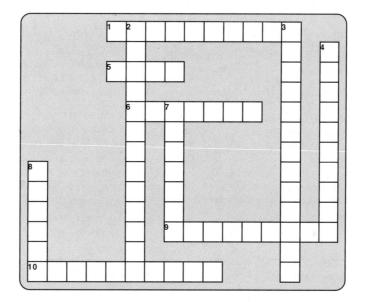

Across

1. Generalized expectation about behavior by members of a particular group *(96)*
5. Shares biologic physical characteristics *(96)*
6. Nation, community, or broad group of people who establish particular aims, beliefs, or standards of living and conduct *(95)*
9. Common social and cultural heritage based on shared traditions, national origin, and physical and biologic characteristics *(97)*
10. Shares characteristics with primary culture, but behaviors and ideals distinguish it from the rest of a cultural group *(95)*

Down

2. Understanding cultural variables and integrating that understanding during interaction *(96)*
3. Belief that own beliefs and cultural practices are the best *(96)*
4. Implies that future activities are possible to recover but not present ones *(101)*
7. Learned beliefs, customs, and practices shared by a group and passed to another generation *(95)*
8. Accepted traditional customs, moral attitudes, or manners of a particular social group *(96)*

MULTIPLE CHOICE

Directions: Select the best answer(s) for each of the following questions.

2. The nurse observes a young, friendly unlicensed assistive personnel (UAP) giving the "thumbs up" hand gesture as he passes by the doorway of his assigned patients. What should the nurse do **first**? *(100)*
   1. Ask the patients what they think about the "thumbs up" gesture.
   2. Suggest that the UAP talk to the charge nurse before someone complains.
   3. Observe the UAP for evidence of additional culturally biased behavior.
   4. Ask the UAP about the hand gesture and the response from the patients.

3. A nursing student has to rely on public transportation and she is late several times for class and clinical. The instructor is very unhappy with the tardiness. What should the student do **first**? *(101)*
   1. Promise never to be late for the remainder of the semester.
   2. Ask for a transfer to another instructor and a different clinical site.
   3. Explain transportation issues and ask for help to problem-solve.
   4. Ask for lenience and offer to do additional make-up assignments.

4. Which behavior **most** strongly suggests that the patient has a future time orientation? *(101)*
   1. Patient declines a recommended cancer screening test because she has no family history of cancer.
   2. Patient goes to the emergency department for acute-onset abdominal pain.
   3. Patient asks the nurse if his daughter can stay overnight with him in the hospital.
   4. Patient initiates a program of regular exercise and healthy eating habits.

5. Which situation **most** strongly indicates a patriarchal family structure? *(101)*
   1. Oldest son makes medical decisions for older adult father and provides emotional support for his mother.
   2. Family requests that diagnosis of cancer be withheld from the patient, who is an older adult female.
   3. Female family members sit at the patient's bedside; male members sit in the waiting room.
   4. At immunization clinic, mother gives her son emotional support and comfort.

6. Based on the nurse's knowledge of health disorders found among persons of Native American ancestry, which question is the nurse **most** likely to ask? *(107)*
   1. "Have you experienced any unintentional weight loss?"
   2. "Has anyone in your family ever been told they have diabetes?
   3. "When was the last time you had a complete physical?"
   4. "Do you know if you have a family history of sickle cell disease?"

7. The nurse is assisting a patient to change position in bed. The patient has a limited understanding of English. What should the nurse do? *(98)*
   1. Speak loudly to emphasize key information.
   2. Keep instructions brief and simple.
   3. Wait for an interpreter.
   4. Provide directions with detailed rationale.

8. What cultural difference(s) does the nurse need to be aware of when caring for an older adult? **Select all that apply.** *(98)*
   1. They are usually more tolerant of other cultures.
   2. They may say hurtful things if cognitive impairment is present.
   3. They are more likely to be rigid in their practices.
   4. They are less likely to use home remedies.
   5. They rely more on traditional religious practices.
   6. They are less likely to be well-educated.

9. The surgeon informs the patient that there is a risk of blood loss during the planned surgical procedure, but the patient is a Jehovah's Witness, so she refuses to sign the consent form. Which nursing action is in the **best** interest of the patient? *(104)*
   1. Support the patient's decision to refuse the procedure.
   2. Discuss realistic alternatives to blood transfusion with the surgeon.
   3. Document the patient's decision in the medical record.
   4. Contact the risk manager for advice about convincing the patient.

10. A patient who is Muslim dies during the night. To respect the patient's religious beliefs, what should the nurse do **first**? *(103)*
    1. Contact the family before giving any post-mortem care.
    2. Stay with the deceased until a family member arrives.
    3. Wait at least 30 minutes before giving post-mortem care.
    4. Contact the organ transplant team because donation is likely.

11. The nurse is from a small town in the United States and is starting a new job in a large urban area with a diverse population. What strategies can the nurse use to develop cultural competence? **Select all that apply.** *(96)*
    1. Perform a self-assessment of beliefs and practices.
    2. Adapt personal beliefs to match those of individual patients.
    3. Keep an open mind about cultural differences.
    4. Treat everyone equally and act the same toward all patients.
    5. Ignore the differences and focus on exhibiting kindness and care.
    6. Understand own values, preferences, and cultural heritage.

12. The nurse is caring for a patient who is dying. What does evidence-based practice indicate about cultural beliefs and rituals that surround death? *(97)*
    1. The family should be encouraged to pray at the bedside.
    2. Respect and protection of the dying person's soul are important.
    3. Lack of religious preference increases problems with coping.
    4. Rituals and ceremonies to delay or ward off death should be discouraged.

13. The patient, who is in no apparent distress, is accompanied to the clinic by several family members who cluster around. All are attempting to talk to each other and the nurse at the same time. The nurse can hear a mixture of English and another language being spoken. What should the nurse do **first**? *(101)*
    1. Try to determine who speaks the best English.
    2. Take only the patient to an examination room and shut the door.
    3. Project calm energy and try to identify the leader of the family.
    4. Physically assess the patient and take vital signs to ascertain stability.

14. A male patient says to the nurse regarding the UAP, "That young Asian woman who helped me with my bath was really nice, but she seemed scared and never looked up; just kept her head down. Did I do something to scare or offend her?" What should the nurse do **first**? *(96)*
    1. Find the UAP and ask her to explain her behavior to the patient.
    2. Reassure him that he did nothing wrong and that the UAP's behavior is cultural.
    3. Tell the patient that you will check with the UAP and then get back to him.
    4. Apologize to the patient and give then give feedback to the UAP.

15. The nurse is a happy and outgoing person, and comes from a family where hugging, touching, patting, or playfully punching are part of normal everyday interaction. What is the **best** strategy for the nurse to combine her personal style with giving culturally appropriate care? *(96)*
    1. Assess her own behaviors and try to understand the origin of her personal style.
    2. Consider different patient care settings and observe interactions.
    3. Learn which cultures can accept touch by health care personnel.
    4. Request to care for patients who are from her own culture.

16. The nurse is working in an assisted-living facility and most residents take their meals in a common dining area. What is the **best** method for seating the residents? *(99)*
    1. Assign seating so that each resident has a consistent place at mealtimes.
    2. Encourage the residents to continuously sit with someone new for stimulation.
    3. Observe how self-mobile and ambulatory residents seat and group themselves.
    4. Ask each resident where he/she would like to sit at the beginning of each meal.

17. The nurse is trying to give all of his patients the 9:00 AM medications. An older Hispanic woman needs 15 medications every morning but is consistently preoccupied whenever the nurse enters the room. What should the nurse do? *(101)*
    1. Administer the medications to other patients first and then help this patient.
    2. Give the patient a 15-minute warning and then stick to the promised time.
    3. Try to find out why the woman is so consistently preoccupied.
    4. Start giving this patient the medications at 8:00 AM so there is extra time.

18. The nursing student is trying to explain the importance of taking blood pressure medication every day to an older patient who is on a fixed income. Which question from the patient is the **best** indication that his perception of time tends to be present-oriented? *(101)*
    1. "Can I save the medication on the days when I feel okay?"
    2. "What should I do if I am running out of medication and have no money?"
    3. "My wife takes blood pressure medication too. Can I share her pills?"
    4. "Would you take this medication if you were in my position?"

19. The nurse is discussing the parents' beliefs and use of folk medicine, which they would like to use to treat their child's respiratory infection. Which health care practice is the cause for **greatest** concern? *(107)*
    1. Placing a religious medal on the bedside table
    2. Having a folk healer come to heal with touch and faith
    3. Giving the child an herbal tea that gives strength and health
    4. Bathing at night instead of in the morning

20. On visiting the patient at home, the nurse finds that the patient is not following the dietary instructions. The nurse discovers that the wife, who shops and cooks, believes that her husband needs "nutritious home-cooked meals from his native country." What should the nurse do **first**? *(107)*
    1. Change the dietary plan to meet the patient's and family's cultural preferences.
    2. Consult a nutritionist for ways to adapt the wife's cooking to the dietary plan.
    3. Revise the patient's nutritional goal to incorporate the cultural dietary patterns.
    4. Ask the wife to describe a typical 24-hour day of meal preparation and snacks.

21. The nurse is assessing a patient who reports, "It feels like there is something inside me that wants to come out." Which questions would the nurse ask to assess the patient's belief system? **Select all that apply.** *(97)*
    1. "When did you first notice the feeling?"
    2. "Why do you think this is happening right now?"
    3. "What do you think is causing the problem?"
    4. "Why do you think this is happening to you?"
    5. "What do you think will help clear up the problem?"
    6. "How long does the feeling last?"

CRITICAL THINKING ACTIVITIES

22. The nurse is caring for an older patient who has recently emigrated from another country. The patient's family is at the bedside and the nurse overhears them speaking in English and Spanish. The nurse's first language is English and she understands and speaks a little Spanish.

    a. Identify nursing interventions that may be used to communicate with a non–English-speaking patient. *(98)*

    _____

    _____

    b. Discuss the advantages and disadvantages of using a family member to translate and communicate with the patient. *(99)*

    _____

    _____

    _____

    _____

    _____

    _____

    _____

c. How should the nurse ask the patient about the following? *(97)*

    i. Language: _____

    ii. Health: _____

    iii. Family structure:_____

    iv. Dietary practices: _____

    v. Use of folk medicine: _____

23. Every morning the same day-shift nurse is late for work, so giving handover report is always delayed. The night-shift nurses have mentioned this to the nurse manager, who has promised to take care of the problem, but the late behavior continues. One of the night nurses tries to talk to the day-shift nurse about her behavior, but the nurse says, "Oh, you Americans are always so worried about time. Just relax. You know I will always be here." Analyze this situation and make suggestions about how the problem can be addressed. Ask your clinical instructor if you can discuss this topic in a postconference. *(101)*

_____

_____

_____

_____

_____

24. Nursing students who grow up and work in the United States sometimes have difficulty describing their own culture and identifying how "American" culture is viewed by people who did not grow up in the United States. *(95)*

a. If you are an American who grew up in the United States, describe the how "American" culture affects your values and belief system.

_____

_____

_____

_____

_____

_____

_____

b. If you are not originally from the United States, discuss how you view "American" culture and how being in that culture is currently affecting you.

_____

_____

_____

_____

_____

_____

_____

_____

Asepsis and Infection Control

SHORT ANSWER

Directions: Using your own words, answer each question in the space provided.

1. Identify four major classifications of pathogens and one example of a microorganism for each. *(121)*

   _____

   _____

   _____

   _____

2. Discuss disinfection and nursing implications for using disinfectants. *(152)* _____

   _____

   _____

3. Identify at least five miscellaneous guidelines for Standard Precautions. *(128)* _____

   _____

   _____

   _____

   _____

4. What is the proper method for disposal of sharps? *(136)*_____

   _____

5. Describe the procedure for gowning for contact isolation. *(134)*_____

   _____

   _____

6. Review the following nursing tasks and identify whether medical asepsis (MA) or surgical asepsis (SA) is necessary to prevent the spread of infection. Label each task as MA or SA. *(118, 140)*

   _____ a. Assisting patient with meal tray

   _____ b. Helping patient brush teeth

   _____ c. Obtaining a urine specimen from an existing catheter

   _____ d. Obtaining a throat swab for a culture

   _____ e. Inserting a urinary catheter

   _____ f. Changing the bed linens

_____ g. Replacing a colostomy bag
_____ h. Drawing up medication in a syringe
_____ i. Removing medication from a bubble pack
_____ j. Dressing change of a new surgical incision
_____ k. Suctioning the lower airway
_____ l. Suctioning the oral cavity

7. Place steps 1-7 of opening a wrapped sterile package in the correct order. *(146)*

_____ Grasp the outer surface of the last and innermost flap; pull the flap back, allowing it to fall flat.

_____ Place the wrapped sterile package flat in the center of the work surface.

_____ Grasp the outside surface of the first side flap; open the side flap; allow it to lie flat on the table surface.

_____ Grasp the outer surface of the tip of the outermost flap; open the outer flap away from your body.

_____ Grasp the outside surface of the second side flap; allow it to lie flat on the table surface.

_____ Remove the tape or seal indicating the sterilization date.

_____ Perform hand hygiene.

MULTIPLE CHOICE
Directions: Select the best answer(s) for each of the following questions.

8. The patient has a large midline abdominal incision. With the specific purpose of reducing a possible reservoir of infection, what would the nurse do? *(122)*
   1. Wear gloves and mask at all times.
   2. Isolate the patient's personal articles.
   3. Direct the patient to cover mouth when coughing.
   4. Change the dressing when it becomes soiled.

9. What should be included in the care of a patient with incontinence and rotavirus? *(137)*
   1. A private room with negative air flow
   2. Hand hygiene after filtration masks are removed
   3. Use of gloves and gown upon entering the room
   4. Use of a surgical mask on the patient during transfers

10. A patient with rubella needs to be transported to the radiology department. What should the nurse do to prepare the patient for transport? *(137)*
    1. Advise the patient to immediately wash hands after returning from procedure.
    2. Call the radiology department and inform them to wear gloves at all times.
    3. Dress the patient in an isolation gown and then apply a mask.
    4. Instruct the patient to wear a mask and follow cough etiquette.

11. Which action by the nursing student requires correction because it contributes to the potential transmission of pathogens? *(123)*
    1. Uses a dampened cloth to wipe off the overbed table
    2. Shakes linens to remove debris and then places them in laundry bag
    3. Holds soiled linens at a distance to prevent touching uniform
    4. Washes hands with soap and water after emptying and cleaning a bedpan

12. When caring for a patient with tuberculosis who is on airborne precautions, what should the nurse routinely use? *(136)*
    1. Regular mask and eyewear
    2. Gown and gloves
    3. Surgical handwashing and gloves
    4. Particulate respirator mask

13. The nurse is observing a nursing student who is preparing to do a sterile dressing change. Which action requires correction and additional instruction? *(146)*
    1. Opening the outer flap of the sterile package by moving it towards the body
    2. Placing the cap of the sterile solution inside up on a clean surface
    3. Opening sterile items and dropping them directly onto the sterile field
    4. Maintaining a 1-inch border around the sterile drape

14. The nurse is aware that the body has normal defenses against infection. Which medication can affect the acidic environment, which is one defense mechanism? *(124)*
    1. Ciprofloxacin
    2. Aluminum/magnesium antacid
    3. Doxycycline
    4. Chlorhexidine gluconate

15. The patient has been receiving antibiotic therapy. Which laboratory result indicates the need to contact the provider for a reevaluation of prescribed therapy? *(125)*
    1. Sensitivity results are positive.
    2. Blood titer is positive for antibodies.
    3. White blood cell count is elevated.
    4. Blood cultures are negative for growth.

16. For what circumstance would it be appropriate to contact the infection-control nurse for assistance? *(126)*
    1. Results of a blood culture are needed to validate antibiotic therapy.
    2. Contaminated waste material needs to be properly disposed.
    3. An unusual cluster of infection is seen in the emergency department.
    4. A newly admitted patient requires droplet and isolation precautions.

17. What is the **best** rationale for the consistent use of Standard Precautions? *(127)*
    1. Centers for Disease Control and Prevention (CDC) recommend "universal blood and body fluid precautions."
    2. It is difficult to accurately identify all patients infected with blood-borne pathogens.
    3. Studies show that infection rates are unaffected by use of protective measures.
    4. Hand hygiene, gloves, masks, eye protection, and gowns are appropriate for patient contact.

18. The patient has tuberculosis and has been placed in a negative-pressure isolation room with airborne precautions. Despite patient education, he sneaks out of his room and goes outside to smoke cigarettes. What should the nurse do **first**? *(138, 139)*
    1. Obtain an order for an around-the-clock sitter.
    2. Report the patient's behavior to the infection-control nurse.
    3. Ask the provider to prescribe a nicotine patch.
    4. Discuss the behavior with the patient.

19. Which patient needs to be placed into contact precautions? *(137)*
    1. Has a draining wound colonized with multidrug-resistant bacteria
    2. Has cancer and currently has leukopenia
    3. Has meningitis caused by invasive *Neisseria meningitidis*
    4. Has tuberculosis caused by *Mycobacterium tuberculosis*

20. A patient comes into the clinic and tells the nurse that he has a sore throat and would like to see a provider. For which tasks does the nurse need to wear gloves? **Select all that apply.** *(127)*
    1. Interview and taking a history
    2. Taking the patient's radial pulse
    3. Measuring an oral temperature
    4. Taking a throat swab for culture
    5. Reviewing the patient's home medications
    6. Using a tongue blade to look at the throat

21. Immediately after donning a pair of gloves, a family member develops red, watery eyes and contact dermatitis with itching of the hands. What should the nurse do **first**? *(133)*
    1. Inform the person that these are the signs/symptoms of latex allergy.
    2. Instruct the person to remove the gloves and wash thoroughly with soap and water.
    3. Contact the provider and observe for any signs of anaphylaxis.
    4. Assess for a personal or family history of latex allergy or other allergies.

22. The nurse sees the unlicensed assistive personnel (UAP) trying to take an overly full laundry bag from the patient's room to the dirty utility room. The UAP is struggling to manage the bag and is partially dragging it on the floor. What should the nurse do? *(123)*
    1. Allow the UAP to continue because she is completing her duties.
    2. Report the UAP for creating a situation where proper handling is impossible.
    3. Assist the UAP to carry the bag and then find out how it got so overfilled.
    4. Remind the UAP that overfilling the bag creates a problem for proper disposal.

23. The nurse is assigned to care for some patients who are in isolation and some who are not. What should the nurse do to meet the needs of all the patients? *(136)*
    1. Provide care for patients who are not in isolation first.
    2. Ask the charge nurse to reassign at least one of the isolation cases to another nurse.
    3. See if patients with same type of isolation can be rearranged to be roommates.
    4. Organize and cluster care of isolation patients to minimize donning and doffing gowns.

24. Which patient is the **most** challenging regarding maintaining sterile technique throughout the procedure? *(140, 141)*
    1. 4-month-old infant is crying and upset, and needs routine immunization
    2. 75-year-old woman is obese and confused and needs an indwelling urinary catheter inserted
    3. 50-year-old man is continuously coughing and needs a dressing change on upper chest
    4. 15-year-old cheerful patient with Down syndrome "wants to help" insert the IV

25. The nurse is assisting a provider by setting up a sterile tray for a procedure at the bedside. When the nurse opens the tray, there is moisture on a piece of equipment. What should the nurse do? *(143)*
    1. Continue to set up the tray, because everything inside the kit is considered sterile.
    2. Return the entire tray to the supply area for resterilization and obtain a new tray.
    3. Put on a sterile glove and remove the moist piece of equipment and set it aside.
    4. Inform the provider about the problem and obtain a new order for additional equipment.

26. The nurse is supervising a nursing student who is setting up a sterile tray to suction a patient. When would the nurse intervene? *(143)*
    1. Student sets up the field on a clean over-bed table that is at waist-level.
    2. Student touches the outside of the sterile wrapper when handling the package.
    3. Student picks up a sterile drape by the corner and lets it unfold by itself without touching any object.
    4. Student puts on sterile gloves, opens the bottle, and sets the cap on the sterile field.

27. A patient is human immunodeficiency virus (HIV)-positive and ready for discharge. He expresses fears about exposure of other family members, particularly young children, to the disease. What is the **best** response to help decrease the patient's fears and concerns? *(121, 122)*
    1. Review general principles of infection control in the home setting.
    2. Review principles of mode of transmission for HIV.
    3. Encourage expression of fears and concerns and validate feelings.
    4. Suggest that the patient maintain contact with family using phone calls, email, or video conferencing.

28. The new nurse observes a provider who routinely comes out of a patient's room, goes to the sink, quickly soaps her hands, rinses, and then shakes water from her hands so that it splashes on the floor, sink, and her uniform. What should the new nurse do? *(126)*
    1. Contact the infection-control nurse for advice.
    2. Do nothing because the provider is not accountable to the nurse.
    3. Check on the patient's status and then write up an incident report.
    4. Offer the provider a paper towel and assess understanding of hand hygiene.

29. Which patient is **most** likely to be susceptible to infection because of factors affecting immunologic defense mechanisms? *(123)*
    1. A 5-year-old child who is not up to date on school immunizations
    2. A 35-year-old woman who has recently returned from Japan
    3. A 73-year-old man who recently had chemotherapy and radiation treatments
    4. A 55-year-old man who has a high-stress job and is overweight

30. The nursing student has been diagnosed with "strep throat." Under what circumstances can the student go to the clinical unit and care for patients and complete the clinical objectives? *(128)*
    1. Has been taking prescribed antibiotics for at least 24 hours
    2. Agrees to wear a mask whenever caring for patients
    3. Cares only for patients who are not susceptible to infection
    4. Can return to clinical if the instructor is aware of the condition

31. Which patient has a condition that will be **most** challenging for the health care team to manage? *(119)*
    1. The patient is immunocompromised and has a wound infected with methicillin-resistant *Staphylococcus aureus*.
    2. The patient has a throat infection and throat culture shows β-hemolytic group A streptococci.
    3. The patient has pelvic inflammatory disease caused by *Neisseria gonorrhoeae*.
    4. The patient handles an exotic animal hide and develops a skin lesion; culture shows *Bacillus anthracis*.

32. Which health care worker is **most** likely to be a vector of infection? *(122)*
    1. A UAP removes a bag full of dirty laundry from a patient's room.
    2. A clinic nurse places a child who was exposed to measles at school in an isolated area.
    3. A nursing student has mild influenza symptoms but feels okay to go to the clinical experience.
    4. A provider sees the last patient at the clinic and forgets hand hygiene before going home.

33. The nurses are assigned a mixture of patients who need isolation or just routine Standard Precautions. Which nurse has exposed her patients to infection via the indirect method of transmission? *(123)*
    1. Nurse A first provides care for all of her patients who are not in isolation.
    2. Nurse B uses her personal stethoscope to assess all of her patients.
    3. Nurse C dons and doffs a new mask, gown, and gloves in caring for all of her patients.
    4. Nurse D washes her hands upon entering and exiting each patient's room.

34. The first-year nursing students are going to the hospital for their first clinical experience. What is the **most** important thing that the students should do to prevent exposing patients to health care–associated infections (HAIs)? *(126)*
    1. Understand how to care for patients who are in different kinds of isolation.
    2. Ensure that personal immunizations are up to date and health status is good.
    3. Know the steps for sterile technique and practice before going to clinical.
    4. Perform hand hygiene using recommendations from the CDC.

35. Which patient is showing signs of an inflammatory response in the absence of infection? *(125)*
    1. The patient has sore throat and hoarse voice that are resolving with antibiotic therapy.
    2. The patient has burning with urination and urine appears cloudy with a strong odor.
    3. The patient's ankle is swollen, red, and tender; symptoms started after falling.
    4. The patient's eye is red and irritated; he wakes with a crusty, yellow drainage.

36. The nurse performs hand hygiene before donning gloves, completes the procedure, and then doffs the gloves. What is the **best** rationale for performing hand hygiene after doffing the gloves and before leaving the patient's room? *(132)*
    1. The patient sees that the nurse is cautious and consistent about hand hygiene.
    2. The nurse may suddenly have to attend to another patient immediately upon exiting the room.
    3. The CDC recommends this final step to complete the procedure.
    4. There is a risk of perforating the gloves during use and the perforation may not be obvious.

37. The nurse is supervising a new UAP in performing care for isolation patients. When is the nurse **most** likely to intervene? **Select all that apply.** *(133, 157)*
    1. The UAP wears a mask dangling around the neck and repositions it before entering patient's room.
    2. The UAP changes the mask every 20 to 30 minutes because it takes a long time to assist a patient.
    3. The UAP removes the mask by grasping the front portion that covers the mouth and pulling if off.
    4. The UAP wears an isolation gown over the uniform to provide an extra layer of warmth.
    5. The UAP pushes the sleeves of her isolation gown up while bathing a patient.

38. The nurse is interviewing a patient at a walk-in clinic. The patient reports fatigue, weight loss, dyspnea, fever, night sweats, and coughing up small flecks of blood. What should the nurse do **first**? *(136)*
    1. Put a mask on the patient and escort him to an isolation room.
    2. Don a mask, gown, and gloves and put a mask on the patient.
    3. Assess for history of respiratory disease or family history of cancer.
    4. Alert the provider about the patient's symptoms.

39. Which actions require intervention? **Select all that apply.** *(152)*
    1. A nursing student uses hot water to clean fecal material from a bedpan.
    2. A new nurse uses a mask, protective eyewear, fluid-resistant gown, and gloves when handling a bedpan.
    3. A UAP dons gloves before performing perineal care.
    4. A provider puts a blood-encrusted instrument into the patient's sink.
    5. A nurse uses a small brush and applies friction to remove dried blood in the grooves of an instrument.

40. The patient has a urinary tract infection. Which nursing intervention would enhance the normal defense mechanism of the urinary system? *(124)*
    1. Instruct the patient to complete the prescription of antibiotics.
    2. Direct the patient to drink extra fluids to flush the urinary system.
    3. Monitor for and report fever and pain in the back or lower abdomen.
    4. Tell the patient that she will be notified about the urine culture.

CRITICAL THINKING ACTIVITIES

41. The nurse is caring for several patients. The patients include a frail 87-year-old woman with a hip fracture; a 78-year-old woman with advanced Alzheimer's disease who is being treated for dehydration secondary to incontinence of watery diarrhea; and a 60-year-old man who sustained a small perforation during a routine colonoscopy, which was recommended as part of his annual physical examination.

    a. Explain conditions that promote the onset of HAIs for these patients. *(126, 127)* _____

    _____

    _____

    b. What measures can be used to prevent HAIs? *(126)* _____

    _____

    _____

    _____

    _____

    c. Although the provider has not currently ordered isolation precautions for any of these patients, the nurse should consider initiating isolation precautions for which patient? Identify the type of isolation that the nurse would choose and give the rationale that supports the decision. *(136)*

    _____

    _____

    _____

42. The nurse is caring for a 35-year-old patient who sustained a penetrating abdominal wound and multiple bruises and contusions in a farming accident. The abdominal wound was very contaminated, but cleaned before and during surgery. The wound-care specialist has been consulted and has taught the nursing staff how to do the dressing changes. The patient has a peripheral IV and is receiving IV antibiotics and pain medication. The nurse identifies that the patient is at risk for infection.

    a. Give examples of questions that the nurse could use to collect data about factors that would affect the patient's immunologic defense mechanisms. *(123)*

    _____

    _____

    _____

    _____

    _____

b. Explain why this patient is likely to have an inflammatory response and describe the physiologic process that will occur. *(125)*

_____

_____

_____

c. Describe the signs and symptoms that would occur if the patient developed a localized infection at the abdominal wound site or at the IV site. *(125)*

_____

_____

d. Describe the signs and symptoms that the nurse would be alert for that would signal a systemic infection. *(125)*

_____

_____

_____

_____

_____

Body Mechanics and Patient Mobility

MULTIPLE CHOICE

Directions: Select the best answer(s) for each of the following questions.

1. A nurse walks into the patient's room and notices that the patient is having trouble breathing. Which position will the nurse use to help relieve the patient's respiratory distress? *(165)*
    1. Lower the head of the bed and place the patient in a supine anatomical position.
    2. Position the patient on the side with knee and thigh drawn up toward the chest.
    3. Lower the patient's head and place the body and legs on a slightly inclined plane.
    4. Raise the head of the bed to 90 degrees and have the patient lean forward on the overbed table.

2. Which position would be **most** comfortable for the patient and provide the **best** access for the nurse to insert a rectal suppository? *(165)*
    1. Sims
    2. Lithotomy
    3. Trendelenberg
    4. Orthopneic

3. Which medications are **most** likely to contribute to orthostatic hypotension? *(162)*
    1. Medications used to treat osteoporosis
    2. Medications used to prevent thrombophlebitis
    3. Medications used to reduce high blood pressure
    4. Medications used to treat arthritis pain

4. The nurse is working with a patient who has poor balance to move from the bed to the chair. What is included in the correct technique for assisting the patient to stand and pivot to the chair? *(163)*
    1. Keep the knees slightly bent.
    2. Maintain a narrow base with the feet.
    3. Keep the stomach muscles loose.
    4. Stand at arm's length from the patient.

5. The patient had a surgical procedure and is getting up to ambulate for the first time. While ambulating down the hallway, the patient says, "I'm going to faint." What should the nurse do **first**? *(168)*
    1. Call out for someone to obtain a wheelchair.
    2. Pull the patient close and lower him gently to the floor.
    3. Lean the patient against the wall until the episode passes.
    4. Support the patient and move quickly back to the room.

6. The patient will be immobilized for an extended period due to extensive injuries. Which intervention will the nurse use to prevent respiratory complications? *(168)*
    1. Suction the airway every hour.
    2. Change the patient's position every 4-8 hours.
    3. Use oxygen and nebulizer treatments regularly.
    4. Encourage deep-breathing and coughing every hour.

7. Patients who are immobilized in health care facilities require that their psychosocial needs be met along with their physiologic needs. Which statement by the nurse acknowledges these needs? *(167)*
   1. "Visiting hours will be limited so you can rest."
   2. "We will help you do everything so you don't have to worry."
   3. "Let's talk about what you used to do at home during the day."
   4. "A private room can be arranged for you."

8. The patient experienced a stroke that left her with severe left-sided paralysis and very limited mobility. Which device would prevent plantar flexion? *(169)*
   1. Footboard
   2. Bed board
   3. Trapeze bar
   4. Trochanter roll

9. When assessing the neurovascular status of a patient, what is an expected finding? *(170)*
   1. Capillary refill after 8 seconds
   2. Pulses strong and easily palpated
   3. Loss of sensation to an affected area
   4. Mild localized discomfort

10. Which range-of-motion (ROM) exercises can be safely performed on the neck? **Select all that apply.** *(171)*
    1. Flexion
    2. Supination
    3. Lateral flexion
    4. Rotation
    5. Hyperextension

11. Which patient has a contracture? *(167)*
    1. Patient has abnormal extension of a finger joint.
    2. Patient's wrist is abnormally flexed and joint is fixed.
    3. Patient's knee is hyperextended.
    4. Patient has abnormal lateral movements of ankle joint.

12. What is the **most** likely complication when an older adult patient gets pulled across the bed when changing wet linens? *(162)*
    1. Dislocation of a joint
    2. Increased stress to the joints
    3. Abnormal hyperextension of a joint
    4. Shearing or tearing of the skin

13. For an older female patient who is at risk for osteoporosis, which associated complication can be minimized by participating in a regular exercise program as prescribed by the provider? *(162)*
    1. Bone loss that results in fractures
    2. Immobility secondary to joint degeneration
    3. Tissue ischemia and pressure injuries
    4. Thrombophlebitis secondary to blood clots

14. The nurse is preparing to assist the patient to transfer from the bed to the chair. Which action demonstrates the nurse's proper use of body mechanics? *(161, 162)*
    1. Stands by the chair and reaches out to guide the patient toward the chair
    2. Stands by the side of the patient and pulls up on the stronger arm
    3. Stands directly in front of the patient and places hands at the patient's waist level
    4. Stands to the side of patient and assists as the patient pivots

15. Which situation is the **best** example of proper ergonomic principles? *(160)*
    1. Nurse A raises the head of the bed, supports the patient's shoulders, and helps to swing the legs around and off the bed using a pivoting motion.
    2. Nurse B rolls the patient onto his/her side. The nurse then stoops, and when standing, brings the patient along with the nurse.
    3. Nurse C gradually lowers the patient into the chair; the nurse bends her hips and knees as the patient leans slightly forward and sits down.
    4. Nurse D assesses for equipment such as IV lines, urinary catheters, or tubes and positions them to avoid tension during the transfer.

16. Which patient behavior should be corrected to reduce the risk of thrombophlebitis? *(167)*
    1. The patient gets out of bed and forgets to put on slippers.
    2. The patient sits in chair and crosses legs while reading a book.
    3. The patient forgets to rise slowly when getting out of bed.
    4. The patient sits in a slouched position on a soft couch.

17. The patient has a cast on the left lower leg. Which assessment is performed to prevent compartment syndrome? *(169)*
    1. Assess the patient's ability and willingness to assist with mobility.
    2. Assess muscle strength, activity tolerance, body position, and ROM.
    3. Assess skin color, temperature, movement, sensation, pulses, capillary refill, and pain.
    4. Assess patient's understanding of cast care and complications of immobility.

18. Which health care facility is using evidence-based practice to protect patients and health care workers from musculoskeletal injuries? *(161)*
    1. Hires unlicensed assistive personnel (UAP) who have at least 3 years experience and demonstrate proficiency in transferring and moving patients
    2. Has mechanical lifts available for use; there is at least an 80% compliance rate and nurses and UAP are trained in the use of devices
    3. Uses National Institute for Occupational Safety and Health (NIOSH) Division of Safety Research guidelines for designing exercise programs for older adults
    4. Places any patient who takes blood pressure medication on fall precautions and UAPs help those patients to ambulate

19. Which nurse is using the **key** factor in body mechanics? *(161)*
    1. Nurse A keeps head aligned and bends straight over at the waist to assist the patient to tie his shoelaces.
    2. Nurse B puts one leg slightly behind other, bends knees, and uses large leg muscles to boost a box to a high shelf.
    3. Nurse C reaches across the bed to support patient's back and shoulders as he dangles his feet for several minutes.
    4. Nurse D keeps head erect and aligns and balances weight on both feet when assisting a patient to stand up.

20. The nurse had a previous back injury and knows that she should avoid twisting her spine as she cares for patients. What is the **best** strategy for the nurse to use? *(161, 162)*
    1. Ask to be assigned to patients who are self-mobile.
    2. Direct the UAP to do any heavy lifting.
    3. Stand directly in front of the person or object being worked with.
    4. Take antiinflammatory pain medication before assisting patients.

21. What is an **early** sign of acute compartment syndrome? *(170)*
    1. Pain upon stretching
    2. Numbness
    3. Paralysis
    4. Cold, pale skin

22. Which patient is the **most** likely candidate for active assisted ROM exercises? *(174)*
    1. Patient A is difficult to arouse but is responsive to painful stimuli.
    2. Patient B is able to move but is very depressed and reluctant to participate.
    3. Patient C has right-sided weakness in the upper body due to a stroke.
    4. Patient D is alert and oriented but is very frail and debilitated.

23. The nurse is helping plan an activity schedule for an older adult resident at a long-term care facility who is at risk for disuse syndrome. Which plan is the nurse **most** likely to suggest? *(174)*
    1. Ten minutes of warmup and stretching, followed by 45 minutes of mild aerobic exercise, followed by 10 minutes of cool-down exercises performed 3 days a week
    2. Twenty minutes of walking on Mondays, Wednesdays, and Fridays and 10-15 minutes of moderate weight training on Tuesdays and Thursdays
    3. Patient participation in active assisted ROM for uninvolved joints for 10 minutes; alternate every 2 hours with passive assisted ROM on involved joints for 10 minutes
    4. Patient participation in activities of daily living (ADLs) (e.g., combing hair, walking to bathroom) for 10-15 minutes every 2-3 hours while awake for a total of 2 hours of activity per 24 hours

24. What instructions should the nurse give to a new home health aide about helping the patient who has problems with immobility? **Select all that apply.** *(180)*
    1. Ensure that the patient wears shoes with a nonslip sole during ambulation and transfer.
    2. Assist the patient to make slow, gradual position changes.
    3. If the patient has orthostatic hypotension, assist him to return to bed and call the provider.
    4. If the patient becomes faint or dizzy when walking, ease him to the floor or a chair.
    5. Be sure the home is free of clutter, wet areas, or rugs that may slide.

CRITICAL THINKING ACTIVITIES

25. The nurse is caring for a patient who has had a stroke with right-sided impairment. The patient has a problem with physical mobility related to right-sided paresis. He has difficulty moving his right arm and leg and this interferes with ADLs.

    a. Before turning or transferring this patient, what patient assessment and preparations should be made? *(180)*

    _____

    _____

    b. Identify the appropriate nursing action to assist the patient to move from the bed to a chair. *(178)*

    _____

    _____

    _____

    c. While transferring the patient from the bed to a chair, the patient starts to fall. What should the nurse do? *(168)*

    _____

    _____

    d. The patient is unable to perform ROM on the right upper and lower extremities. What can the nurse do to help the patient accomplish the ROM exercises? *(174)*

    _____

    _____

26. The nurse is caring for a patient who is comatose after sustaining a severe head injury several months ago. He is breathing on his own and his vital signs are stable but he shows no purposeful movements.

    a. What are the complications of immobility for this patient? *(167)* _____

    b. What nursing interventions may be implemented to prevent the occurrence of complications of immobility? *(167)*

    _____

    _____

    _____

    c. During morning hygiene, the nurse notes a reddened area on the patient's sacrum. What nursing interventions can be used to address this finding? *(168)*

    _____

    _____

    _____

Hygiene and Care of the Patient's Environment

chapter

9

MULTIPLE CHOICE

Directions: Select the best answer(s) for each of the following questions.

1. The nurse is teaching a patient who has diabetes about foot care. What should be included in the self-care instructions? *(217)*
   1. Carefully cut corns and apply moleskin.
   2. Inspect feet daily for breaks in the skin.
   3. Wear loose shoes or sandals to air the feet.
   4. Use alcohol on a gauze pad to clean between toes.

2. The nurse will delegate denture care to the unlicensed assistive personnel (UAP). What instructions should the nurse give to the UAP about the patient's dentures? *(230)*
   1. Use hot water and a mild soap.
   2. Let the patient wear them at night.
   3. Brush dentures with a soft toothbrush.
   4. Wrap them in a soft towel when not worn.

3. In delegating the early morning care that should occur before breakfast, what does the nurse remind the UAP to do for the patient? *(189)*
   1. Shampoo the patient's hair and comb it.
   2. Assist the patient with a bath and clean gown.
   3. Offer the patient a backrub with warmed lotion.
   4. Help the patient wash hands and face.

4. A patient who is paralyzed from the waist down is at risk for developing a pressure injury on the sacral area. Which intervention would the nurse use for this patient? *(205)*
   1. Frequently check and change the bed linens.
   2. Teach to shift weight every 15 minutes.
   3. Obtain an order for a donut cushion for sitting.
   4. Keep skin moist and frequently reapply lotion.

5. The nurse notices a reddened area on the patient's sacrum. What should the nurse do **first**? *(205)*
   1. Cleanse the skin with alcohol.
   2. Wash the area with warm water and soap.
   3. Massage the area to stimulate blood flow.
   4. Assess for other areas of erythema.

6. The nurse is assessing the oral cavity of an unconscious patient and sees tenacious, dried exudate on the tongue, teeth, and gums. What instructions should be given to the UAP? *(231)*
   1. Use a moistened sponge applicator and gently clean crusts several times per shift.
   2. Spray the mouth with a bulb syringe and use oral suction to remove the fluid.
   3. Use a toothbrush with paste and scrub the area until the crusts are removed.
   4. Wrap a gauze sponge around a tongue blade and apply hydrogen peroxide.

7. The nurse is evaluating the eye care that has been delegated to and is being provided by a new staff member. Which action is appropriate? *(220)*
   1. Removing dried secretions with moist gauze
   2. Using soap and water on a washcloth
   3. Cleansing the eyes from the outer to the inner canthus
   4. Wiping plastic eyeglasses with a clean paper towel

8. The nurse observes the patient performing ear care. Which behavior indicates a need for additional teaching? *(221)*
   1. Cleans the pinna with a cotton-tipped swab
   2. Turns the hearing aid off when not in use
   3. Leaves the hearing aid by a sunny window
   4. Rotates a clean washcloth to clean ear canal

9. The nurse is caring for a postpartum patient. Which assessment should the nurse perform **first** before starting perineal care? *(214)*
   1. Note presence of accumulated secretions.
   2. Evaluate the appearance of the perineum.
   3. Assess ability to perform own care.
   4. Ask about burning with urination.

10. The nurse is caring for an older adult patient who requires assistance with elimination. He can walk very slowly, but is frequently incontinent of urine before he can get to the toilet. What should the nurse do to help the patient with elimination? **Select all that apply.** *(228)*
    1. Instruct the UAP to be alert for the call signal and answer promptly.
    2. Obtain an order for an indwelling catheter until bladder training is achieved.
    3. Show the patient how to use a urinal and place it within his reach.
    4. Obtain an order for a commode chair and place it close to the bed.
    5. Restrict fluids to exact intervals to establish a voiding pattern.
    6. Make a plan with the patient to call sooner, rather than delaying.

11. The nursing student is told to observe the bowel movements of an adult patient and report any abnormalities to the nurse. What should the student report as an **unexpected** finding? *(226)*
    1. Stool was a dull clay color.
    2. Stool had soft, formed consistency.
    3. Patient had two bowel movements.
    4. Stool had the shape of the rectum.

12. The nurse is caring for an obese patient who needs assessment of skin and self-care abilities. The patient also needs perineal care, partial bath, and the bed linen changed. What is the **best** strategy to meet the needs of the patient? *(192)*
    1. Instruct the UAP to perform all tasks except the skin assessment.
    2. Ask the UAP to call when the patient's back is positioned for assessment.
    3. Assess skin and self-care abilities while working with the UAP to complete care.
    4. Assess skin and self-care abilities, then tell the patient to perform her own care.

13. Which patient is **most** likely to request that the room temperature be turned down? *(188)*
    1. Has chronic obstructive pulmonary disease
    2. Has alternating chills and fever
    3. Has peripheral vascular disease
    4. Has end-stage pancreatic cancer

14. The nurse is caring for older adult residents in an assisted-living facility. What is the **best** strategy to prevent skin breakdown among this vulnerable group? *(190)*
    1. Make daily rounds and assess skin condition.
    2. Instruct UAP to help residents out of bed as much as possible.
    3. Plan a toileting schedule for the residents at greatest risk.
    4. Ask the dietary department to serve high-quality protein foods.

15. A family member tells the nurse that the staff is spending too much time laughing and chatting at the nurses' station and it is disturbing the patient's rest and comfort. What should the nurse do **first**? *(189)*
    1. Instruct the staff to be more discreet and move conversation to the breakroom.
    2. Assess other environmental factors that are interfering with patient's comfort.
    3. Apologize to the family member and assure that the situation will be corrected.
    4. Assess the patient's discomfort and ask what other things are interfering with rest.

16. The nurse is supervising a nursing student who is giving a patient a bed bath. The nurse would intervene if the student performed which action? *(191)*
    1. Lowers the side rail to perform care
    2. Raises the head of the bed to a semi-Fowler's position
    3. Bathes arms using long, firm strokes
    4. Puts up all four side rails after completing the bath

17. The care plan indicates that all caregivers should encourage the patient's independence in accomplishing activities of daily living (ADLs). What is the **best** indication that the nurses and UAP are successful with this part of the care plan? *(230)*
    1. The UAP waits until the patient uses the call light for assistance.
    2. The nurse sees that the commode chair is close to the bed.
    3. The nurse observes that the patient is brushing his own teeth.
    4. The UAP tells the patient to independently complete ADLs.

18. An unconscious patient needs oral care. What instructions should the nurse give to the UAP to ensure the safety of the patient? **Select all that apply.** *(212)*
    1. Put the patient in a side-lying position; use pillows for support as needed.
    2. Report bleeding, sores in the mouth, or obvious problems with teeth or gums.
    3. Check for gag reflex by gently inserting a tongue blade into the throat.
    4. Use a soft toothbrush to clean inner and outer surfaces of teeth; swab mouth and tongue
    5. Have an oral suction device ready and check function prior to starting.
    6. Perform hand hygiene before donning clean gloves.

19. A neighbor tells the nurse that he has muscle soreness and stiffness after performing a new exercise program. What would the nurse recommend? *(193)*
    1. A tub bath with the proper temperature of 113° to 115° F (45° to 46° C).
    2. A bath with the water temperature at a tepid 98.6° F (37° C).
    3. A sitz bath that lasts 20-30 minutes for soaking and relaxing.
    4. A shower with a recommended water temperature of approximately 110° F (43° C).

20. A patient with dementia needs assistance with bathing. What strategies are **best** to help the patient accomplish this task? **Select all that apply.** *(201)*
    1. Maintain a relaxed demeanor, smile frequently, and use a calm tone of voice.
    2. Demonstrate and explain the desired behavior, such as how to turn on the water.
    3. Reassure frequently and say things such as, "You are doing well. We are almost done."
    4. Try to repeat the same hygiene pattern every day and wash the same body parts.
    5. Use distraction rather than trying to negotiate or making demands.
    6. Attempt to have the same caregivers as often as possible for hygienic care.

21. What is a general principle to consider when using heat and cold therapy for patients? *(208-210)*
    1. Application usually lasts only 10-20 minutes.
    2. The patient should adjust the temperature settings for comfort.
    3. The patient should move the application around for relief.
    4. Application is positioned for convenient observation.

22. A cold application is ordered for the patient. What is a positive effect of this treatment? *(211)*
    1. Vasodilation
    2. Local anesthesia
    3. Reduced blood viscosity
    4. Increased metabolism

23. The nurse applies heat to a large area on the patient's trunk. The patient reports feeling slightly dizzy and his pulse is rapid. What is the **best** physiologic explanation for this systemic reaction? *(206)*
    1. The heat application has triggered a fever.
    2. The trunk contains some large blood vessels.
    3. The application is causing vasodilation.
    4. Antibodies and leukocytes are activated.

24. What instructions should the nurse give to the UAP about applying a warm, moist compress to a small abscess in the patient's axilla? **Select all that apply.** *(207)*
    1. Compress should be 105° to 110° F.
    2. Apply for 30-40 minutes.
    3. Report pain, exudate, or redness.
    4. Notify about completion of therapy.
    5. Evaluate the response to therapy.

25. The home health nurse is observing a family member assist the patient with a heating pad. The nurse would intervene if the family member performs which action? *(209)*
    1. Assists the patient to lie on the heating pad
    2. Adjusts the pad to the lowest temperature setting
    3. Places a cloth between the skin and the heating device
    4. Checks electrical cord for fraying or kinks

26. The patient was diagnosed with a sprained ankle and the provider recommended a cold application for 20 minutes. Which condition would cause the nurse to question the order? *(206)*
    1. The patient's ankle is already slightly swollen.
    2. The pain medication has not had time to work.
    3. The patient has a history of peripheral vascular disease.
    4. The patient tells the nurse that 20 minutes is too long.

27. With appropriate instructions and supervision, which tasks related to hygienic care could be delegated to experienced UAP? **Select all that apply.** *(192)*
    1. A patient with diabetes wants to soak his feet in warm water.
    2. A patient with an indwelling urinary catheter needs assistance with pericare.
    3. A patient who is bedridden would like to have his legs massaged after a bed bath.
    4. A patient on anticoagulant therapy is too unsteady to hold his disposable razor for shaving.
    5. A patient who is unconscious has secretions along the margins of the eyelids.
    6. A patient with peripheral vascular disease would like to have her toenails trimmed.

28. What is an expected change related to aging that necessitates more frequent oral hygiene for older adults? *(190)*
    1. Older adults don't recognize that good dental health helps preserve their ability to eat.
    2. There is a decreased production of saliva and commonly an alteration in the sense of taste.
    3. Older adults tend to have more dental caries because teeth are less resistant to bacteria.
    4. There is a decreased ability to chew and digest raw fruits and vegetables that contribute to dental health.

29. A new resident has been admitted to a long-term care facility. What is the **most** important thing for the nurse to assess before delegating oral hygiene to the UAP? *(192)*
    1. Does the resident have adequate supplies, such a soft-bristle toothbrush and nonalcohol-based mouthwash?
    2. Does the UAP understand how to assist the resident and maximize the resident's independent efforts?
    3. Does the resident actually want and need assistance or is self-care more appropriate?
    4. Does the resident have a gag reflex and is he able to spit out residue from toothpaste and mouthwash?

30. The nurse is assessing a patient who is immobile because of injuries sustained in a car accident. What areas does the nurse pay special attention to for the prevention and early detection of pressure injuries? **Select all that apply.** *(202)*
    1. Sacrum
    2. Scapulae
    3. Trochanteric areas of the hips
    4. Heels
    5. Back of the head
    6. Sternum

CRITICAL THINKING ACTIVITIES

31. For the following patients, identify how bathing may be affected or altered.
    a. The patient is extremely fatigued. *(222)* _____

    b. The patient is on complete bedrest. *(212)* _____

    c. The patient has right-sided paralysis following a stroke. *(229)* _____

    d.   The patient has inflammation of the perianal tissue. *(193)* _____

_____

    e.   The patient is an East Indian Hindu. *(188)* _____

_____

    f.   The patient is an older adult who is incontinent. *(192)* _____

_____

32. A 30-year-old female patient has quadriplegia secondary to a diving accident that occurred 5 years ago. She was very healthy and athletic prior to the accident, but within the last several months, she has been hospitalized several times for recurrent urinary tract infections and significant weight loss. She currently has a poor appetite.

    a.   Identify possible risk factors that will contribute to development of pressure injuries for this patient. *(202)*

_____

_____

    b.   The nurse observes a stage I pressure injury on the patient's sacral area. Describe the criteria for a stage I pressure injury. *(203)*

_____

_____

_____

    c.   The nurse observes suspected deep tissue injury on the patient's right heel. Describe the criteria for suspected deep tissue injury. *(203)*

_____

_____

    d.   How can the nurse prevent the development of pressure injuries? *(203)* _____

_____

_____

    e.   Identify general guidelines for care of pressure injuries. *(205)* _____

_____

_____

_____

_____

Safety

chapter

10

ABBREVIATIONS

Directions: For each abbreviation, write out the full term or phrase.

1. RACE: *(249)* _____

2. CDC: *(246)* _____

3. OSHA: *(247)* _____

4. PASS: *(249)* _____

5. SRD: *(236)* _____

MULTIPLE CHOICE

Directions: Select the best answer(s) for each of the following questions.

6. The older adult tells the nurse that he is having trouble reading the labels on his medication bottles. What is the **best** strategy that the nurse could suggest to reduce the risk of an accidental medication error? *(242)*
   1. Recommend that a younger family member assist in handling the pills.
   2. Teach the patient to use a medication organizer to manage the medication.
   3. Tell the patient to have the pharmacist read the label information to him.
   4. Assist the patient to memorize the shape and color of each pill.

7. In which clinic setting is the nurse **most** likely to need knowledge of how to apply safety reminder devices (SRDs) and manage the care of these patients? *(241)*
   1. Pediatric walk-in clinic
   2. Outpatient surgery clinic
   3. Mental health walk-in clinic
   4. Adult ambulatory care clinic

8. A confused patient is yelling at the unlicensed assistive personnel (UAP). As the nurse enters the room, the patient throws the food tray at the UAP. What should the nurse do **first**? *(246)*
   1. Ask the UAP to explain what is happening with the patient.
   2. Instruct the UAP to move towards the door and then slowly shut it.
   3. Slowly walk towards the patient and use a gentle touch to soothe him.
   4. Calmly talk to the patient and respectfully address him by name.

9. The nurse is teaching a new group of UAP how to evacuate residents from a long-term care facility in case of a fire or other emergency. What piece of equipment for the universal carry method does the nurse need to teach about? *(248)*
   1. A blanket
   2. A wheelchair
   3. A stretcher
   4. A mechanical lift

10. The older adult residents in a nursing home must be evacuated because the facility is at risk for flooding and damage due to a hurricane that will pass through the area in several days. The nurse is assigned to keep a log to document the events. What information is **most** important to record? **Select all that apply.** (253)
    1. How each resident was transported
    2. Name of residents
    3. Where the residents were sent
    4. What personal belongings were sent
    5. Who transported each resident
    6. Notification of family members and health care providers

11. In the event of a mercury spill, what is the **priority** nursing action? (245)
    1. Evacuate everyone from the room.
    2. Close the interior doors and open windows.
    3. Vacuum the mercury and the glass shards.
    4. Mop the floor with hot water and soap.

12. The nurse is caring for a patient who relies on mechanical ventilation. The nurse hears a fire alarm and flames are visible in a back corridor. What should the nurse do **first**? (249)
    1. Seek assistance to move the patient and the ventilator to safety.
    2. Turn off the oxygen supply and provide manual respiratory support.
    3. Close the patient's door, call 911, and fight the fire in the corridor.
    4. Delegate the UAP to move ambulatory patients toward the exit.

13. The nurse is planning to teach a community group about fire safety in the home. What information should be included in the presentation? **Select all that apply.** (251)
    1. No smoking by the patient, family, or visitors in areas where oxygen is used.
    2. Use safety matches to light candles or fireplaces.
    3. Install fire alarms, smoke detectors, and carbon monoxide detectors.
    4. Practice fire escape routes from each room and practice exit drills.
    5. Use one electrical circuit to facilitate monitoring of cords and appliances.
    6. Cover electrical cords with a secure carpet to prevent falls.

14. An older adult patient in a long-term care facility has been wandering around outside of the room during the late evening hours. The patient has a history of falls. How should the nurse intervene? (242)
    1. Obtain an order for a bed and chair alarm.
    2. Keep the light on and play the television all night.
    3. Put up the side rails and frequently check on the patient.
    4. Have the family come to check on the patient at night.

15. The nurse applies a gait belt to a male patient of average build who has some weakness on the left side. How does the nurse position herself before assisting the patient to ambulate down the hall ? (236)
    1. On the patient's left side and holding the weak left arm.
    2. On the patient's right side and holding the front of the gait belt.
    3. On the patient's left side and holding the back of the gait belt.
    4. On the patient's right side and holding one arm around his waist.

16. The nurse is considering the use of an SRD to prevent a patient from self-injury. When using an SRD, what should the nurse do? **Select all that apply.** (238)
    1. Obtain a provider's order for the SRD.
    2. Explain the purpose of the SRD to the patient.
    3. Explain the purpose of the SRD to the family.
    4. Obtain consensus of nursing staff for type of SRD.
    5. Exhaust all alternatives before using an SRD.

17. The nurse notices smoke coming from the wastebasket in a patient's room. Upon entering the room, the nurse sees a fire that is starting to flare up. What should the nurse do **first**? (249)
    1. Extinguish the fire.
    2. Remove the patient from the room.
    3. Close the door to the room.
    4. Turn off all electrical equipment.

18. Which occurrence is **most** likely to be investigated as a "sentinel event"? (236)
    1. Patient leaves the hospital against medical advice because she gets angry with the nurse.
    2. An older patient sustains a broken arm related to the use of an SRD.
    3. A nurse is 2 hours late administering routine scheduled medications.
    4. During a follow-up phone call, a patient reports that care in the hospital was poor.

19. The nurse is conducting a fall risk assessment on an older adult patient who is moving into an assisted-living center. Which questions would the nurse ask? **Select all that apply.** *(236)*
    1. "Have you had any falls in the past year?"
    2. "Are you able to independently get up after a fall?"
    3. "Do you feel unsteady when you stand up?"
    4. "Are you able to independently walk from room to room?"
    5. "Have you ever lost consciousness before or after a fall?"
    6. "Do you use a cane or other assistive device?"

20. The nurse is giving instructions to the UAP about patient safety and fall prevention. What should the nurse tell the UAP about helping the patient to go to the bathroom? *(242)*
    1. "Help the patient whenever she needs help."
    2. "Ask her if she wants to walk or use the bedpan."
    3. "Have her sit up slowly and dangle her legs before standing."
    4. "Help her to the commode chair if she seems weak."

21. For the care of a patient who has an SRD in place, which task can be delegated to a UAP? *(240)*
    1. Observe for circulation distal to the SRD.
    2. Check for respiratory effort and breathing.
    3. Change position every 2 hours.
    4. Determine when the SRD can be removed.

22. Which instructions should be given to the UAP who is assigned to assist in the care of a patient who is being treated with internal radiation? *(237)*
    1. "Do not go into the room unless the patient uses the call bell."
    2. "Help children to don a lead shield apron before entering the room."
    3. "Wear a mask, eye shield, and isolation gown when entering the room."
    4. "Wear your personal dosimeter during care or when handling patient items."

23. A patient begins to have a grand mal seizure. What is the **priority** action? *(237)*
    1. Monitor the patency of the airway.
    2. Protect against falls and other injuries.
    3. Suction the mouth to prevent aspiration.
    4. Gently insert an oral airway between the teeth.

24. The nurse is talking to a young mother who has an infant who has just started to crawl. Based on knowledge of growth and development, which safety issue is currently the **most** important to discuss with the mother? *(237)*
    1. What to do when using pots and pans on the stove
    2. How to ensure backyard pool safety measures
    3. How to manage electrical sockets and cords
    4. Where to obtain safety labels for cleaning products

25. Which newly obtained piece of equipment creates the **greatest** risk for falls for an older adult? *(242)*
    1. Gait belt
    2. Prescription lenses
    3. Safety bar in shower
    4. Walker

26. The postoperative patient demonstrates some mild dizziness and mild shortness of breath when moving from sitting to standing position. What action would the nurse perform **first**? *(237)*
    1. Assist the patient to get into bed.
    2. Assist the patient to sit back down.
    3. Check vital signs and assess symptoms.
    4. Call the provider for an order for oxygen.

27. The patient reports dizziness when standing up too fast. Which over-the-counter medication is **most** likely to be contributing to the patient's orthostatic hypotension? *(242)*
    1. Nonaspirin pain reliever
    2. Antihistamine
    3. Vitamin supplement
    4. Medicated cough drop

28. An infant has a wound with a dressing on the left upper arm. He repeatedly attempts to remove the dressing. Which SRD would the nurse select? *(238)*
    1. Mummy wrap
    2. Wrap jacket
    3. Bilateral wrist SRDs
    4. Right elbow SRD

29. A mother brings her alert and playful child to the clinic because she "found him playing with this empty bottle of baby aspirin." Which question is the **most** important to ask the mother? *(252)*
    1. "Has he ever done anything like this before?"
    2. "How many times has he vomited since the ingestion?"
    3. "How many pills do you think were in the container?"
    4. "Did you contact poison control before you drove to the clinic?"

30. A patient with a latex allergy is exposed to latex. Which sign or symptom is cause for the **greatest** concern? *(245)*
    1. Hives
    2. Laryngeal edema
    3. Runny eyes and nose
    4. Localized swelling

31. Before the nurse can intervene, the UAP pushes contaminated material into an over-filled sharps container and sustains a puncture wound. What should the nurse do **first**? *(247)*
    1. Tell the UAP to immediately report to the infection-control nurse.
    2. Assist the UAP to scrub the wound with copious amounts of soap and water.
    3. Report the UAP for improper handling of hazardous material.
    4. Dispose of the sharps container to prevent any additional injuries to others.

32. The nurse started a new job in a small long-term care facility in a rural area. The back exit hallway is being used as a storage area while a new storage area is being planned. What should the nurse do **first**? *(249)*
    1. Report the facility for unsafe conditions.
    2. Express unwillingness to work in unsafe conditions.
    3. Review the facility's policies/procedures for emergencies.
    4. Check the building for other safety issues.

33. The nurse is sitting at the front desk at a walk-in clinic. A patient comes in and reports fever, malaise, and muscle aches with a rash on the tongue, mouth, and throat. The nurse notes pustules on the patient's palms. What should the nurse do **first**? *(254)*
    1. Notify the public health department.
    2. Put on personal protective equipment.
    3. Take vital signs and a complete history.
    4. Call the provider to triage the patient.

34. It is suspected that a patient has been exposed to cyanide gas. The nurse is alert for which symptom? *(256)*
    1. Erratic behavior
    2. Nausea and vomiting
    3. Respiratory distress
    4. Vesicle formation

35. The nurse is reviewing the disaster preparedness plan for a small nursing home. What should be included in the plan? **Select all that apply.** *(253)*
    1. Emergency treatment for the most critically injured
    2. Possible admission to a hospital or transfer to a temporary shelter
    3. Log to document residents' names and locations
    4. System to notify families and providers
    5. Designation of an area for decontamination
    6. Method of patient identification, such as a bracelet or picture ID

36. The nurse is working in a local health department and there has been an unusually large number of phone calls about food-borne illness. Which question is the nurse **most** likely to ask callers to differentiate the possible involvement of the bioterrorist agent that causes botulism from other more common causes of food-borne illness? *(254)*
    1. In addition to gastrointestinal symptoms, have you had drooping eyelids or difficulty swallowing or speaking?
    2. Have you experienced a low-grade fever, sweating, fatigue, and a nonproductive cough?
    3. How soon after eating did the abdominal cramping, vomiting, and diarrhea start?
    4. Have you had fever, malaise, and muscle aches with a rash on the tongue, mouth, throat, and palms?

CRITICAL THINKING ACTIVITIES

37. The nurse is caring for a patient in a long-term care facility. The patient has a history of falls in the home.

   a. To prevent falls, identify a patient outcome and three nursing interventions. *(236, 237)*

_____

_____

_____

_____

   b. Describe how the nurse can promote safe ambulation for the patient in a health care facility. *(236)*

_____

_____

_____

_____

   c. Identify three additional factors that influence the safety of the older adult in the home or health care environment. *(242)*

_____

_____

_____

38. The nurse is working in a small urban outpatient clinic. The nurse manager has just informed the staff that the disaster plan may have to be activated because the emergency department of a nearby hospital has identified a possible bioterrorism-related event.

   a. What is the role of the nurse in a disaster event? *(253)* _____

_____

_____

   b. What indications would alert the nurse to a possible bioterrorism-related event? *(255)* _____

_____

_____

39. List your personal fears or concerns about safety for family, friends, and self that might occur during a bioterrorism event. Discuss these fears and concerns with a classmate or your instructor.

_____

_____

_____

_____

Admission, Transfer, and Discharge

IDENTIFYING PATIENTS' REACTIONS TO ADMISSION TO A HEALTH CARE FACILITY

1. Directions: Identify and record the patient's reaction to admission to a health care facility in the blanks provided; then on the figure below (use a, b, c, or d), indicate where each patient would be on Maslow's Hierarchy. The first item is completed for you as an example. *(13, 260)*

   a. Patient appears anxious as he enters the exam room for the first time. He nervously begins to ask the nurse a series of questions about what will happen to him. Reaction: Fear of the unknown

   b. A preschooler who is admitted to the hospital is happily engaged in playing with the toys that the nurse has provided, but when her parents prepare to leave, she begins to cry and clings to them. Reaction: _____

   c. An older adult woman who has just moved into an assisted-living facility seems to need a lot of social interaction. She becomes very talkative when the nurse tries to leave the room. Reaction: _____

   d. An adolescent is admitted to the hospital, but refuses to take off his clothes and put on a hospital gown. Reaction: _____

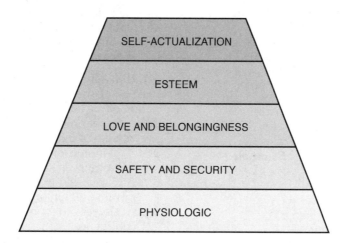

SELF-ACTUALIZATION

ESTEEM

LOVE AND BELONGINGNESS

SAFETY AND SECURITY

PHYSIOLOGIC

MULTIPLE CHOICE

Directions: Select the best answer(s) for each of the following questions.

2. The nurse is admitting a new patient to the diagnostic and surgical center. What should the nurse do **first**? *(262)*
   1. Assess immediate needs.
   2. Take vital signs.
   3. Check identification band.
   4. Orient patient to the facility routines.

3. An experienced LPN/LVN is working on a medical-surgical unit. The LPN/LVN sees that a new RN has not completed the admission assessment on a patient who arrived 20 hours ago. What should the LPN/LVN do **first**? *(265)*
   1. Wait to see if the new RN completes the admission assessment.
   2. Mention the incomplete admission assessment to the nurse manager.
   3. Remind the RN that the Joint Commission requires admission assessment within 24 hours.
   4. Offer to collect data so that the new nurse can complete the admission assessment.

4. An older adult patient is postoperative for hip surgery. He is transferred by ambulance from the hospital to a rehabilitation (rehab) unit. One hour after he is assisted into bed at the rehab unit, he dies in his sleep. Which documentation provides the **best** legal protection for the transferring nursing staff? *(269)*
   1. The provider's discharge summary and order to transfer the patient to the rehab unit
   2. The discharge assessment that was performed just before the patient left the hospital
   3. The assessment that was performed by the ambulance team in route to the rehab unit
   4. The partially completed admission assessment performed by the rehab unit nurse

5. The patient is being transferred from the medical-surgical unit to a long-term care center. What tasks can be delegated to the unlicensed assistive personnel (UAP)? **Select all that apply.** *(269)*
   1. Change soiled dressings.
   2. Bathe an incontinent patient.
   3. Assist to collect personal items.
   4. Take a final set of vital signs.
   5. Review transfer details with family.

6. A rational patient wishes to leave the hospital against medical advice (AMA), despite the nurse's best attempt at therapeutic communication. What is the nurse's **first** responsibility? *(274)*
   1. Notify the provider.
   2. Document the incident.
   3. Detain the patient.
   4. Obtain an AMA form.

7. The patient has an old head injury and demonstrates occasional intermittent episodes of belligerence and confusion interspersed with appropriate behavior. He is currently angry and wants to leave AMA. The nurse is unable to reach the provider. What should the nurse do **first**? *(275)*
   1. Explain the AMA form and consequences to the patient.
   2. Call the supervising RN, because the patient now has acute needs.
   3. Notify the family and ask them to take responsibility.
   4. Contact the risk manager and ask for permission to detain.

8. During the admission of a patient to a health care facility, what are the responsibilities of the admission department representative? **Select all that apply.** *(261)*
   1. Obtaining identifying information
   2. Giving information on the Health Insurance Portability and Accountability Act
   3. Placing the correct identification band on the patient's wrist
   4. Obtaining a list of current medications
   5. Obtaining emergency contact information
   6. Gathering insurance information

9. Which newly admitted patient is **most** likely to need and benefit from an individualized explanation of the bathroom facilities? *(263)*
   1. A 75-year-old woman with advanced Alzheimer's disease
   2. A 20-month-old child who has just started toilet training
   3. A 65-year-old man who is from a rural farming region of China
   4. A 50-year-old woman who has stress incontinence

10. The nurse is placing an identification band on a patient who was admitted through the emergency department. What is **best** to say as the band is applied? *(261)*
    1. "This is your assigned hospital identification number."
    2. "The primary purpose of the band is to maintain safety."
    3. "All patients have to wear these; it's standard procedure."
    4. "We don't want to lose you while you are in the hospital."

11. The patient is newly admitted and seems anxious, but also appears very hesitant to ask questions. Which statement by the nurse **best** demonstrates empathy? *(263)*
    1. "Call me if you need anything; I'll be happy to help you."
    2. "There's nothing to worry about; we'll take good care of you."
    3. "I know you must have a lot of questions; I know I would."
    4. "You seem a little uncertain; do you have some questions?"

12. The nurse is trying to explain the bed controls and the call button and other items related to hospitalization, but the older adult patient keeps telling the nurse to "wait for my son to get here." What should the nurse do **first**? *(263)*
    1. Go find the son or other available family members.
    2. Leave written information at the bedside.
    3. Give brief information using very simple language.
    4. Offer comfort measures and ensure patient safety.

13. Which tasks related to admitting a new patient can be delegated to the UAP? **Select all that apply.** *(262, 265)*
    1. Obtain personal care items, such as water pitcher or packaged cleansing cloths.
    2. Position the bed for transfer from stretcher or wheelchair.
    3. Hang signs above the bed related to care, such as "nothing by mouth."
    4. Ask the patient if he/she needs special equipment, such as a walker.
    5. Store belongings, such as jewelry, watch, or wallet, in bedside table.
    6. Assist the patient to arrange desired items, such as eyeglasses, within reach.

14. The patient tells the nurse that he would like to be transferred to hospital X, because his cardiologist doesn't come to hospital Y. What should the nurse do? *(269)*
    1. Obtain an AMA form and have the patient sign it.
    2. Call hospital X and advise that the patient desires transfer.
    3. Advise the patient that the cardiologists in hospital Y are good.
    4. Advise the patient that a transfer requires an order from the provider.

15. A patient with Alzheimer's disease is being transferred from a long-term care facility to an acute care hospital for possible sepsis and change in mental status. Which question is the **most** important to ask the nurse who is giving the report? *(268, 269)*
    1. "Has the family been advised about the reason for the transfer?"
    2. "What is the patient's baseline mental status and behavior?"
    3. "When is the patient scheduled to be transferred?"
    4. "Will the patient be accompanied by a nurse or family member?"

16. Which patient is likely to have the **most** complex discharge plan? *(273)*
    1. A 73-year-old man with chronic disease who has no family in the area
    2. A 23-year-old mother who just delivered her first healthy baby
    3. A 17-year-old adolescent who broke his leg during a ski trip
    4. A 35-year-old woman who had an emergency appendectomy

17. The nurse is giving instructions to a family caregiver of an older patient who will need help after discharge from the hospital. The nurse senses tension, resentment, and unwillingness from the caregiver. What should the nurse do **first**? *(273)*
    1. Continue to give the instructions and ask for feedback from the caregiver.
    2. Notify the provider for an order for home health nursing.
    3. Get a social service consult to resolve family tensions and problems.
    4. Assess the caregiver's attitude toward the patient and the circumstances.

CRITICAL THINKING ACTIVITIES

18. The patient is admitted through the emergency department for an exacerbation of a chronic respiratory disorder. When the patient arrives at his room on the medical-surgical unit, he appears very tired. He has oxygen per nasal cannula and demonstrates labored breathing. He is able to speak, but his sentences are short and he takes a breath after every few words. How would the nurse modify the nursing actions related to the admission to meet the needs of this particular patient? *(265)*

    a. Checking and verifying the identification band: _____

    _____

    b. Assessing immediate needs: _____

    _____

    c. Explaining hospital routines, such as visiting hours, mealtime, and morning wake-up: _____

    _____

    d. Orienting the patient to the room:_____

    _____

    _____

19. A 45-year-old woman was admitted to the hospital for chronic infection of a stasis ulcer on her leg. She will be discharged after completing antibiotic therapy and consultation with the wound care specialist.

    a. Identify examples of health care disciplines other than nursing that are involved in referrals and explain their role in the discharge process. *(273)*

    _____

    _____

    _____

    _____

    b. Discuss the importance of discharge instructions for patients who have chronic conditions. *(273)*

    _____

    _____

    _____

Vital Signs

WORD SCRAMBLE

Directions: Unscramble the words that are related to taking and interpreting vital signs and then match the term to the correct definition or characteristic listed below.

Scrambled Term	Unscrambled Term	Definition or Characteristic
1. cardiaydarb *(290)*		
2. dysaenp *(295)*		
3. pertherhymia *(282)*		
4. pneabrady *(295)*		
5. ssylicto *(296)*		
6. achypneat *(295)*		
7. yyhhdrstmia *(290)*		
8. pohymiather *(283)*		
9. diacartachy *(290)*		
10. sionpertenhy *(279)*		

Definition or characteristic of terms related to taking and interpreting vital signs

a. Irregularity in the normal rhythm of the heart
b. Normal finding for well-conditioned athlete
c. Represents the ventricles contracting, forcing blood into the aorta and the pulmonary arteries
d. Expected respiratory pattern while exercising
e. Laboring with difficulty to get enough oxygen
f. Slow respiratory rate, fewer than 10 per minute
g. Above-normal body temperature
h. Expected heart rate if very frightened or angry
i. The silent killer
j. Occurs more frequently in cold weather

FIGURE LABELING

11. Directions: Label the figure below with the names and sites for assessment of peripheral pulses. *(293)*

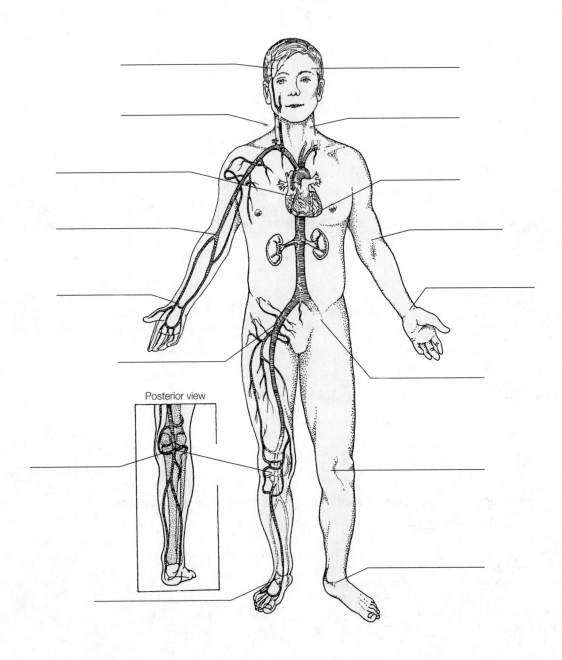

Posterior view

FIGURE LABELING

12. Directions: Identify on the aneroid gauge where the Korotkoff's sounds are heard for a blood pressure of 136/78 mm Hg. *(290)*

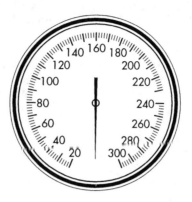

TABLE ACTIVITY

13. Directions: Complete the table below with the expected vital signs for different age groups. *(281)*

Age Group	Heart Rate (per Minute)	Respiratory Rate (per Minute)	Blood Pressure (mm Hg)
Neonate			Systolic:
Infant			Systolic:
Toddler			Systolic:
School-age (6-10 years)			Systolic: Diastolic:
Adolescent (10-18 years)			Systolic: Diastolic:
Adult			Systolic: Diastolic:
Older adult			Systolic: Diastolic:

MULTIPLE CHOICE
Directions: Select the best answer(s) for each of the following questions.

14. The nurse is taking blood pressures (BP) at a community health fair and screening people for risk factors for hypertension. Which person has the **most** risk factors for developing hypertension? *(298)*
    1. 23-year-old athletic Asian American woman with a BP of 120/80 mm Hg and a family history of hypertension
    2. 32-year-old African American mother of two children with a BP of 134/70 mm Hg who exercises regularly
    3. 66-year-old thin Jewish American male with a BP of 124/80 mm Hg; he regularly drinks alcohol and has a sedentary lifestyle
    4. 45-year-old African American man with a BP of 130/80 mm Hg who smokes, is overweight, and eats a vegetarian diet

15. The unlicensed assistive personnel (UAP) just reported patients' vital signs to the nurse. For which patient is an increased pulse an expected finding? *(280)*
    1. Patient received antihypertensive medications 4 hours ago.
    2. Patient needs scheduled routine medication for hypothyroidism.
    3. Patient who has a fever had a dose of antipyretic medication 6 hours ago.
    4. Patient's medications are being managed by the cardiac rehabilitation team.

16. The nurse needs to get an apical pulse on an older woman who has large, sagging breasts. What should the nurse do **first**? *(282)*
    1. Lift the left breast and place the bell or diaphragm at the fifth intercostal space.
    2. Lift the breast and place palm of hand over the point of maximal impulse.
    3. Use the bell of the stethoscope to make a tight seal against the lateral chest wall.
    4. Obtain the ultrasonic Doppler and position it where breast tissue is most flattened.

17. The nurse observes that the patient has an elevated temperature. What questions would the nurse ask to collect data about a systemic infection? **Select all that apply.** *(283)*
    1. Do you feel thirsty?
    2. Do you have a headache?
    3. Are you having trouble resting or getting comfortable?
    4. Would you like some medication to reduce your fever?
    5. Have you experienced any chills?

18. The UAP reports to the nurse that the "pulse oximeter might be broken" because some of the patients had low readings. What should the nurse do **first**? *(296)*
    1. Instruct the UAP to go back and retake the readings on any patient who had a low value.
    2. Ask the UAP if the patients who had a low reading were having any problems breathing.
    3. Examine and troubleshoot the pulse oximeter and test it on several healthy staff members.
    4. Assess the patients who had low readings and determine if extraneous factors are present.

19. The nurse hears in report that the patient has peripheral arterial disease that affects his lower extremities. What would the nurse expect to find during assessment? *(293)*
    1. Popliteal pulses are full and bounding and there is some mild edema in the posterior calf.
    2. Dorsalis pedis and posterior tibial pulses are weak, and toes are cooler than upper leg.
    3. Patient reports severe pain with loss of sensation and decreased strength and movement in legs.
    4. Brachial and radial pulses are weak compared to dorsalis pedis and posterior tibial pulses.

20. The nurse notes that a patient occasionally sighs during the morning assessment. What is the clinical significance of occasional sighing? *(295)*
    1. The patient had trouble breathing during the night and sighing is related to lower blood oxygen levels.
    2. This is a behavior that many people demonstrate when they are bored or frustrated.
    3. The patient has a chronic lung disease and deep breathing is characteristic of the disorder.
    4. Occasional sighing is considered normal and allows all alveoli to be aerated.

21. An experienced UAP reports that the patient is alert and asking for breakfast. Vital signs have been completed and recorded as follows: axillary temperature of 100.6° F, pulse of 80 beats/min, respirations 16/min, and BP 120/70 mm Hg. What is the nurse's **first** action? *(288)*
    1. Instruct the UAP to obtain a breakfast tray for the patient.
    2. Ask the UAP to repeat the temperature using the oral or tympanic method.
    3. Direct the UAP to repeat all of the vital signs and observe technique.
    4. Ask the UAP to explain the choice of axillary method to measure the temperature.

22. A new nurse has taken a job on a medical-surgical unit. According to the shift report, the four assigned patients are stable and should have a predictable clinical stay. Based on the report, how often does the nurse plan to take the vital signs? *(280)*
    1. Every hour until the nurse verifies for self that the patients are stable.
    2. Before and after administering any oral or intravenous medications.
    3. According to facility policy for frequency unless status changes.
    4. At the beginning and end of the shift, unless the provider orders otherwise.

23. The nursing student takes a BP on a patient who has been in a coma for several months. The student reports to the nurse that the BP seems too low. What would the nurse do **first**? *(280)*
    1. Direct the student to retake the BP on the opposite extremity.
    2. Go with the student and assess the patient for other signs/symptoms.
    3. Instruct the student to check the chart to see what is baseline for the patient.
    4. Remind the student that a prolonged coma will cause changes in vital signs.

24. A patient who is brought to the emergency department was discovered lying in an alley. He is cold and wet and demonstrates slurred speech. His temperature is 94° F. How does his condition affect his pulse rate? *(290)*
    1. Tachycardia is likely due to the stress of cold exposure.
    2. Since he is conscious, there should be no effects on pulse.
    3. A decreased heart rate reflects lowered metabolism.
    4. Palpating pulses will be impossible because of vasoconstriction.

25. The UAP takes vital signs at 3:00 AM and reports to the nurse that the patient's temperature is 97.6° F (36.4° C). The nurse sees that the patient's temperature at 6:00 PM was 99.6° F (37.5° C) and at 11:00 PM was 98.2° F (36.8° C). What should the nurse do? *(283)*
    1. Thank the UAP and explain that lower temperatures occur between 1 AM and 4 AM.
    2. Repeat the temperature, but use a different method than what the UAP used.
    3. Tell the UAP to document the temperature and not to worry about it.
    4. Ask the UAP to get the patient a warm blanket and increase the room temperature.

26. Two nurses simultaneously assess to determine if a patient has a pulse deficit. One nurse counts the apical pulse at 105 beats/min. The other nurse takes the radial pulse and counts 96 beats/min. What is the pulse deficit? *(293)*

_____

27. When assessing the apical pulse, how does the nurse count the pulse rate? *(293)*
    1. Counts for 20 seconds and multiplies by 3
    2. Counts for 60 seconds and does not multiply
    3. Counts for 30 seconds and multiplies by 2
    4. Counts for 15 seconds and multiplies by 4

28. The nurse is supervising a first-year nursing student who is checking the patient's peripheral pulses. The nurse would intervene if the student performed which action? *(291)*
    1. Palpated all of the pulses, including carotids and femorals bilaterally
    2. Positioned the patient in the prone position to assess the popliteal artery
    3. Palpated the point of maximal impulse and assessed the apical pulse for 60 seconds
    4. Palpated the radial pulse with the pads of the index and third fingers

29. Which factor/condition is **most** likely to increase the patient's respiratory rate? *(296)*
    1. Opioid medication
    2. Acute pain
    3. Hypothermia
    4. Brainstem injury

30. The nurse counts respirations immediately following measurement of the radial pulse while the fingers are still in place over the artery. What is the **best** rationale for this technique? *(296)*
    1. Rapport has been established so the patient is likely to be less anxious.
    2. Therapeutic touch of the nurse's fingers on the patient's wrist is soothing.
    3. Patients may voluntarily alter respiratory rate if they know they are being monitored.
    4. Counting respirations immediately after pulse check is an efficient timesaver.

31. A nursing student is preparing to take the BP on a patient who has excessive adipose tissue on the upper arm. If the student uses a normal-sized cuff, what is likely to occur? *(302)*
    1. The BP will be falsely elevated.
    2. The patient will be uncomfortable during the procedure.
    3. The systolic pressure will be artificially lower.
    4. The BP is likely to be very close to baseline.

32. The nurse receives the end-of-shift report from the off-going nurse. Based on the vital sign information for the assigned adult patients, which patient should the nurse check on **first**? *(281)*
    1. BP 120/80, P 68, R 16
    2. BP 110/74, P 72, R 14
    3. BP 130/90, P 80, R 18
    4. BP 120/90, P 62, R 9

33. The nurse sees in the patient's documentation that the patient has a radial pulse of 4+. What assessment would the nurse plan to make for this patient? *(290)*
    1. Doppler assessment of pulses for hands and feet
    2. Observe for pallor or cyanosis in the hands
    3. Assess BP for hypertension
    4. Assess apical and radial pulse for a pulse deficit

34. The patient's pulse oximetry reading appears to be lower than expected. The patient is breathing easily, the lungs are clear, the oxygen is delivered as ordered, and the patient reports, "feeling fine." What would the nurse do **first**? *(282)*
    1. Check the position of the pulse oximeter.
    2. Feel the patient's fingers for coolness or warmth.
    3. Apply the pulse oximeter to own finger to test function.
    4. Ask the patient if he has any circulation problems.

35. The nurse needs to take the temperature of a baby who was brought to the clinic for his 6-month well-baby visit. Which method of measuring the temperature is the **best** choice for this patient? *(288)*
    1. Oral
    2. Axillary
    3. Rectal
    4. Temporal arterial

36. The nurse received a new stethoscope as a graduation present. What will he/she do to care for and appropriately use the stethoscope? *(290)*
    1. Drape the stethoscope around the neck to have it readily available.
    2. Clean the tubing with alcohol swabs after every patient contact.
    3. Remove the earpieces regularly and clean off cerumen, dust, and oils.
    4. Frequently rub the tubing between the palms to keep it soft.

37. The nurse is caring for a patient who is several days postoperative for major abdominal surgery. The UAP reports that the pulse is 120 beats/min. The nurse rechecks the pulse and gets 122 beats/min. What will the nurse assess for? **Select all that apply.** *(290)*
    1. Pain
    2. Infection
    3. Anxiety
    4. Hemorrhage
    5. Substance abuse
    6. Hypothermia

38. The patient has a sudden deterioration in condition with confusion; diaphoresis; pallor; and cold, clammy skin. Which peripheral pulse site is the **best** to quickly determine the pulse rate? *(293)*
    1. Radial
    2. Femoral
    3. Carotid
    4. Brachial

39. The nurse hears in report that the patient has bilateral dorsalis pedis pulses 3+. How does the nurse use this information in planning care? *(291)*
    1. Allots time to check circulation and sensation on both feet every 2 hours
    2. Plans to follow up and ensure that the provider is aware of the finding
    3. Instructs UAP to do range-of-motion exercises to hands every 3 hours
    4. Plans to do routine change-of-shift assessment and observe as needed

40. The UAP tells the nurse that the patient has a respiratory rate of 40/min and "is having trouble breathing." What additional signs or symptoms is the nurse **most** likely to observe? **Select all that apply.** (295)
    1. Pursed-lip breathing
    2. Flared nostrils
    3. Epistaxis
    4. Costal retractions
    5. Fatigue
    6. Shortness of breath

41. The nurse checks the patient's BP and obtains a reading of 160/90 mm Hg. What is the pulse pressure? _____ (297)

42. The nurse hears in report that the patient has an auscultatory gap. The nurse plans to adapt the technique for measuring which vital sign? (300)
    1. Temperature
    2. Pulse
    3. Respiratory rate
    4. BP

MATH AND CONVERSION

43. Convert the following temperature readings (282)

    a. 37° C   =   _____ ° F

    b. 101.2° F   =   _____ ° C

    c. 39.2° C   =   _____ ° F

    d. 97.8° F   =   _____ ° C

44. Convert weight in pounds to the equivalent in kilograms. (306)

    a. A patient who weighs 44 lbs weighs _____ kg.

    b. A patient who weighs 210 lbs weighs _____ kg.

45. Convert weight in kilograms to the equivalent in pounds. (306)

    a. A patient who weighs 6 kilograms weighs _____ lbs.

    b. A patient who weighs 16 kilograms weighs _____ lbs.

46. Convert height in feet and inches to the equivalent in centimeters. (306)

    a. A patient who is 5 feet 9 inches tall is _____ centimeters.

    b. A patient who is 2 feet 3 inches tall is _____ centimeters.

47. Fluid balance may be assessed by weighing the patient. If the patient weighs 2 kg less today than yesterday, how much fluid was lost? _____ mL (306)

CRITICAL THINKING ACTIVITIES

48. A 58-year-old female patient was admitted with pneumonia 2 days ago. The nurse recognizes that the patient must be monitored for signs of worsening infection. The patient's temperature, taken at 7:00 AM, is 101.2° F.

    a. Discuss factors that may be affecting the body temperature of this patient. (283) _____
    _____
    _____

    b. What systemic signs and symptoms are associated with an elevated temperature? (283)_____
    _____
    _____

    c. What should the nurse do if the patient's temperature is above normal? (283) _____
    _____
    _____

49. The nurse is caring for a patient who was admitted for a chronic respiratory problem. Upon entering the room, the nurse observes that the patient is struggling to move from a supine position to a sitting position and breathing is rapid and labored. The nurse notes tension in neck and shoulder muscles with each inspiration. The patient is anxious and repeatedly apologizes for "being a bother" while trying to explain why he came to the hospital and how his disease is affecting his life and his family.

a. For this patient, what factors may be contributing to the increased respiratory rate? *(296)* _____

_____

_____

_____

b. What should the nurse do if the patient's respirations are rapid and labored? *(296)* _____

_____

_____

_____

c. Write a response that the nurse could use to help this patient deal with the immediate respiratory problem. *(296)*

_____

_____

_____

50. Discuss how the nurse uses clinical judgment to determine the frequency, method, and interpretation of vital signs. *(307)*

_____

_____

_____

_____

_____

_____

_____

_____

_____

Physical Assessment

TABLE ACTIVITY

1. Directions: Complete the table by supplying the correct terms that you would use to document the physical assessment findings described on the right. Aim for correct spelling! *(314)*

Term	Description
	Lack of appetite resulting in the inability to eat
	Heart rate of less than 60 beats per minute
	Difficulty passing stools or infrequent passage of hard stools
	Bluish discoloration of the skin and mucous membranes
	Profuse sweating
	Shortness of breath or difficulty breathing
	Extravasation of blood into the subcutaneous tissues
	Abnormal accumulation of fluid in interstitial spaces
	Redness or inflammation of the skin or mucous membranes
	The protective response of the tissues of the body to irritation or injury
	Yellow tinge to the skin
	State or quality of being indifferent, apathetic, or sluggish
	Sensation often leading to the urge to vomit
	Must sit upright or stand to breathe comfortably
	Unnatural paleness or absence of color in the skin
	Itching and an uncomfortable sensation leading to an urge to scratch
	Creamy, viscous, pale yellow, or yellow-green exudate; liquefied necrosis of tissues
	Unhealthy yellow color; usually said of a complexion or skin
	Heart rate greater than 100 beats per minute
	Abnormally rapid rate of breathing
	Expel the contents of the stomach out of the mouth

MULTIPLE CHOICE
Directions: Select the best answer(s) for each of the following questions.

2. The patient sprains his ankle. During the inflammatory response, damaged tissue releases chemicals that increase the permeability of the capillary walls, which allows white blood cells and plasma to move into the area. What does the nurse expect to be included in the subjective and objective data? *(314)*
   1. Patient reports pain and obvious swelling around ankle.
   2. Patient reports numbness and skin is cool and pale.
   3. Patient reports pruritus and there is a fine red rash.
   4. Patient reports weakness and peripheral pulses are weak.

3. The nurse is almost finished doing a routine head-to-toe assessment on a newly admitted patient. Suddenly, the patient starts coughing and reports "trouble breathing." What should the nurse do **first**? *(316)*
   1. Quickly complete the head-to-toe assessment and then call the provider.
   2. Switch to a focused respiratory assessment and listen to lung sounds.
   3. Assist the patient to sit upright and give oxygen per mask or nasal cannula.
   4. Stay with the patient and reassure him that the coughing episode will pass.

4. The nurse needs to assess a patient who had a head injury. Which neurologic assessment would the nurse perform **first**? *(325)*
   1. Vital signs
   2. Motor function
   3. Pupillary response
   4. Level of consciousness

5. The nurse hears in shift report that an older patient has "tenting" over the sternum. Based on this information, what is **most** important for the nurse to monitor and assess? *(327)*
   1. Auscultate lung sounds and respiratory status.
   2. Monitor intake and output and check electrolyte values.
   3. Observe the anterior trunk for redness or ecchymoses.
   4. Monitor for tenting on other areas of the body.

6. An older adult woman walks into the interview room. She smiles at the nurse and looks around the room. The nurse says, "Please take a seat," and the woman takes a brochure from the display case. The nurse says, "Why have you come to see us today?" The woman says, "Yes dear, tea is fine. Thank you." Based on this interaction, what assessments will the nurse perform **first**? *(328)*
   1. Head-to-toe assessments to detect any problems
   2. Mental status and family structure/support
   3. Cultural, age, and gender influences on behavior
   4. Auditory sensory perception and cognitive function

7. The patient is diagnosed with sickle cell trait. Based on the nurse's knowledge of pathophysiology, which intervention is **most** likely to be recommended for the patient? *(312)*
   1. Review of allergens in the home environment
   2. Referral for genetic counseling
   3. Dietary evaluation to identify deficiencies
   4. Prescription for broad-spectrum antibiotics

8. The nurse is examining the patient's eyes. Which finding is the **most** important to report to the provider? *(328)*
   1. Eyes appear asymmetric; left eyelid has a fold, right eyelid does not.
   2. Sclerae of both eyes are white and the conjunctivae are pink.
   3. Right pupil constricts when light is applied and left pupil also constricts.
   4. There is similar puffiness and periorbital edema around both eyes.

9. The nurse hears in report that the patient had a Glasgow Coma Scale score of 15 during the night shift. What is an **early** sign that indicates a deterioration in neurologic status? *(326)*
   1. Patient knows his own name, but does not recognize his spouse.
   2. Patient is unable to move hands or fingers on command.
   3. Patient's right pupil is slightly larger and more sluggish than the left.
   4. Patient has widening pulse pressure, bradycardia, and irregular breathing.

10. To decrease the risk for lung disease, which lifestyle modification is the **most** important to recommend to patients? *(313)*
    1. Seek cancer screening.
    2. Exercise regularly.
    3. Stop smoking.
    4. Limit dietary fats.

11. While obtaining the vital signs of an adult, the nurse observes that the patient is diaphoretic and flushed. Which change in vital signs would the nurse expect to accompany this observation? *(314)*
    1. Respiratory rate of 10/min
    2. Pulse of 65 beats/min
    3. Blood pressure of 100/60 mm Hg
    4. Temperature of 101° F (38.3° C)

12. The nurse hears in report that the patient has had occasional episodes of cyanosis and dyspnea. Which physical assessment does the nurse plan to frequently perform during the shift? *(314)*
    1. Check for abdominal pain.
    2. Assess respiratory effort.
    3. Monitor urinary output.
    4. Assess for headache.

13. While assessing the patient, the nurse observes that the patient experiences orthopnea. What instruction will the nurse give the unlicensed assistive personnel (UAP) about assisting the patient? *(315)*
    1. The patient is too weak to walk to the bathroom.
    2. Dizziness will occur if the patient stands up too quickly.
    3. Keep the head of the bed elevated at all times.
    4. The dominant hand is not functioning properly.

14. The patient's oral temperature is 101.2° F (38.4° C). The patient tells the nurse that he doesn't feel well, but has no known health conditions. What question would the nurse ask **first** to try to localize the source of infection? *(320)*
    1. "What other symptoms are you having?"
    2. "Do you have any known allergies?"
    3. "Have you ever felt like this before?"
    4. "When did you first notice the fever?"

15. The nurse hears in report that a patient who has cancer is experiencing anorexia. Which assessment does the nurse plan to conduct during the shift? *(332)*
    1. Assess need for supplemental oxygen.
    2. Evaluate ability to independently ambulate.
    3. Review efficacy of PRN pain medication.
    4. Assess need for supplemental nutrition.

16. The nurse is interviewing an older patient and notices that the patient is slumping and irritable and frequently sighs. Which question would the nurse ask to validate the **most** likely interpretation of the patient's behavior? *(324)*
    1. "Are you short of breath?"
    2. "Are you feeling tired?"
    3. "Would you like some water?"
    4. "Are you having pain?"

17. A patient tells the nurse that she is "afraid of the doctor." How could this affect the objective data? *(312)*
    1. Description of pain will be exaggerated.
    2. Patient is likely to experience nausea
    3. Blood pressure could be higher than expected.
    4. Pupils will be constricted and nonreactive.

18. The provider tells the nurse that the patient has pruritus. Which objective finding is the nurse **most** likely to observe? *(315)*
    1. Scratch marks on skin
    2. Abdominal distention
    3. Abnormal breath sounds
    4. Low-grade temperature

19. The nurse uses the OPQRSTUV method of obtaining the most information about the patient's pain. Which question addresses the P in the OPQRSTUV? *(320)*
    1. On a scale of 1 to 10, what number is the pain?
    2. What causes the pain to increase or decrease?
    3. When did you first notice the pain?
    4. Is the pain spreading out to other areas?

20. The nurse reads in the patient's chart that the patient has crackles in the posterior lower lobes. What does the nurse expect to hear during auscultation if the patient's condition is unchanged? *(329)*
    1. Short, discrete, bubbling sounds on inspiration
    2. High-pitched, musical sounds on inspiration
    3. Grating sounds on expiration
    4. Coarse gurgling on expiration

21. Which evaluation statement indicates that the antibiotic therapy has successfully resolved the patient's leg infection? *(314)*
    1. The patient reports that pain is decreased compared to previously.
    2. The patient is observed independently ambulating in hallway.
    3. The wound site shows no signs of erythema; white cell count is normal.
    4. The wound site shows edema, redness, and white cell count is elevated.

22. Which method would be **best** to assess an older patient's ability to accomplish activities of daily living ? *(322)*
    1. Accompany the patient during ambulation to the bathroom.
    2. Ask the patient what he normally eats during the day.
    3. Take a full set of vital signs and include pain assessment.
    4. Observe the patient's level of consciousness and orientation.

23. The nurse is assessing an older patient. Which explanation should the nurse use? *(316)*
    1. "I am going to auscultate the posterior lung fields."
    2. "I will be checking your motor function."
    3. "I would like to check your perineal area."
    4. "I am going to listen to your heartbeat."

24. The nurse is **most** likely to use the Glasgow Coma Scale for which patient? *(326)*
    1. Recently had a myocardial infarction
    2. Sustained a serious head injury
    3. Shows some signs of septic shock
    4. Has risk for respiratory failure

25. The nurse observes jugular venous distention on a patient who is sitting in the interview chair. What other signs or symptoms would the nurse check to validate suspicion of heart failure? *(327)*
    1. Low heart rate
    2. Increased urinary output
    3. Dependent edema in legs
    4. Jaundice of sclera

26. A new nurse documents PERRLA in the patient's chart. When the preceptor nurse asks her to describe the findings, the new nurse is unable to explain. What should the preceptor nurse do **first**? *(328)*
    1. Show the new nurse how to perform the assessment.
    2. Ask the new nurse how she knew to document PERRLA.
    3. Instruct the new nurse to seek out the nurse educator.
    4. Report the new nurse for falsifying the documentation.

27. The nurse is assessing the patency of the nostrils. What is the **best** method to use? *(328)*
    1. Use a penlight and observe for blockage or excess mucus.
    2. Press against one nostril and ask the patient to breathe.
    3. Give the patient a tissue and instruct to blow the nose.
    4. Ask the patient to breathe quietly and listen for air movement.

28. What is the UAP's role in assessing the respiratory system? *(329)*
    1. Observe and report changes in rate and depth.
    2. Determine a position that accommodates orthopnea.
    3. Auscultate the lung sounds every 4 hours or as needed.
    4. Monitor and interpret the pulse oximeter readings.

29. What would be considered a normal finding when assessing the patient's spine? *(330)*
    1. A gentle inward curvature of the lumbosacral curve
    2. A large posterior curvature of the thoracic spine
    3. An increased curvature of the lumbar spine
    4. A right or left lateral spinal curvature

30. The nurse is unable to palpate the popliteal pulse. Which pulse would the nurse assess before informing the provider? *(331)*
    1. Femoral pulse
    2. Dorsalis pedis pulse
    3. Brachial pulse
    4. Apical pulse

CRITICAL THINKING ACTIVITIES

31. A 40-year-old man comes to the clinic. He desires a general physical check-up and reports, "not feeling quite 100%." This is the patient's first visit to the clinic, so there are no medical records available for comparison. Provide examples of questions that the nurse could ask to obtain information during a review of systems. *(321, 322)*

   a. Respiratory: _____

   _____

   b. Endocrine: _____

   _____

   c. Gastrointestinal: _____

   _____

   d. Cardiac: _____

   _____

   e. Neurologic: _____

   _____

   f. Genitourinary: _____

   _____

32. A 30-year-old woman comes to the emergency department. She reports pain in the lower abdomen. She appears very uncomfortable and is walking in a slightly bent-over position. Her hands are supporting her lower abdomen as she moves toward the examination room.

   a. Use the OPQRSTUV method to elicit information about the abdominal pain. *(320)* _____

   _____

   _____

   _____

   _____

   _____

   b. Describe how the nurse performs the physical assessment of the abdomen. *(333)*_____

   _____

   _____

   _____

   _____

33. How does the nurse generate subjective and objective data when the patient says, "I have a really bad headache"? *(320, 321)*

   _____

   _____

   _____

   _____

   _____

34. The nurse is conducting an interview with a patient who was just admitted to the medical-surgical unit. The nurse stands at the bedside and initially smiles at the patient, but as she is asking the questions, the nurse frequently glances out the window and shifts restlessly back and forth. She diligently fills out the admission form while reading the questions from the form. When the patient tries to explain a point, she cuts him off and moves on to the next question. She checks the equipment necessary for the patient's care while the patient is trying to explain his symptoms. Discuss this nurse-patient interaction from the patient's point of view. *(319, 323)*

_____
_____
_____
_____
_____
_____
_____
_____
_____
_____
_____

Oxygenation

SHORT ANSWER

Directions: Using your own words, answer each question in the space provided.

1. List five teaching points that the nurse will review with patients who are on oxygen therapy. *(340)*

    a. _____

    b. _____

    c. _____

    d. _____

    e. _____

2. List three patient problem statements that are used for patients who are having problems with adequate oxygenation. *(341)*

    a. _____

    b. _____

    c. _____

MULTIPLE CHOICE

Directions: Select the best answer(s) for each of the following questions.

3. In performing nursing skills and procedures for patients, which nursing action demonstrates the nurse's understanding and use of Standard Precautions? *(339)*
    1. Always checks the patient's armband and asks the patient to state his or her name
    2. Assesses the patient's understanding and teaches accordingly
    3. Performs hand hygiene before and after every patient encounter
    4. Evaluates the patient's response to and tolerance of the procedure

4. The patient requires suctioning of pulmonary secretions. What is the most accurate problem statement for this patient's condition? *(341)*
    1. Potential for fluid volume excess
    2. Inability to maintain breathing pattern
    3. Potential for inadequate tissue perfusion
    4. Inability to clear airway

5. What is included in the preparation for tracheostomy care in the acute care environment? *(342)*
    1. Using clean technique and supplies for cleaning
    2. Preparing cotton balls to clean inside the ostomy
    3. Removing and cleaning the outer cannula
    4. Placing the patient in a semi-Fowler's position

6. The nurse is caring for a patient who is on 3 L oxygen per nasal cannula. What tasks can be delegated to the unlicensed assistive personnel (UAP)? **Select all that apply.** *(340)*
   1. Ensuring that the oxygen flow is set at 3 L/min throughout the shift
   2. Helping the patient to clean area around nares and ears
   3. Counting the respiratory rate and taking the pulse oximeter reading
   4. Listening to breath sounds before and after the patient coughs
   5. Assisting the patient to a semi-Fowler's position
   6. Observe the nares, external nasal area, and ears for breaks in skin integrity

7. The nurse is reviewing laboratory results and sees that the PaO$_2$ level for a 75-year-old patient is 80 mm Hg. What should the nurse do **first**? *(344)*
   1. Notify the provider about the unusually low level.
   2. Contact the clinical laboratory to verify the low result.
   3. Check the previous laboratory values for comparison.
   4. Assess patient for signs/symptoms of respiratory distress.

8. Which patient is the **most** likely candidate for an endotracheal tube? *(346)*
   1. The patient is discovered in the bathroom, unresponsive and pulseless.
   2. The patient is choking on a foreign body that cannot be dislodged.
   3. The patient needs long-term mechanical ventilation for oxygenation.
   4. The patient needs precise, controlled concentration of oxygen.

9. The nurse walks into the room and notices that the patient is anxious, demonstrates labored breathing, and seems to be struggling to get out of bed. What should the nurse do **first**? *(342)*
   1. Gently advise the patient to calm down, then and ask him what is wrong.
   2. Count the respiratory rate, note rhythm, and auscultate breath sounds.
   3. Assist him to sit upright and calmly instruct him to take slow, deep breaths.
   4. Stay with the patient, apply oxygen, and have another nurse call the provider.

10. The nurse must be vigilant for signs of hypoxia in an older patient who has dementia and also has risk for decreased oxygenation because of chronic respiratory disease and immobility. What is an **early** sign that warrants additional assessment of respiratory status? *(341)*
    1. Lips are cyanotic, fingers are cool, and capillary refill is sluggish.
    2. Respirations are slow and shallow.
    3. Patient seems restless and anxiously picks at linens.
    4. Pulse is slower than normal and is thready and weak.

11. The nurse is caring for a patient with a tracheostomy. What signs/symptoms indicate the need for suctioning? **Select all that apply.** *(353)*
    1. Fine crackles in posterior lobes
    2. Gurgling sounds heard during respiration
    3. Restlessness or anxiety
    4. Emesis in the oral cavity
    5. Drooling excessive secretions
    6. Patient indicates need for suctioning

12. The patient had an uneventful hip surgery several days ago and will soon be transferred to a rehabilitation unit. The patient says to the nurse, "I feel silly complaining about this, but I feel a little short of breath and I feel a little anxious and fuzzy-headed." The patient has no known history of respiratory or cardiac problems. What should the nurse do **first**? *(342)*
    1. Reassure the patient that she is not being silly, and that anxiety is normal.
    2. Take the vital signs, apply a pulse oximeter, and listen to breath sounds.
    3. Ask the patient to describe what she is feeling and what she thinks is going on.
    4. Apply oxygen per nasal cannula, notify the charge nurse, and call the provider.

13. In caring for a patient with a tracheostomy, what interventions will the nurse use to reduce the risk for infection? **Select all that apply.** *(346)*
    1. Evaluate the patient for excess secretions and suction as often as necessary.
    2. Provide constant airway humidification.
    3. Provide frequent mouth care.
    4. Wear a mask when performing routine tracheostomy care.
    5. Remove water that condenses in equipment tubing.
    6. Change or clean all respiratory therapy equipment every 8 hours.

CRITICAL THINKING ACTIVITIES

14. Identify how the nurse achieves the following before, during, and after the performance of a procedure. *(338, 339)*

    a. Identify the patient: _____

    _____

    b. Reduce the spread of microorganisms: _____

    _____

    c. Provide privacy:_____

    _____

    d. Ensure the patient's safety:_____

15. The nurse is caring for an older patient who has chronic obstructive pulmonary disease (COPD). The family comes in and spends several hours with him. The patient is in good spirits and introduces the nurse to his family when she comes in to give him his medication. The family leaves and the nurse observes that the patient is resting and assumes that he is very tired after the long visit. Two hours later, the nurse goes into check on the patient; his breathing is very shallow and he is very difficult to arouse. The nasal cannula is in place and the oxygen is flowing at 7 L/min. *(344, 345)*

    a. What does the nurse suspect? _____

    _____

    b. What should the nurse do? _____

    _____

    c. What should the nurse have done to prevent this situation? _____

    _____

    d. Discuss how the "hypoxic drive" affects patients with COPD. _____

    _____

    _____

    _____

    _____

Elimination and Gastric Intubation

CLINICAL APPLICATION OF MATH AND CONVERSION

Directions: Calculate or make the necessary conversions for math problems encountered in performing skills for patients.

1. At the beginning of the shift, the nurse inserts a urinary catheter and observes 300 mL of urine output into the drainage bag. One hour later, there is an order to send a urine sample, so the nurse uses the appropriate sterile technique and draws 20 mL from the port. At that time, the nurse notes 350 mL of urine in the bag, empties the bag, and records the urine output. At the end of the shift, the drainage bag contains 500 mL. How many mL of urine are recorded as the total output for the shift? *(368)* _____ mL

2. The patient vomits 200 mL of green bile drainage. Twenty minutes later, he vomits 100 mL. The provider orders the insertion of a nasogastric tube to decompress the stomach. During the procedure, the patient vomits 50 mL. At the end of the shift there is 150 mL in the drainage container. What does the nurse record as the output of emesis for the shift? *(378)* _____ mL

3. Using sterile technique, the nurse inserts a straight catheter into the patient, allows some urine to pass into the drainage container, then collects 15 mL in the specimen container (midstream sample), then allows the bladder to empty by placing the end of the catheter in the drainage container. The nurse removes the catheter and measures the urine in the drainage container at 750 mL. What does the nurse record as output? *(368)* _____ mL

4. The patient is receiving continuous bladder irrigation through a three-way indwelling urinary catheter. Prescribed and administered: 350 mL of normal saline irrigating solution. There are 475 mL in the urinary drainage bag. What is the patient's urinary output? *(372)* _____ mL

5. The provider has ordered nasogastric tube irrigation with 100 mL of normal saline. After confirming tube placement and assessing bowel sounds, the nurse instills 30 mL of normal saline and then withdraws the fluid and measures 25 mL. The nurse instills another 30 mL and withdraws and measures 20 mL. The nurse instills another 30 mL and withdraws 30 mL. The nurse instills the last 10 mL and withdraws and measures 10 mL. How does the nurse record the intake and output? *(379)* _____ mL

6. The nurse is irrigating a nasogastric tube to maintain the patency of the tube. The nurse instills 30 mL of normal saline and withdraws 35 mL. How does the nurse record intake and output? *(379)* _____ mL

FIGURE LABELING

7.   Directions: label the figure below with the names of the three landmarks that are used to measure the length of insertion of a nasogastric tube. *(376)*

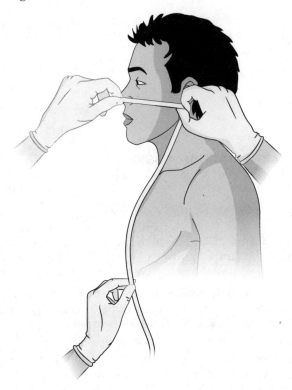

MULTIPLE CHOICE
Directions: Select the best answer(s) for each of the following questions.

8.   The nursing student has the opportunity to perform urinary catheterization on a patient. What should the student do **first**? *(360)*
   1.   Perform hand hygiene and don gloves.
   2.   Explain the procedure to the patient.
   3.   Obtain the necessary equipment.
   4.   Check the provider's order.

9.   The nurse must perform catheter care. Prior to starting the procedure, the nurse raises the bed and lowers one side rail. What is the **best** rationale for this action? *(360)*
   1.   Ensures patient safety and comfort
   2.   Promotes good body mechanics
   3.   Facilitates visualization of the patient's body
   4.   Adheres to standard procedure

10.   The nurse has inserted the urinary catheter into the patient and while the balloon is being inflated, the patient expresses discomfort. What should the nurse do? *(367)*
   1.   Remove the catheter and begin the procedure again.
   2.   Pull back on the catheter to determine tension.
   3.   Draw fluid out of the balloon and move the catheter forward.
   4.   Continue to inflate the balloon since discomfort is expected.

11.   Which instruction will the nurse give to the unlicensed assistive personnel (UAP) about catheter care for the patient? *(368)*
   1.   Maintain continuous tension on the external catheter tubing.
   2.   Empty the drainage bag once a day or sooner if necessary.
   3.   Attach the drainage bag to the side rails, below the level of the bladder.
   4.   Clean the urinary meatus and 2 inches down the catheter.

12. The charge nurse delegates the removal of an indwelling urinary catheter to a new staff member. Which action requires correction? *(364)*
    1. Explaining the burning sensation with the first voiding
    2. Obtaining a final urine specimen from the drainage bag
    3. Deflating the balloon and pinching the catheter
    4. Using clean gloves and performing perineal care

13. The home health nurse is assessing whether a patient with a spinal cord injury would be a candidate for intermittent self-catheterization. Which criteria would support this choice for this patient? **Select all that apply.** *(364)*
    1. The patient and family understand the use and cost of sterile supplies.
    2. The patient understands how to recognize signs/symptoms of infection.
    3. The patient has the manual dexterity to perform the cleaning and insertion.
    4. The patient and family are seeking ways for the patient to maintain independence.
    5. The family wants noninvasive and natural methods to maintain bodily functions.

14. The nurse has just removed a urinary catheter from a postsurgical patient. What is the **most** important instruction to give the UAP? *(361)*
    1. Be especially gentle when performing perineal care, because area is likely to be irritated.
    2. Report the amount of food and fluids that the patient consumes for the remainder of the shift.
    3. Measure the amount of the first voiding and report the time and amount to the nurse.
    4. Assist the patient to ambulate because the patient is likely to be sore and uncomfortable.

15. What is the **most** important thing for the nurse to assess for in caring for an older patient who has a condom catheter? *(362)*
    1. Inspect the skin underneath the catheter.
    2. Monitor for a urinary tract infection.
    3. Measure the daily urinary output.
    4. Assess for urinary retention.

16. The patient has an indwelling urinary catheter. The UAP reports that no new urine is collecting in the bag since it was measured and discarded at the beginning of the shift. What should the nurse do **first**? *(362)*
    1. Irrigate the system using sterile closed technique.
    2. Call the provider for an order to discontinue the catheter.
    3. Give the patient oral fluid to flush the bladder and catheter.
    4. Check for kinks in the tubing system and reposition the patient.

17. The nurse is assessing the insertion site of the patient's indwelling urinary catheter and notices exudate. What other assessments is the nurse **most** likely to perform before notifying the provider? *(369)*
    1. Look at the trends of intake and output for the past several days.
    2. Gently palpate the patient's suprapubic area to assess for bladder distention.
    3. Check the patient's temperature and draw fresh urine from the drainage port.
    4. Observe the clarity, odor, and color of urine in the collection bag.

18. The student nurse is obtaining a urine specimen from a patient who has had an indwelling catheter for several days. Which action(s) require(s) correction? **Select all that apply.** *(362, 364)*
    1. Disconnects the catheter from tubing and collects urine in a sterile container
    2. Obtains the urine from the collection bag using the drainage tube on the bag
    3. Draws urine directly from the catheter by using a sterile small-gauge needle
    4. Applies clean gloves and scrubs the drainage port with an alcohol swab
    5. Uses a sterile needle and syringe and collects 10 mL from the drainage port

19. For a patient on a bladder retraining program, which dietary/fluid intervention is the **best**? *(364)*
    1. Encourage black coffee for breakfast.
    2. Help the patient identify high-fiber foods.
    3. Restrict fluid intake to control bladder.
    4. Encourage at least 2000 mL of fluid each day.

20. An older adult resident in a long-term care facility is incontinent of urine. The nurse observes that the resident always asks for assistance to go to the toilet after eating breakfast. Based on this observation, what would the nurse do **first**? *(373)*
    1. Instruct UAP to apply incontinence pants before breakfast.
    2. Note times that the resident asks for help to the bathroom or requires changing of underwear.
    3. Suggest that the health care team plan and initiate a bladder training program.
    4. Obtain an order for a condom catheter or an indwelling urinary catheter.

21. The nurse hears in report that a patient receiving tube feedings has been having trouble with dumping syndrome. Based on the report, which action is the nurse **most** likely to perform? *(375)*
    1. Ensure that the feeding is administered very slowly.
    2. Auscultate bowel sounds before and after the feeding.
    3. Stay with the patient while the feeding is infusing.
    4. Offer the feeding through a straw instead of the tube.

22. The postsurgical patient has a Salem sump tube for decompression of the stomach. The nurse observes fluid leaking out of the pigtail. What should the nurse do? *(379)*
    1. Remove the tube and reinsert it.
    2. Introduce 30 mL of air into the pigtail.
    3. Pull the tube back a few centimeters.
    4. Increase the pressure of the wall suction.

23. Which evaluation statement indicates that the polystyrene sulfonate enema was a successful therapy? *(382)*
    1. The patient evacuated 300 mL of light-brown fluid after the third enema.
    2. Removal of hard fecal mass was followed by a small, soft, brown stool.
    3. The patient reports resumption of normal bowel pattern after enema.
    4. The patient's serum potassium level is within normal limits.

24. Which patient is **most** likely to need extra teaching about how to protect the skin around an ostomy? *(383)*
    1. The patient has a colostomy of the transverse colon.
    2. The patient has an ileostomy.
    3. The patient has a colostomy of the descending colon.
    4. The patient has a urostomy.

25. The patient tells the home health nurse that he is doing fine and has been irrigating his colostomy 5-6 times a week with 2000 mL each time. What is the **immediate** concern that needs to be followed up? *(388, 389)*
    1. The patient needs to have blood drawn for possible low electrolyte levels.
    2. The patient needs review of teaching points about colostomy care.
    3. The patient needs to have laboratory studies to rule out peritonitis.
    4. The patient needs to have psychological evaluation for failure to cope.

26. The patient begins to cough and gag when the nurse inserts a nasogastric tube. The nurse instructs the patient to breathe easily and take a few sips of water, but the patient continues to cough. What should the nurse do **first**? *(377)*
    1. Remove the tube and let the patient rest before reinsertion.
    2. Attach a syringe to the tube and aspirate for stomach contents.
    3. Use a flashlight and tongue blade to look at the throat.
    4. Pull the tube back just slightly and instruct the patient to breathe slowly.

27. Before the digital removal of a fecal impaction, the nurse checks the medical record. Which part of the patient's history alerts the nurse to be especially observant during the procedure? *(382)*
    1. Cardiac disease
    2. Hysterectomy
    3. Urinary infection
    4. Diabetes mellitus

28. The nurse has just inserted a nasogastric tube. The patient is coughing and gagging. The nurse takes a small amount of clear aspirated material and tests it with color-coded pH paper and the pH is 8. What should the nurse do **first**? *(377)*
    1. Call the provider to obtain an order for an x-ray to confirm placement.
    2. Ask the patient to speak his name and state his full address.
    3. Pull the tube out and tell the patient it was probably down his airway.
    4. Ask the RN to come and verify the tube placement before use.

CRITICAL THINKING ACTIVITIES

29. The nurse must insert an indwelling urinary catheter in a female patient who is very obese.

   a. Discuss the challenges of maintaining sterility while inserting a urinary catheter in obese female patients. *(365, 367)*

   _____
   _____
   _____
   _____
   _____

   b. What steps can the nurse take to maintain sterility? *(365)* _____
   _____
   _____
   _____
   _____

30. The nurse sees that the provider has ordered a straight catheter urine specimen from a patient who is transgender (male to female). What should the nurse assess before starting the procedure? (Note to student: If you are unsure about how to answer this question, have a discussion with your instructor and classmates.) *(365)*

   _____
   _____
   _____
   _____
   _____
   _____
   _____
   _____

Care of Patients Experiencing Urgent Alterations in Health

SHORT ANSWER

Directions: Using your own words, answer each question in the space provided.

1. The nurse is at a community event and several people are injured when a large tent structure is blown over by the wind. What information is essential to convey when calling the emergency medical system for help? *(394)*

_____

_____

_____

2. The provider directs the nurse to call Poison Control to get advice for a patient who comes to the health care facility for "feeling sick after spraying the yard with insect spray." What information is necessary to report when calling Poison Control? *(410)*

_____

_____

_____

3. Identify areas that should be included in a teaching plan for safety and response to an emergency in the home environment. *(418)*

_____

_____

_____

4. Directions: Refer to the figure and use the Rule of Nines to determine how much of the body surface is burned for an adult patient who has severe burns to the anterior and posterior thorax and both upper extremities. _____% *(417)*

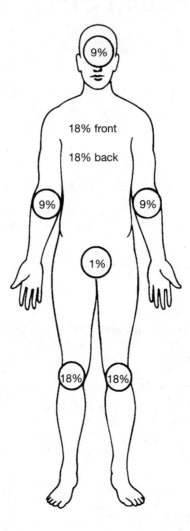

MULTIPLE CHOICE
Directions: Select the best answer(s) for each of the following questions.

5. Which patient has the **best** chance to fully recover because of the nurse's actions? *(395)*
   1. 4-year-old drowns; nurse starts cardiopulmonary resuscitation (CPR) within 4 minutes of clinical death
   2. 32-year-old with brain death has a cardiac arrest; nurse starts CPR within 2 minutes
   3. 17-year-old with biologic death has a respiratory arrest; nurse immediately delivers rescue breaths
   4. 55-year-old is electrocuted; nurse starts CPR within 10 minutes of clinical death

6. Which patient has a condition that could resemble brain death? *(396)*
   1. The patient has a blood alcohol level of 80 mg/dL.
   2. The patient has a core temperature below 30° C (86° F).
   3. The patient has oliguria secondary to hypovolemic shock.
   4. The patient fainted and was unconscious for 5 minutes.

7. The nurse is teaching basic CPR to a new group of unlicensed assistive personnel (UAP). When would the nurse intervene? *(397)*
   1. The UAP leans forward over the mannikin and creates pressure to depress the sternum at least 2 inches (5 cm).
   2. The UAP compresses at a rate of 100 to 120 compressions per minute without pausing between compressions.
   3. The UAP places the heel of one hand over the lower end of the sternum and places heel of the other hand on top.
   4. The UAP interlaces fingers to keep them off the chest and keeps hands in contact with the chest.

8. The nurse initiates CPR on a frail older woman who has cardiac arrest. During the compressions, the nurse hears and feels the cracking of the ribs. What should the nurse do? *(397)*
   1. Change hand position and then continue compressions.
   2. Stop compressions and assess for crepitus or flail chest.
   3. Stop compressions, but continue to deliver the rescue breaths.
   4. Verify correct hand position and continue compressions.

9. The nurse is caring for a patient who may have a cervical spine injury. The patient is lying flat and begins to vomit. What should the nurse do? *(416)*
   1. Immediately use an oral suction catheter to remove vomitus and direct the patient to hold breath during suctioning.
   2. Direct the patient to look straight ahead and not move his neck, then sit him upright using the bed mechanism.
   3. Direct several people, acting together as one unit, to help logroll the victim onto his side to allow drainage.
   4. Immediately report vomiting to the provider and ask if cervical spine injuries have been ruled out.

10. The nurse notes heavy spurting of bright-red blood from the patient's groin area after he returns from an arteriogram procedure. The nurse dons clean gloves and applies gauze and direct pressure. The gauze is quickly saturated. What should the nurse do **first**? *(404)*
    1. Increase the patient's IV fluid, take vital signs, monitor bleeding, and notify the provider.
    2. Place an additional layer of gauze on top of the saturated dressing and continue to hold pressure.
    3. Elevate the hips and apply more pressure over the groin area; ask someone to check a distal pulse.
    4. Apply a pressure bandage and monitor distal pulses, sensation, and temperature of the skin.

11. The nurse arrives outside of the public library and finds a person lying on the ground. What is the **first** action to take? *(394)*
    1. Check if the victim is unconscious.
    2. Check the carotid or brachial pulse.
    3. Move the victim to a flat, hard surface.
    4. Direct someone to call 911.

12. A patient is unresponsive to normal verbal stimuli and not breathing. How does the nurse assess for a carotid pulse? *(394)*
    1. Assess the location of the pulse for a maximum of 5 seconds.
    2. Check strength of the pulse for 5 seconds and then compare it to the opposite side.
    3. Assess the pulse rate for 10 seconds and then check for 3-second capillary refill.
    4. Check the rate, rhythm, and strength of the pulse for a maximum of 10 seconds.

13. Which sign or symptom of a foreign body airway obstruction is of **greatest** concern? *(400)*
    1. Says, "I think I swallowed something."
    2. Is coughing so hard that he can't speak.
    3. Makes a wheezing sound between coughs.
    4. Demonstrates a high-pitched inspiratory noise.

14. The person gives the universal sign for choking. How does the nurse prepare to perform abdominal thrusts? *(401)*
    1. By instructing the person to lean over the back of a chair
    2. By placing the fist over the sternum
    3. By placing the fist slightly above the navel
    4. By putting the heel of the hand over the xiphoid process

15. For an unconscious adult victim with a foreign body airway obstruction, what should the nurse do? *(401)*
    1. Apply a series of three quick chest thrusts.
    2. Repeat 10 abdominal thrusts and attempt to ventilate.
    3. Perform finger sweeps between abdominal thrusts.
    4. Visually look for object each time before providing a breath.

16. Which interventions are appropriate for a victim who is in hypovolemic shock at the scene of an accident? **Select all that apply.** *(403)*
    1. Establish airway.
    2. Control bleeding.
    3. Keep the head elevated.
    4. Cover with a blanket or coat.
    5. Provide oral fluids, such as water.
    6. Administer over-the-counter analgesics.

17. During a camping trip, a person who is allergic to bee stings is stung by a bee. The nurse immediately scrapes the skin to remove the stinger. Which question should the nurse ask **first**? *(411)*
    1. "What happens when you get stung by a bee?"
    2. "Do you want to go to the hospital?"
    3. "Where is your epinephrine pen?"
    4. "Do you have any diphenhydramine?"

18. The nurse finds a person lying at the bottom of a long staircase. The person is conscious but appears dazed and confused. There are no obvious injuries or signs of bleeding. What should the nurse do **first**? *(394)*
    1. Assist the person to sit up and suggest that he rest on a step.
    2. Instruct the person to remain still and ask for permission to assist.
    3. Initiate spinal cord precautions and hold head and neck in alignment.
    4. Ask the person what happened and if he is having pain or distress.

19. Two nurses are shopping together in a mall and they witness a person collapse and become unresponsive. Based on assessment, they initiate two-rescuer CPR. Under which circumstances can the two nurses discontinue the CPR? **Select all that apply.** *(394)*
    1. A relative of the unresponsive person tells them to stop.
    2. Mall personnel arrive with the automated external defibrillator.
    3. The curious crowd pushes in and bystanders are loud and unruly.
    4. Trained medical personnel arrive and take over CPR.
    5. The person remains unconscious but spontaneous pulse and breathing occur.
    6. A layperson offers to take over the role of doing compressions.

20. The provider informs a patient's wife that her husband has suffered brain death and is in an irreversible coma, even though his heart is still beating. Which comment indicates that the wife has understood what the provider said? *(395, 396)*
    1. "His heart is still beating, so there is still a chance he'll recover."
    2. "He is in a coma, but do you think that he can hear what I say?"
    3. "I must notify the family so that everyone can come and say goodbye."
    4. "How long do you think he will have to stay in the intensive care unit?"

21. Which assessment finding confirms cardiac arrest? *(396)*
    1. Absence of radial pulse
    2. Absence of carotid pulse
    3. Absence of spontaneous respirations
    4. Unresponsiveness to normal stimuli

22. The latest recommendation for CPR is to go "hard and fast" when performing chest compressions. What is the **best** rationale for maintaining the recommended 100 compressions/minute? *(397)*
    1. The rescuer will become fatigued if compressions exceed 100/minute.
    2. Lacerations of the liver or spleen are more likely to occur if speed is excessive.
    3. Releasing external chest compression allows time for blood to flow back into the heart.
    4. A smooth motion is required to prevent rocking and rolling that decrease the force.

23. The nurse is performing CPR on an infant. What is the **most** common event that could occur? *(399)*
    1. Fracture of the rib
    2. Gastric distention
    3. Aspiration of emesis
    4. Laceration of spleen

24. An infant is observed picking up something from the floor and putting it into his mouth before the mother can stop him. He demonstrates coughing, gagging, stridor, and respiratory distress. What should the nurse do **first**? *(401)*
    1. Instruct the mother to hold the child and look into the mouth with a flashlight.
    2. Place the infant in a supine position and deliver five chest thrusts.
    3. Place two fingers just above the navel and deliver five abdominal thrusts.
    4. Hold the infant with the head lower than trunk and deliver five back blows.

25. The nurse is assessing a trauma patient who was treated for shock in the emergency department. Oliguria is noted and immediately reported to the provider. Which complication is **most** related to this finding? *(402)*
    1. Right-sided heart failure
    2. Kidney failure
    3. Paralytic ileus
    4. Electrolyte imbalance

26. The nurse hears a scream; a patient has slipped in the bathroom. There is bright-red blood spurting from her forearm. What should the nurse do **first**? *(404)*
    1. Don sterile gloves and apply firm pressure using a sterile gauze pad.
    2. Use layers of sterile dressing material and wrap them snugly with an elastic bandage.
    3. Don clean gloves and use a clean towel to apply direct pressure; elevate the arm.
    4. Locate the brachial artery and use the heel of the hand to compress the artery.

27. Under what circumstances would the nurse use a tourniquet? *(404)*
    1. The nurse is acting in good faith and conforms to Good Samaritan principles.
    2. The provider gives a telephone order to apply a tourniquet.
    3. The victim tells the nurse to apply a tourniquet.
    4. Pressure and elevation have failed to control life-threatening bleeding.

28. An older patient comes to the clinic for epistaxis. It is readily controlled with steady pressure applied to the bridge of the nose. What additional assessment is **most** important for this patient? *(405)*
    1. Measuring the blood pressure
    2. Understanding of self-care measures
    3. First-aid attempts performed by the patient
    4. Checking an oral temperature

29. Which patient has the **greatest** risk for internal bleeding? *(406)*
    1. A 20-month-old child who stumbled and struck his forehead on a coffee table
    2. A 70-year-old woman sustained a hip fracture and takes an anticoagulant
    3. A 25-year-old man who was punched and kicked in the stomach
    4. A 30-year-old woman who was admitted for postpartum hemorrhage

30. A young man who is injured is brought to the clinic by his friends. They are all very excited, but they are able to point out that he has a stick poking out of the anterior chest wall. Which symptoms indicate that the patient has a pneumothorax? **Select all that apply.** *(407)*
    1. Pain worsens with inspiration and expiration efforts.
    2. Breathing is labored and difficult.
    3. A hissing sound is audible as air flows in and out of his chest.
    4. The patient is unconscious and unresponsive to normal stimuli.
    5. Pulse is weak, rapid, and thready.
    6. His chest does not expand on the side of injury during inspiration.

31. The home health nurse sees the patient lying on the floor. On entering the house, the nurse can smell a strong odor of gas and the house is extremely hot. What should the nurse do **first**? *(410)*
    1. Step out of the house and call 911.
    2. Call Poison Control and describe situation.
    3. Establish responsiveness and start cooling measures.
    4. Open the windows and move the patient out of the house.

32. The nurse comes home and finds that her teen-age son and his friends have been challenging each other to chug large shots of whiskey. Which adolescent needs to be taken to the hospital for serious alcohol intoxication? *(411)*
    1. Face appears flushed and seems sleepy.
    2. Demonstrates slurred speech and continuously giggles.
    3. Is loudly singing and starting to remove clothes.
    4. Is incontinent of bowel and bladder and is hallucinating.

33. It's the Fourth of July and the nurse is working at a walk-in clinic. Several people who were viewing a parade come in and report abdominal cramps, headache, weakness, nausea, and diaphoresis. All are alert and oriented. Which intervention would the nurse use **first**? *(413)*
    1. Establish peripheral intravenous sites on everyone.
    2. Give everyone several cool compresses.
    3. Assist everyone to remove constrictive clothing.
    4. Move everyone into a cool environment.

34. A person sustains full-thickness burns to both forearms while lighting an outdoor grill. The nurse would intervene if a bystander attempts to perform which action? *(417)*
    1. Removes smoldering clothing
    2. Removes victim's wedding ring
    3. Applies an antiseptic cream to the burns
    4. Places forearms in cold water

35. Which patient is **most** likely to need a tetanus toxoid injection? *(406)*
    1. Patient fell off a bike and has abrasions on the knee, last known tetanus shot was several years ago.
    2. Patient sustained a puncture wound from stepping on a nail that went through his workboots.
    3. Patient was elbowed during a basketball game and has swelling and ecchymoses on right lateral chest.
    4. Patient sustained a deep cut on the hand while washing a drinking glass; there was extensive bleeding.

36. The patient has a sutured laceration on the palmar surface of the hand. When will the supervising nurse intervene? *(409)*
    1. The student nurse positions the hand in the anatomical position before applying the bandage.
    2. The student nurse covers the entire wound with the dressing and roller gauze is applied uniformly.
    3. The student nurse applies roller gauze with a number of evenly spaced overlapping turns.
    4. The student nurse covers the tips of the fingers with the gauze bandage and secures roller gauze with tape.

37. The nurse is on a hiking trip and one of the children finds an injured bat and picks it up. The bat bites the child before any of the adults can intervene. What should the nurse do **first**? *(411)*
    1. Monitor for shock and seek medical attention immediately.
    2. Capture the bat and observe for injury or signs and symptoms of disease.
    3. Immediately wash the bite area with soap and water for 5 minutes.
    4. Assess for and control bleeding and apply a thick gauze bandage.

CRITICAL THINKING ACTIVITIES

38. The nurse comes upon the scene of a motor vehicle accident. Several people are standing around a woman who is lying on the ground in a supine position. She is crying and trying to sit up. The right sleeve of her blouse is torn and blood is pooling on the asphalt underneath her arm.

    a. How does the Good Samaritan law affect the nurse in the situation? *(394)* _____

    _____

    _____

    b. What actions should the nurse take first to help this victim? *(394)* _____

    _____

    _____

c. What assessments would lead the nurse to believe the victim is in shock? *(402)* _____

_____

d. What interventions are appropriate for a victim in shock at the scene of an accident? *(395)* _____

_____

39. The nurse is hiking with a group of friends on a cool, windy autumn day. They come across a man who is sitting in the middle of the trail. He is alert, but his speech is slurred. His clothes are wet and muddy and he is not wearing any shoes. Others in the group look around to see if they can find any additional clues about what happened to the man. The nurse starts to assess the man and notes that he is shivering and decides to assess him for additional signs of hypothermia.

a. What factors in the scenario helped the nurse to identify that hypothermia might be occurring? *(413)*

_____

_____

_____

b. What are the signs and symptoms of hypothermia? *(413)* _____

_____

_____

c. For the conscious victim with hypothermia, what interventions can be provided at the scene? *(413, 414)*

_____

_____

_____

40. Review Box 16.2 and think about the events that necessitate CPR. Select one (or two) of the events that you are most likely to encounter because of your work or family/home situation and mentally "rehearse" how you would respond. Based on your mental rehearsal of the event, identify information, equipment, skills, or safety precautions that you want to have if the actual event happens. *(395)*

_____

_____

_____

_____

_____

_____

_____

_____

_____

Student Name_____ Date_____

Dosage Calculation and Medication Administration

chapter 17

BASIC MATH REVIEW

Directions: Use basic math functions (e.g., addition, subtraction, conversion, rounding, etc.) to solve the review problems.

1. Change the improper fraction to a mixed number: $\frac{8}{5} =$ _____ *(424)*

2. Change the mixed number to an improper fraction: $7\frac{5}{8} =$ _____ *(425)*

3. Reduce the fraction to the lowest term: $\frac{25}{100} =$ _____ *(425)*

4. Add the fractions and reduce the sum to its lowest term: $2\frac{1}{3} + 5\frac{1}{4} =$ _____ *(426)*

5. Subtract the fractions and reduce the answer to its lowest term: $\frac{1}{2} - \frac{1}{3} =$ _____ *(426)*

6. Multiply the fractions and reduce the product to its lowest term: $\frac{1}{3} \times \frac{3}{12} =$ _____ *(426)*

7. Divide the fractions and reduce the answer to its lowest term: $\frac{3}{10} \div \frac{5}{25} =$ _____ *(427)*

8. Add the decimals: $57.629 + 14.22 =$ _____ *(428)*

9. Subtract the decimals: $0.089 - 0.0057 =$ _____ *(428)*

10. Round the decimal to hundredths and then to tenths: $5.753 =$ _____ _____ *(424)*

11. Multiply the decimals: $64.75 \times 22.9 =$ _____ *(428)*

12. Divide the decimals and round to the nearest hundredth: $2.9 \div 0.218 =$ _____ *(428)*

13. Convert the fraction into a decimal: $\frac{1}{2} =$ _____ *(428)*

14. Convert the fraction into percent: $\frac{75}{100} =$ _____ *(429)*

15. Solve for X: $20 : 40 = X : 5$ $X =$ _____ *(429)*

TABLE ACTIVITY

16. Directions: In the table below, fill in the metric measures that are equivalent to the amount given as apothecary measures, according to the conversion information in your textbook. *(423, 424)*

Equivalents for Metric and Apothecary Measures

Metric	Apothecary
_____ milligrams	1 grain
_____ kilograms	1 pound
_____ kilograms	2.2 pounds
_____ milliliters	1 fluid ounce
_____ milliliters	1 pint
_____ milliliters	1 quart

17. Directions: Convert and calculate the following equivalents using the equivalent measure information from your textbook for conversion. *(423, 424)*

   a. 30 mL = _____ ounces

   b. 1000 mL = _____ liters

   c. 1 L = _____ quarts

   d. 500 mL = _____ pints

   e. 60 mg = _____ grains

   f. 1 kg = _____ pounds

   g. 400 mL = _____ liters

   h. 2 mcg = _____ milligrams

   i. 4 mg = _____ grams

   j. 44 pounds = _____ kilograms (round to whole number)

   k. 5 mg = _____ micrograms

   l. 1 inch = _____ centimeters

   m. 25 inches = _____ centimeters

   n. 225 pounds = _____ kilograms (round to whole number)

   o. 8 ounces = _____ milliliters

   p. 24 ounces = _____ milliliters

   q. 250 mcg = _____ milligrams

   r. 3 teaspoons = _____ milliliters

   s. 2 tablespoons = _____ milliliters

CLINICAL APPLICATION OF MATH

Directions: Calculate the math problems using the equivalent measures from your text (i.e., 1 inch = 2.5 centimeters, 1 pound = 2.2 kilograms, 30 milliliters = 1 ounce, etc.).

18. The patient's height is 25 inches. What is the patient's height in centimeters? *(423)* _____ centimeters

19. The patient's height is 36 inches. What is the patient's height in centimeters? *(423)* _____ centimeters

20. The patient's abdominal girth is 38 inches. What is the patient's abdominal girth in centimeters? *(420)* _____ centimeters

21. The patient weighs 158 pounds. What is the patient's weight in kilograms? *(424)* _____ kilograms (round to whole number)

22. The patient weighs 57 pounds. What is the patient's weight in kilograms? *(424)* _____ kilograms (round to whole number)

23. The patient weighs 12.2 kilograms. What is the patient's weight in pounds? *(424)* _____ pounds (round to whole number)

24. Calculate the patient's total fluid intake for breakfast: 8 ounces of milk, 6 ounces of juice, and 10 ounces of coffee. *(424)* _____ mL

25. Calculate the patient's total fluid intake for 24 hours: 16 ounces of milk, 10 ounces of coffee, 6 ounces of juice, 2 liters of water, 500 mL of IV fluid. *(424)* _____ mL

26. Calculate the patient's total fluid intake and output for 24 hours: 6 ounces of milk, 16 ounces of coffee, 3 liters of water, 250 mL of IV fluid. *(424)* Intake _____ mL
Urine 2950 mL, wound drainage 200 mL. Output _____ mL

27. The prescription is for carbamazepine 200 mg po tid. *(430)*
Available—carbamazepine 100-mg tablets
How many tablets should be given per dose? _____ tablets

28. The prescription is for methyldopa 250 mg po bid. *(430)*
Available—methyldopa 125-mg tablets
How many tablets should be given per dose? _____ tablets

29. The prescription is for penicillin suspension 500,000 units po. *(430)*
Available—penicillin suspension 200,000 units/5 mL
How much should be prepared? _____ mL

30. The prescription is for morphine 4 mg IM PRN for pain. *(430)*
Available—morphine 10 mg/mL
How much should be prepared? _____ mL

31. The prescription is for heparin 5000 units subQ. *(430)*
Available—heparin 10,000 units/mL.
How much should be given? _____ mL

32. The prescription is for methylprednisolone sodium succinate 50 mg IV. *(430)*
Available—methylprednisolone sodium succinate 125 mg/2 mL
How much is prepared? _____ mL

33. Using Young's rule, identify the dose for a child who is 3 years old when the adult dose is 75 mg. *(431)* _____ mg

34. Using Clark's rule, identify the dose for a child who weighs 30 pounds when the adult dose is 50 mg. _____ mg *(431)*

35. Using Fried's rule, identify the dose for a child who is 10 months old when the adult dose is 100 mg. _____ mg *(431)*

36. Using the body surface area calculation, identify the dose for a child with a body surface area of 1.1 when the adult dose is 10 mg. _____ mg *(431, 432)*

37. An IV is prescribed to infuse at 75 mL/hr. The drip factor is 10 gtt/mL. The rate of infusion should be _____ gtt/min. *(477)*

38. An IV is prescribed to infuse at 125 mL/hr. The drip factor is 10 gtt/mL. The rate of infusion should be _____ gtt/min. *(477)*

39. An IV is prescribed to infuse at 30 mL/hr with a microdrip set. The rate of infusion should be _____ gtt/min. *(477)*

40. An IV of 1000 mL is to infuse over 6 hours. The drip factor is 15 gtt/mL. The rate of infusion should be _____ gtt/min. *(477)*

41. An IV of 1000 mL is to infuse at 125 mL/hour and the nurse will use an infusion pump that can be set to deliver fluid in mL/hour. What is the pump setting? _____ mL/hour *(477)*

42. An IV of 250 mL contains potassium to be infused over 2 hours. The nurse will use an infusion pump that can be set to deliver fluid in mL/hour. What is the pump setting? _____ mL/hour *(477)*

43. An IV of 100 mL contains an antibiotic to be infused over 30 minutes. The nurse will use an infusion pump that can be set to deliver fluid in mL/hour. What is the pump setting? _____ mL/hour *(477)*

44. An IV of 250 mL contains an antibiotic to be infused over 1 hour and 30 minutes. The nurse will use an infusion pump that can be set to deliver fluid in mL/hour. What is the pump setting? _____ mL/hour *(477)*

45. The provider prescribes an IV infusion of dextrose 5% and normal saline to infuse at 125 mL/hour for 8 hours. The nurse uses an electronic infusion pump to alarm every 2 hours. How many mL should the patient receive in each 2-hour period? _____ mL *(477)*

SHORT ANSWER

46. What are the six rights of medication administration? *(438, 439)* _____

_____

_____

47. What are the three label checks of medication administration? *(438)* _____

_____

_____

MULTIPLE CHOICE
Directions: Select the best answer(s) for each of the following questions.

48. A patient needs a PRN dose of pain medication. The provider's prescription reads: 2 mg oral MS PRN for severe pain. The pharmacy sends magnesium sulfate. What should the nurse do **first**? *(439)*
   1. Ask the patient if he has ever taken magnesium sulfate for relief of pain.
   2. Call the provider and ask for clarification of the prescription.
   3. Use a drug reference and see if magnesium sulfate is a pain medication.
   4. Call the pharmacy and ask for clarification of what was sent.

49. A new nurse is working in a small rural long-term care facility. An older provider routinely directs the care of the residents and he prefers to handwrite his notes and orders, rather than use a computer. What should the new nurse do **first** if the provider's handwriting is illegible? *(442)*
   1. Consult the director of nursing services about the provider's behavior.
   2. Call the provider for clarification whenever it is necessary.
   3. Ask the charge nurse for assistance in interpreting the handwriting.
   4. Gently offer to help the provider learn how to use the computer.

50. Based on Joint Commission requirements, under what circumstances must the nurse perform medication reconciliation? **Select all that apply.** *(438)*
    1. The patient has just been admitted to the medical-surgical unit.
    2. The provider has just made morning rounds and several new medications are prescribed.
    3. The patient's daughter is taking her father home after a prolonged hospitalization.
    4. The patient is being transferred to a rehabilitation unit after having hip surgery.
    5. The patient has just finished a complete course of prescribed antibiotics.

51. The nurse is assigned to give routine immunizations to infants who are seen in the well-baby clinic. In addition to standard medication documentation, what must be recorded when giving immunizations? *(439)*
    1. Duration and course of postinjection observation time
    2. Lot number of vial, manufacturer, and expiration date of vaccine
    3. Age of the child at time of any previous immunizations or vaccinations
    4. Informed consent with signatures from both parents or any guardians

52. The nurse is reviewing the prescriptions that the provider wrote for several patients. Which one will the nurse attend to **first**? *(433)*
    1. A prescription for a PRN stool softener
    2. A dose of antipyretic medication now
    3. A stat dose of IV epinephrine
    4. A one-time only dose of an anxiolytic

53. A prescription for codeine gr ½ is written for the patient. The medication is supplied in mg. What should the nurse administer? *(424)*
    1. 3 g
    2. 30 g
    3. 3 mg
    4. 30 mg

54. An IV of 500 mL D₅W is to infuse over 4 hours. The administration set is 15 gtt/mL. What is the correct number of gtt/min? *(477)*
    1. 19 gtt/min
    2. 24 gtt/min
    3. 31 gtt/min
    4. 42 gtt/min

55. The nurse determines the location for an injection by identifying the greater trochanter of the femur, the anterosuperior iliac spine, and the iliac crest. Which injection site has the nurse located? *(471)*
    1. Rectus femoris
    2. Ventrogluteal
    3. Dorsogluteal
    4. Vastus lateralis

56. Upon getting the assignment for the evening, the nurse notices that two patients on the unit have the same last name. What is the **best** way to prevent medication errors for these two patients? *(439)*
    1. Ask the patients their names.
    2. Check the patients' identification bands.
    3. Ask another nurse about their identities.
    4. Verify their names with the family members.

57. The nurse is working in the newborn nursery and will be giving vitamin K injections to the babies. What is the preferred site for these injections? *(470)*
    1. Deltoid
    2. Dorsogluteal
    3. Ventrogluteal
    4. Vastus lateralis

58. When preparing an opioid medication, the nurse drops the pill on the floor. What should the nurse do? *(437)*
    1. Discard the medication in the biohazard container.
    2. Notify the pharmacy for a replacement dose.
    3. Wipe off the medication and administer it.
    4. Have another nurse witness the disposal of the pill.

59. When would the nurse use the Z-track technique? *(470)*
    1. The patient is extremely obese.
    2. The child is younger than 5 years old.
    3. The prescribed medication can irritate tissue.
    4. The prescribed dose of medication is very large.

60. A tuberculin test will be given to the patient. What site would the nurse select for this intradermal injection? *(475)*
    1. Upper outer aspect of the arm
    2. Anterior aspect of the forearm
    3. Middle third of the anterior thigh
    4. A 2-inch diameter around the umbilicus

61. How does the nurse determine what the drip factor is for an IV set? *(477)*
    1. Ask the charge nurse.
    2. Calculate the IV rate.
    3. Look in a reference book.
    4. Check the IV tubing box.

62. The nurse is observing the patient self-administer medication with a metered-dose inhaler (MDI). What action by the patient requires correction and further instruction? *(462)*
    1. Shakes canister to determine how much is left
    2. Inhales one puff with one inspiration
    3. Inhales medication slowly and deeply
    4. Waits 2-5 minutes between puffs

63. What types of medications cannot be crushed for ease of administration? **Select all that apply.** *(443)*
    1. Extended-release capsules
    2. Tablets
    3. Sublingual tablets
    4. Enteric-coated tablets
    5. Sustained-release capsules

64. The nurse identifies that a patient is having an idiosyncratic reaction to a medication. Which patient's report is consistent with the nurse's analysis? *(433)*
    1. Hypnotic medication causes him to be awake most of the night.
    2. Antianxiety medication seems to make the pain medication more effective.
    3. Previous dosage of pain medication does not seem to be working like it used to.
    4. Antibiotic medication seems to cause an uncomfortable, itchy rash.

65. Which route of drug administration will achieve the **fastest** onset of action? *(434)*
    1. Intravenous
    2. Buccal
    3. Rectal
    4. Oral

66. The nurse has five stable patients and each needs many medications. All of the medications are scheduled to be administered at 9:00 AM. What should the nurse do **first**? *(438)*
    1. Inform the RN that some of the medications were given late, despite best efforts.
    2. Start at 08:30 AM and give medications to the most cooperative patients first.
    3. Administer as many medications at 9:00 AM as possible and then write an incident report.
    4. Ask the RN to change patient assignments so that medications are given on time.

67. An IV of 1000 mL 5% dextrose and 45% saline is to infuse over 8 hours. The IV fluid is started at 0800 hours. At 1400 hours, how much IV fluid has the patient received if the nurse correctly set the flow rate? *(477)*
    1. 1000 mL
    2. 750 mL
    3. 625 mL
    4. 500 mL

68. The nurse hears in report that 1000 mL of normal saline was started at 3:00 AM to infuse at 125 mL per hour. At 7:30 AM, the nurse evaluates the patient and the IV infusion, which is running by gravity; the IV fluid bag shows that approximately 200 mL has been infused. What should the nurse do **first**? *(477)*
    1. Calculate the amount of fluid that should have infused and then give it.
    2. Report the error to the charge nurse and write an incident report.
    3. Document the amount of fluid infused and the appearance of the site.
    4. Recalculate the drops/minute and reset the rate of flow to 125 mL/hour.

69. The provider prescribes two medications and suggests to the nurse that they could be mixed together in the same syringe to prevent the patient from having to get two separate injections. The nurse mixes the drugs, but a precipitate forms in the syringe. What should the nurse do? *(433)*
    1. Ask the provider to verify the request to mix the drugs.
    2. Gently rotate the syringe between the palms of the hands to mix the solution.
    3. Discard the syringe and call the pharmacy for information about compatibilities.
    4. Administer the medications as prescribed and document the injection site.

70. The nurse is giving a patient the morning medications. The patient says, "I don't recognize this pill." What should the nurse say? *(438)*
    1. "The medications that you will get in the hospital may be different than the ones you take at home."
    2. "Medications are made by different manufacturers. They can be chemically identical but have a different appearance."
    3. "Let me review the list of your home medications and I'll find out if anything new was prescribed for you."
    4. "I carefully checked all of your medications against the provider's prescriptions and these are correct."

71. The patient reports having an anaphylactic reaction to an IV medication but cannot remember the name. The nurse informs the provider and the provider tells the nurse to go ahead and administer the prescribed medication. What should the nurse do? *(478)*
    1. Refuse to administer the medication because the allergy history is not clarified.
    2. Take baseline vital signs and recheck the patient frequently during the infusion.
    3. Inform the charge nurse or RN about the potential for an adverse reaction.
    4. Call the pharmacy and see if they have any records of the patient's allergies.

72. The nurse has performed a medication calculation and has determined that to give the prescribed dose, 15 tablets would have to be administered to the patient. The nurse has asked two other nurses to recheck the calculations and the answer is always 15. What should the nurse do **first**? *(438)*
    1. Give the 15 tablets because the calculations have been checked and rechecked.
    2. Call the pharmacy and ask if the medication comes in a different strength.
    3. Call the provider and ask for verification of the prescription.
    4. Consult a reliable drug reference to see if the prescribed dose is within safe range.

73. Two nurses are standing in the medication area. Nurse A is preparing medication, but hears an alarm indicating that an unstable patient needs help right away. She hands the prepared medication to Nurse B and asks her to give it to the correct patient. What should Nurse B do **first**? *(438)*
    1. Go ahead and give it because she witnessed all of the preparations that Nurse A made.
    2. Inform the charge nurse that Nurse A needs assistance because of a critical patient.
    3. Give the medication, but later indicate to Nurse A that she should do the documentation.
    4. Discard the prepared medication and prepare another dose and give it to the patient.

74. The nurse is supervising a nursing student who must give several medications. The nurse would intervene if the student performed which action? *(444)*
    1. Puts a suppository in a uniform pocket
    2. Used aseptic technique to handle pills
    3. Looked at the meniscus when pouring a liquid
    4. Read the label of the bottle as she took it off the shelf

75. The patient has an order for a medication that is to be delivered via an MDI. Which chronic health condition is the patient **most** likely to have? *(458)*
    1. Hypertension
    2. Chronic bronchitis
    3. Diabetes mellitus
    4. Arteriosclerotic heart disease

76. Which factor would be the **most** important in the nurse's decision to choose an 18-gauge needle? *(467)*
    1. Viscosity of solution
    2. Age of patient
    3. Length of needle
    4. Weight of patient

77. The nurse is assessing an existing IV that seems to have stopped infusing. What should the nurse do **first**? *(468)*
    1. Recalculate the drip rate and then count the number of drops per minute.
    2. Discontinue the IV and inform the RN or provider.
    3. Check for infiltration and ask the patient about pain or discomfort.
    4. Try repositioning the patient's extremity or adjusting the height of the IV bag.

78. The nurse is performing an intradermal injection for an allergy test. He does not aspirate for this type of injection. What is the **best** rationale for the nurse's technique? *(472)*
    1. This is standard procedure and he is following the procedure manual.
    2. Aspirating can cause bruising and the patient will receive many allergy tests.
    3. There are no major veins or arteries in the intradermal tissues.
    4. The needle is so fine and short that it is unlikely to cause tissue damage.

79. The nurse is assessing a patient who is receiving IV fluid and medication. Which finding is the **most** serious? *(478)*
    1. The patient complains of pain at the insertion site.
    2. The patient is dyspneic and has a weak, thready pulse.
    3. The patient's arm is swollen and the skin is cool to the touch.
    4. The patient is very scared and upset because the IV bag is empty.

80. An older patient is receiving a medication that is potentially nephrotoxic. Which assessment is the **most** relevant to potential nephrotoxicity? *(479)*
    1. Change of mental status
    2. Reduced urinary output
    3. Nausea and vomiting
    4. Increased blood pressure

81. Upon assessment of the IV insertion site, the nurse suspects that the patient has phlebitis. Which assessment finding supports the nurse's analysis? *(478)*
    1. Edema at the site
    2. Erythema along the vein
    3. Cool skin around site
    4. Sluggish flow of IV fluid

82. The nurse is at home and her husband accidentally gets a caustic chemical splash in his eyes. What should the nurse do **first**? *(449)*
    1. Drive him to the hospital and flush his eyes with sterile normal saline.
    2. Call Poison Control and ask for advice about the specific chemical.
    3. Gently flush his eyes with tap water for at least 15 minutes.
    4. Assess him for burning, changes in visual acuity, or pain.

83. Which patient is the **most** likely candidate for the use of a Morgan lens to flush the eye? *(455)*
    1. Patient has allergic conjunctivitis in both eyes.
    2. Patient was sprayed in the eyes with pepper spray.
    3. Patient needs frequent eye irrigations at home.
    4. Patient has pain after prolonged use of contact lenses.

84. Which patient is **most** likely to need an ear irrigation? *(455)*
    1. A child who inserted a dried pinto bean into the ear canal
    2. A toddler who has a severe ear infection with exudate
    3. A teenager who has bleeding from the ear after a fight
    4. An older patient who reports a crackling noise in ear

CRITICAL THINKING ACTIVITIES

85. Identify home health safety information that should be included in a teaching plan for medication administration. *(442)*

    _____

    _____

    _____

86. Discuss ways to prevent medication errors and maximize safety in medication administration. *(442)*

    _____

    _____

    _____

87. Look at the medication prescription below for patient John Smith and identify what parts of the prescription are missing. *(436)*

    John Smith: BD 6/9/51
    Penicillin G potassium 1.2 million units
    Dr. James Jones

    _____

    _____

88. The patient needs a medication; however, to deliver the correct dose, the nurse has to perform some calculations because the amount of medication in the vial exceeds the prescribed dose. It's a very busy day. The nurse is trying to train a new nurse, there is a call light on, a provider wants to ask about a patient, the nurse left his calculator at home, and suddenly a patient falls on the floor. The nurse instructs the new nurse to perform the calculation and after a while they go to give the medication. The patient sustains no harm, but later the nurse thinks about his day and realizes that this situation could have harmed the patient. Analyze factors that could contribute to potential errors and discuss what the nurse should have done in this situation. *(442)*

_____

_____

_____

_____

89. The provider prescribes 0.07 mg of epinephrine. Epinephrine Injection, USP 1:1000 (1 mg/mL) is supplied in a 1-mL ampoule single-dose container. Indicate on the tuberculin syringe how many mL the nurse will draw up. *(466)*

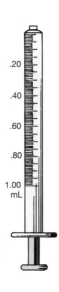

Fluids and Electrolytes

chapter
18

TABLE ACTIVITY

1. Directions: List the normal value range for the electrolytes.

Electrolyte	Normal Value Range
Sodium *(487)*	a.
Potassium *(489)*	b.
Chloride *(490)*	c.
Calcium *(491)*	d.
Phosphorus *(493)*	e.
Magnesium *(493)*	f.
Bicarbonate *(494)*	g.

CLINICAL APPLICATION OF MATH AND CONVERSION

Directions: Calculate or make the necessary conversions for math problems encountered in performing skills for patients.

2. Diet and fluid restriction and medications have been administered to the patient to decrease excess fluid volume. On the first day, the patient's weight was 150 pounds. After therapy, the patient's weight is 145.5 pounds. Assuming that the weight change represents fluid loss, how much fluid did the patient lose? _____ L *(485)*

3. A patient with chronic renal failure is having difficulty adhering to the dietary and fluid recommendations. At the last visit, the patient's weight was 205 pounds. Today, the patient's weight is 214 pounds. Assuming that the weight change represents fluid gain, how much fluid did the patient gain? _____ L *(485)*

4. The nurse is totaling the intake and output (I&O) at the end of the 8-hour shift. Data from today is recorded on the flowsheet for the patient: *(485)*

Intake	Output
0800: 8 ounces coffee, 6 ounces juice	0700: 300 mL urine
10:00: 300 mL water	0930: 450 mL urine
1200: 12 ounces of chicken broth, 5 ounces Jell-O	1400: 500 mL urine
1430: 200 mL water	1500: 250 mL urine

What is the total intake? _____ mL

What is the total output? _____ mL

5. The nurse is inserting a nasogastric tube into a patient for the purpose of decompressing the stomach. During the procedure, the patient vomits 500 mL of bile emesis. This is recorded on the flowsheet. Immediately after the tube placement is established and hooked to suction, 400 mL of green bile emesis flows through the tube into the collection cannister. At the end of the shift, a total of 600 mL is noted in the cannister, recorded on the flowsheet and then discarded. For the urinary drainage bag, at 0700: 300 mL was recorded and discarded; at 1200: 250 mL was recorded and discarded; and at 1500: 200 mL was recorded and discarded. What was the total output at the end of the shift? _____ mL *(485)*

6. The provider orders strict I&O on a postsurgical patient. The patient has an indwelling urinary catheter; the urinary drainage bag was emptied: 0800 for 400 mL, 1200 for 450 mL, and at the end of the shift there is 700 mL in the drainage bag. The patient had one episode of vomiting clear emesis of 300 mL. The patient also has a Jackson-Pratt drain with 15 mL at the end of the shift. The patient has an IV of normal saline that is infused at 125 mL/hour for the 8-hour shift. The patient is on a clear liquid diet and intake is shown below for the shift.

What is the total intake for the 8-hour shift? _____ mL

What is the total output for the 8-hour shift? _____ mL *(485)*

Intake
0800: 8 ounces diluted apple juice
1000: 200 mL water
1200: 6 ounces broth and 3 ounces diluted juice
1430: 400 mL water

MULTIPLE CHOICE
Directions: Select the best answer(s) for each of the following questions.

7. The patient is experiencing hyperkalemia. What treatment does the nurse anticipate? *(491)*
   1. Intravenous (IV) calcium
   2. Fluid restrictions
   3. Foods high in potassium
   4. Administration of loop diuretics

8. Following thyroid surgery, the patient reports nausea and a tingling sensation around nose, mouth, ears, fingers, and toes. The nurse observes muscle spasms in the patient's feet and hands. What is the **most** important sign/symptom for the nurse to observe for and report? *(492)*
   1. Respiratory distress
   2. Altered mental status progressing to seizure
   3. Polyuria and excessive thirst
   4. Positive Chvostek's sign

9. Which patient has the **greatest** risk for dehydration? *(483)*
   1. 30-year-old female with vomiting and diarrhea
   2. 72-year-old obese male with a fever and anorexia
   3. 2-year-old with an ear infection and vomiting
   4. 45-year-old underweight female with influenza

10. The nurse offers to take an older neighbor to the grocery store. As they are shopping, the neighbor tells the nurse that, "My doctor told me to watch my salt intake." Which items in the shopping cart would the nurse suggest they put back on the shelf? **Select all that apply.** *(487)*
    1. Cheddar cheese
    2. Ketchup
    3. Oranges
    4. Pretzels
    5. Frozen TV dinner

11. The nurse sees that the patient is scheduled to have a potassium supplement. In addition to the last potassium level, what would the nurse assess before administering the potassium? *(489)*
    1. Urinary output
    2. Blood pressure
    3. Respiratory rate
    4. Hematocrit level

12. The nurse notes that a resident who lives in a long-term care center has poor fluid intake and spends most of the day dozing in a chair. Based on this observation, which subjective report is the resident **most** likely to report? *(483)*
    1. Shortness of breath
    2. Constipation
    3. Nausea
    4. Headache

13. A patient who has diabetes reports to the nurse that he feels nauseated and has abdominal pain. The nurse observes that the patient is breathing very deeply and rapidly. Based on the assessment findings and the laboratory results, what does the nurse suspect ? *(498)*

pH	7.30
Pa_{CO_2}	30 mm Hg
Pa_{O_2}	70 mm Hg
O_2 saturation	98%
HCO_3^-	18 mEq
K^+	6.5 mEq/L

1. Metabolic alkalosis
2. Metabolic acidosis
3. Respiratory alkalosis
4. Respiratory acidosis

14. The patient is encouraged by his doctor to eat foods that are rich in potassium. Which lunch tray would be the **best**? *(489)*
    1. Seafood salad with crackers and strawberries with whipped cream
    2. Egg salad on whole grain bread with coffee and potato chips
    3. Grilled white toast with tomato soup and orange juice
    4. Pork cutlet with milk gravy and mushrooms and melon salad

15. The nurse is supervising a new nurse who will administer IV potassium to a patient. When would the supervising nurse intervene? *(490)*
    1. New nurse delegates unlicensed assistive personnel to obtain an infusion controller
    2. New nurse checks the provider's prescription for the dose, route and time of medication
    3. New nurse draws dose with a sterile needle and syringe and scrubs the IV insertion port
    4. New nurse calls pharmacy to find out when the potassium infusion will be ready

16. Earlier in the shift a patient with severe diarrhea seemed irritable, anxious and twitchy. The RN calls from the patient's room and asks that a vial of calcium gluconate be brought to the room immediately. In addition, to the calcium gluconate, what emergency equipment would the LPN/LVN try to quickly obtain for patient with a very low calcium? *(492)*
    1. Chest tube insertion tray and oxygen mask
    2. IV pump and IV normal saline for bolus
    3. Automated external defibrillator
    4. Tracheotomy tray and a resuscitation bag

17. The nurse is assessing an older adult and observes dry mucous membranes, increased heart rate, decreased blood pressure and poor skin turgor. The patient seems mildly confused and continuously asks for water. What would the nurse do **first**? *(483)*
    1. Assess the patient for additional signs of dehydration
    2. Offer the patient a glass of water and reassess in several hours
    3. Count the respirations and assess for additional signs of respiratory acidosis
    4. Call the provider and report the assessment findings.

18. What is the **best** food source for calcium? *(491)*
    1. Milk.
    2. Meat.
    3. Whole grains.
    4. Green leafy vegetables.

19. The patient has experienced a prolonged episode of diarrhea. Which clinical observation is consistent with the development of metabolic acidosis? *(498)*
    1. Increased perspiration
    2. Increased respiratory rate
    3. Increased urinary output
    4. Decreased heart rate

20. The patient has had emphysema for a number of years. Which set of arterial blood gas values indicates that the patient is in respiratory acidosis? *(497)*
    1. pH 7.35, $Paco_2$ 40, HCO_3^- 22
    2. pH 7.40, $Paco_2$ 45, HCO_3^- 30
    3. pH 7.30, $Paco_2$ 50, HCO_3^- 24
    4. pH 7.48, $Paco_2$ 55, HCO_3^- 18

21. While in the delivery room with his wife, the father-to-be begins to develop an anxiety reaction and lightheadedness. Which intervention does the nurse use to prevent respiratory alkalosis? *(498)*
    1. Coach panting respirations.
    2. Provide nasal oxygen.
    3. Have him breathe into a paper bag.
    4. Have him cough and deep-breathe.

22. A child has gotten into the medicine cabinet in the home and ingested the remaining contents of an aspirin (acetylsalicylic acid) bottle. What is the life-threatening condition that can occur as a result of excessive aspirin ingestion? *(498)*
    1. Metabolic acidosis
    2. Metabolic alkalosis
    3. Respiratory acidosis
    4. Respiratory alkalosis

23. The patient has had continuous gastric suction. The nurse recognizes that acid-base imbalances can occur with this treatment. Which laboratory data confirms metabolic alkalosis? *(498)*
    1. pH elevated, $Paco_2$ normal, and HCO_3^- elevated
    2. pH elevated, $Paco_2$ elevated, and HCO_3^- decreased
    3. pH decreased, $Paco_2$ decreased, and HCO_3^- decreased
    4. pH decreased, $Paco_2$ normal, and HCO_3^- decreased

24. What is the **best** way for the nurse to determine the patient's fluid balance? *(485)*
    1. Assess vital signs.
    2. Weigh the patient daily.
    3. Monitor IV fluid intake.
    4. Check diagnostic test results.

25. The patient used excessive antacids, which resulted in a serum sodium level of 150 mEq/L. Why would the provider instruct the nurse to give an IV hypotonic solution? *(486)*
    1. To correct intracellular dehydration
    2. To correct intravascular volume
    3. To increase the sodium level
    4. To pull fluid from the cells

26. The nurse is caring for a postoperative patient. Which solution is the provider **most** likely to order to replace the fluid deficiency related to the patient's NPO (nothing by mouth) status in the pre- and postoperative period? *(486)*
    1. Hypotonic solution
    2. Hypertonic solution
    3. Isotonic solution
    4. Parental nutrition

27. What purposes do the electrolytes serve in the body? **Select all that apply.** *(487, 490)*
    1. Maintenance of normal body metabolism
    2. Regulation of water balance in the body
    3. Regulation of water and electrolyte contents within cells
    4. Formation of hydrochloric acid in gastric juice
    5. Transportation of nutrients to cells and waste products from cells

28. The patient has been placed on a low-sodium diet to assist in the treatment of hypertension. Which patient statement indicates an understanding of the diet teaching? *(487)*
    1. "Cheese is a good between-meal snack for me."
    2. "It is okay for me to eat at my favorite seafood restaurant."
    3. "In order for me to eat enough vegetables, I can prepare canned peas and corn."
    4. "I use a lot of fresh vegetables, although I should give up table salt."

29. Which patient has the **greatest** risk for developing hypokalemia? *(489)*
    1. Has a small bowel obstruction
    2. Has renal failure
    3. Consumes excessive alcohol
    4. Takes prescribed loop diuretic

30. The nurse is monitoring an older patient who is receiving a fluid bolus for dehydration. The nurse notices that the patient suddenly has a slight cough and seems a little short of breath. The patient reports, "I'm okay." What should the nurse do **first**? *(508)*
    1. Notify the RN and the health care provider.
    2. Auscultate the lungs and assess for fluid overload.
    3. Stop the bolus infusion and establish a saline lock.
    4. Weigh the patient and compare to baseline.

31. The nurse receives notification from the laboratory that a patient's potassium level is 6 mEq/L. The nurse has paged the provider and is awaiting a call back. What should the nurse do **first**? *(489)*
    1. Attach the patient to a cardiac monitor.
    2. Encourage foods and fluids that contain potassium.
    3. Ensure that intravenous calcium gluconate is available.
    4. Check medications that could affect potassium levels.

32. The nurse is checking the laboratory data of a woman who is at risk for osteoporosis. Which electrolyte value is **most** relevant to this condition? *(491)*
    1. Sodium level of 145 mEq/L
    2. Calcium level of 3.0 mEq/dL
    3. Potassium 3.5 mEq/dL
    4. Phosphorus of 3.4 mEq/dL

33. The nurse hears in report that the patient has been receiving aluminum hydroxide to correct an electrolyte imbalance. Which electrolyte value indicates that the therapy is working? *(493)*
    1. Phosphorus level of 4.1 mEq/dL
    2. Magnesium level of 1.5 mEq/dL
    3. Bicarbonate level of 22 mEq/dL
    4. Calcium level of 4.5 mEq/dL

34. The nurse is caring for a patient who had surgery on the parathyroid glands. Which electrolyte level in the low-normal range is the **greatest** concern? *(492)*
    1. Calcium level of 4.6 mEq/dL
    2. Sodium level of 127 mEq/dL
    3. Potassium level of 3.7 mEq/dL
    4. Magnesium level of 1.7 mEq/dL

35. The patient has a medical diagnosis of diabetic ketoacidosis. Which clinical manifestation indicates that the blood buffer system is exhausted? *(495)*
    1. Urinary output is decreased.
    2. Respiratory rate is increased.
    3. Heart rate is decreased.
    4. pH is increased.

36. The patient is on mechanical ventilation. The arterial blood gas results indicate that the patient has respiratory alkalosis. What would the nurse do **first**? *(497)*
    1. Suction the airway for excessive secretions or a mucus plug.
    2. Notify the RN or the health care provider.
    3. Check the ventilator settings and compare to the orders.
    4. Deliver breaths using a bag-valve-mask with high-flow oxygen.

CRITICAL THINKING ACTIVITIES

37. The nurse is caring for an older patient who was brought to the hospital for confusion. The family reports that the patient lives alone and is usually alert and independent, but recently complained of stomach cramps, vomiting, and diarrhea. The nurse notes that home medications include a diuretic and blood pressure medication. Mucous membranes are dry. Laboratory results show potassium 3.4 mEq/L and serum sodium 127 mEq/L.

    a. Identify at least two considerations for the older adult patient regarding fluid, electrolyte, and acid-base balance. *(506)*

        _____

        _____

    b. What is the clinical significance of a serum potassium of 3.4 mEq/L? *(489)* _____

        _____

        _____

    c. For this patient, what factors are likely to be contributing to the current serum potassium value? *(490)*

        _____

        _____

    d. What are the **most** common signs/symptoms associated with hypokalemia, and what are the nursing interventions for the imbalance? *(490)*

        _____

        _____

    e. What is the clinical significance of a serum sodium of 127 mEq/L? *(487)* _____

        _____

        _____

    f. Identify the **most** common signs and symptoms of hyponatremia, and nursing interventions for the imbalance. *(488)*

        _____

        _____

    g. The nurse is monitoring the patient's I&O. What should be counted as part of the output? *(485)*

        _____

        _____

38. The nurse is caring for a patient with pneumonia. The patient is having dyspnea. The following laboratory data are available for review.

pH	7.30
$Paco_2$	50 mm Hg
Pao_2	70 mm Hg
O_2 saturation	90%
HCO_3^-	22 mEq

a. What do these laboratory values suggest for this patient? *(497)* _____

_____

b. What signs and symptoms are likely to be associated with the laboratory values? *(497)* _____

_____

_____

_____

c. What treatment does the nurse anticipate will be ordered for this patient? *(497)*_____

_____

_____

Student Name_____   Date_____

Nutritional Concepts and Related Therapies

SHORT ANSWER

Directions: Using your own words, answer each question in the space provided.

1. Identify the six classes of nutrients and their general function. *(526)*_____

    _____

    _____

2. For each vitamin, identify a food source, its function in the body, and signs and symptoms of deficiency and toxicity (if applicable). *(533, 534)*

    a. Vitamin A:_____

        _____

    b. Vitamin D:_____

        _____

    c. Vitamin K:_____

        _____

3. For each mineral, identify a food source, its function in the body, and signs and symptoms of deficiency and toxicity (if applicable). *(536, 537)*

    a. Calcium: _____

        _____

    b. Potassium:_____

        _____

    c. Sodium: _____

        _____

CLINICAL APPLICATION OF MATH AND CONVERSION

4. The provider prescribes an enteral feeding to infuse at 30 mL/hour for 3 hours and then to check the residual and notify with the results. How many mL will the patient receive in 3 hours? *(563)* _____ mL

5. The patient was directed by the provider to consume 1500 kcal/day to achieve weight-loss goals. If the patient consumes 60% carbohydrates, 20% protein, and 20% fats, calculate the total number of grams/day for carbohydrates _____ g; fats _____ g; and protein _____ g. (Recall that carbohydrates and protein will provide 4 kcal/g. Fats provide 9 kcal/g.) *(526)*

6. According to the dietary reference intake (DRI), the protein requirement for healthy adults is 0.8 g/kg of body weight per day. How many grams of protein does a man require if he weighs 185 pounds? *(531)* _____ g

7. According to the DRI, the carbohydrate requirement for healthy adults should be between 45% and 65% of daily kilocalories per day. For a person who is consuming 1500 kilocalories per day, what is the range of kilocalories that should come from carbohydrates? *(527)* _____ kcal to _____ kcal

8. The nutrition label on a jar of peanut butter indicates that there are 16 g of total fat, 8 g of carbohydrates and 7 g of protein per serving. Based on information from the textbook (carbohydrates and protein will provide 4 kcal/g and fats provide 9 kcal/g), calculate how many kilocalories are in a serving of peanut butter. *(526)* _____ kcal

9. Calculate your own body mass index (BMI). _____ *(549, 550)*

10. A patient with end-stage renal disease has the following urinary output from the past 24 hours: 15 mL at 0700, 20 mL at 1200, 30 mL at 1700, 10 mL at 2100, and 5 mL at 0400. The provider's prescription for fluid restriction is 750 mL + urine output from previous 24 hours. How much fluid is the patient allowed to have? *(557)* _____ mL

11. The patient is receiving enteral feedings per nasogastric (NG) tube. The provider prescribes water to infuse at 100 mL/hr every 6 hours. How much water per NG tube should the patient receive every 24 hours? _____ mL *(563)*

TABLE ACTIVITY

12. Directions: Complete the table below with the missing numerical value or the interpretation of the numerical value. The first block is done for you. *(530)*

Numerical Value	Interpretation of Numerical Value
LDL Cholesterol	
<100	Optimal
100-129	
	Borderline high
160-189	
	Very high
Total Cholesterol	
	Desirable
200-239	
≥240	
HDL Cholesterol	
<40 men; <50 women	

FIGURE LABELING

13. Directions: Label the figure below with the correct tube feeding sites. *(559)*

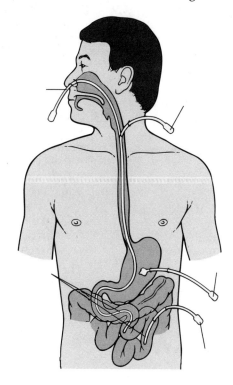

MULTIPLE CHOICE

Directions: Select the best answer(s) for each of the following questions.

14. The nurse is teaching a patient who has heart failure to read nutrition labels on food products. Which nutritional fact is the **most** important for this patient to pay attention to? *(556)*
    1. The total number of kilocalories of fat per serving
    2. The % daily value of fiber provided in a serving
    3. The number of milligrams of sodium per serving
    4. The number of grams of protein per serving

15. The patient has risk for osteoporosis. Which foods is the nurse **most** likely to suggest? *(538)*
    1. Eggs, raw fruits and vegetables
    2. Whole-grain breads and pasta, and poultry
    3. Green leafy vegetables and citrus fruits
    4. Sardines, tofu, cheese, and broccoli

16. Which laboratory result is the nurse **most** likely to examine to determine if the treatment for iron deficiency anemia is effective? *(536)*
    1. Hemoglobin level
    2. Electrolyte values
    3. Blood clotting factors
    4. Albumin level

17. Which patient is **most** likely to benefit from an increase in dietary fiber? *(528, 554)*
    1. Has chronic obstructive pulmonary disease
    2. Has a high risk for metabolic syndrome
    3. Has a high risk for osteoporosis
    4. Has a recent diagnosis of hepatitis

18. A parent tells the nurse, "The school nutritionist advised parents to send packed lunches that include complete proteins, but I'm not exactly sure what that means." What is the **best** response? *(531)*
    1. "What would you normally send in a packed lunch?"
    2. "Just pack a variety of foods that you know your child will eat."
    3. "Complete proteins are generally of animal origin, like eggs or meat."
    4. "Does your child have any dietary restrictions or food allergies?"

19. A patient is interested in adding antioxidants to the diet. What is the **best** advice? *(532)*
    1. Take vitamin supplements, especially A, C, and E.
    2. Eat a wide variety of fruits and vegetables.
    3. Eat dairy products, such as cheese, yogurt, and milk.
    4. Take a multi-vitamin and mineral supplement.

20. According to the National Institute of Health's Office of Dietary Supplements, which patient should be advised to have an additional 35 mg/day of vitamin C beyond the usual recommended adult dose? *(534)*
    1. A patient who was recently diagnosed with cancer.
    2. A patient who has recent onset of cold symptoms.
    3. A patient who drinks alcohol daily.
    4. A patient who smokes cigarettes every day.

21. The patient is interested in lowering his cholesterol levels and reducing the risk of cardiovascular disease. Which breakfast tray offers the **most** water-soluble fiber to help the patient meet his goals? *(528)*
    1. Half a grapefruit with hard-boiled egg
    2. Hash-brown potatoes with sausage patty
    3. Yogurt with honey, granola, and fresh strawberries
    4. Oatmeal topped with cinnamon and raw apple slices

22. Which patients have conditions that would prompt the nurse to monitor serum sodium levels? **Select all that apply.** *(538)*
    1. The patient is having a prolonged high fever.
    2. The patient has severe diarrhea and vomiting.
    3. The patient has iron deficiency anemia.
    4. The patient has chronic renal disease.
    5. The patient has cystic fibrosis.

23. The home health nurse sees that the patient's potassium level is 3.6 mmol/L. There is nothing in the patient's medication or health history that should affect the potassium levels. What will the nurse do? *(537, 539)*
    1. Tell the patient to make an appointment to see the provider as soon as possible.
    2. Suggest that the patient eat sweet potatoes, fruits, vegetables, fresh meat, legumes, and milk.
    3. Take vital signs and assess the patient for signs/symptoms of hyperkalemia.
    4. Instruct the patient to have a potassium test repeated every 12-18 months.

24. The nurse is assessing an older resident at a long-term care center. The resident appears flushed, skin turgor is poor, mucous membranes are dry, and resident seems unusually irritable. What would the nurse do **first**? *(540)*
    1. Test for gag reflex; then offer oral fluids
    2. Obtain an order for electrolyte values
    3. Take vital signs and check urine specific gravity
    4. Check blood sugar and offer a popsicle

25. A woman is in the first trimester of pregnancy. She reports several episodes of nausea and vomiting, a headache, and irritability. The nurse observes shallow breathing and perspiration, and the woman appears shaky and nervous. What would the nurse do **first**? *(542)*
    1. Check blood glucose level
    2. Take the temperature
    3. Check pulse oximeter reading
    4. Attach electrocardiogram monitor

26. The patient is going to be discharged with a prescription for an anticoagulant medication. Which question should the nurse ask? *(535)*
    1. "How many servings of leafy green vegetables would you normally eat in a week?"
    2. "Do you drink at least 8 glasses of fluid every day?"
    3. "What would you typically eat for breakfast every morning?"
    4. "Are you having any problems with constipation or adequate fiber intake?"

27. The patient reports noticing that his gums bleed very easily. If the bleeding is caused by a nutritional deficiency, which types of food will correct the problem? *(533)*
    1. Milk, egg yolks, and liver
    2. Broccoli, peppers, and tomatoes
    3. Cereals, legumes, and nuts
    4. Poultry, fish, and brown rice

28. Which patient is at risk for pernicious anemia and is **most** likely to be prescribed a vitamin B_{12} supplement? *(535)*
    1. Frequently tries different weight-loss plans
    2. Eats small amounts of a variety of foods
    3. Prefers meat and potatoes, with very few vegetables
    4. Adheres to a strict vegan diet

29. The nurse is working with a patient who requires an increase in complete proteins in the diet. Which foods will the nurse recommend? **Select all that apply.** *(531)*
    1. Soy
    2. Eggs
    3. Peanuts
    4. Beans
    5. Fish
    6. Yogurt

30. A patient reports routinely taking high doses of vitamin supplements. Which vitamin has the **greatest** potential for toxic effects related to high dosage? *(532)*
    1. A
    2. B$_1$ (thiamine)
    3. B$_2$ (riboflavin)
    4. C

31. A patient with ascites has fluid restrictions of 1000 mL/per 24 hours. The nurse observes that the patient frequently asks visitors and staff to give him extra fluids. What would the nurse do **first** to improve the patient's compliance? *(557)*
    1. Assess the patient's understanding of the fluid restrictions.
    2. Offer suggestions to decrease sensation of thirst (e.g., chew gum).
    3. Post a sign over the bed that indicates fluid limits.
    4. Instruct family, friends, and staff that fluids are limited and measured.

32. Which item is allowed on a clear liquid diet? *(547)*
    1. Orange juice
    2. Gelatin
    3. Sherbet
    4. Cream soup

33. Which patient is **most** likely to be prescribed a carbohydrate-modified diet? *(551)*
    1. Has heart failure
    2. Has hypertension
    3. Has cirrhosis of the liver
    4. Has diabetes mellitus

34. An Asian American patient reports experiencing nausea, a bloated feeling, and flatulence after eating. Which question is the **most** relevant? *(553)*
    1. "Do you have any food allergies?"
    2. "Are you following the MyPlate guidelines?"
    3. "What did you eat just before the onset of the symptoms?"
    4. "Is anyone who ate the same food having the same symptoms?"

35. Patients with nasogastric (NG) tubes may develop otitis media. What will the nurse do to prevent this occurrence? *(560)*
    1. Increase fluid intake.
    2. Remove and reinsert the tube every 24 hours.
    3. Suction the nose and mouth.
    4. Turn the patient side to side every 2 hours.

36. The nurse is evaluating the performance of a unlicensed assistive personnel (UAP) who is feeding a patient. Which action indicates a need for correction? *(561)*
    1. Offering the patient the bedpan before the meal.
    2. Placing the patient in a recumbent position.
    3. Providing opportunity for hand hygiene before the meal.
    4. Talking with the patient during the feeding.

37. Which admission assessments should be performed for long-term care residents in relation to potential nutritional problems? **Select all that apply.** *(545)*
    1. Problems with fine motor movements
    2. Ability to chew and swallow different textures of foods
    3. Typical daily fluid intake
    4. Ability to obtain and prepare own food
    5. Dietary restrictions related to chronic health problems
    6. Food preferences or rituals related to cultural background

38. The nurse sees an order for "clear liquid diet, advance as tolerated to regular diet." What does the nurse do to get the **best** food selection for the patient? *(547)*
    1. Contact the provider for clarification of the order.
    2. Ask the patient if he is hungry and what he prefers to eat.
    3. Assess the patient's overall response to the clear liquid diet.
    4. Call the nutritionist and ask for an individualized diet plan.

39. The mother asks the nurse about giving strained fruits to her infant. When should this food be introduced? *(543)*
    1. 2 months
    2. 5 months
    3. 8 months
    4. 12 months

40. The patient is taking a diuretic medication every day. Which electrolyte value is the **most** important to monitor? *(546)*
    1. Chloride
    2. Sodium
    3. Phosphorus
    4. Potassium

41. What are nursing responsibilities in promoting nutrition for patients? **Select all that apply.** (524)
    1. Assisting patients to eat or drink
    2. Designing diet plans for patients with chronic health problems
    3. Recording the patient's fluid and food intake
    4. Observing the patient for signs of poor nutrition
    5. Communicating dietary concerns to other members of the health care team
    6. Monitoring laboratory values that are related to nutritional intake

42. The patient has just ordered lunch at a restaurant. According to the USDA MyPlate recommendations, which food item should the patient plan to divide and take a portion home in a carry-out box? (524)
    1. 10 ounces grilled skinless chicken breast
    2. 1 cup of steamed vegetables
    3. ¾ cup of mixed fruit salad
    4. ¾ cup of brown rice pilaf

43. The patient is trying to understand the difference between dietary reference intakes (DRIs) and recommended dietary allowances (RDAs). Which patient statement **best** indicates an understanding of DRIs? (524)
    1. "DRIs replace the RDAs but are similar, so I could use either one to monitor my cholesterol."
    2. "Using DRIs, I could decrease my risk for diabetes and monitor my sugar consumption."
    3. "RDAs apply to healthy adult Americans; but I should rely on DRIs because I am overweight. "
    4. "DRIs are based on disease states; so I can use them as a guideline to control my thyroid problem."

44. Following bariatric surgery, a patient experiences nausea, cramping, diarrhea, sweating, lightheadedness, and palpitations after eating. What is the **most** important self-care measure for the nurse to reinforce? (552)
    1. Immediately report the symptoms to the surgeon; surgical intervention may be necessary.
    2. Be patient and live with the symptoms; they are expected and temporary.
    3. Avoid concentrated sweets and drink fluids 30-60 minutes before and after meals.
    4. When symptoms occur, replace the next meal with extra fluids such as diluted juices.

45. The patient has sustained severe injuries in an accident. Which food sources supply the nutrient that plays the **biggest** role in helping the patient to build and repair injured tissue? (527)
    1. Green vegetables and bright-colored fruits
    2. Pasta and breads made from whole grains
    3. Beans, legumes, and soy products
    4. Lean meats, poultry, and fish

46. The nurse routinely participates in long distance endurance sports, such as running, swimming, and cycling. Which foods should the nurse eat to have energy over a longer period of time? (527)
    1. Corn and potatoes
    2. Milk and citrus fruits
    3. Honey and table sugar
    4. Chocolate and electrolyte drinks

47. The nurse is talking to a patient who has high cholesterol and a family history of cardiovascular disease. Which foods are **most** likely to counteract the high cholesterol? (528)
    1. Wheat bran and celery
    2. Orange juice and white rice
    3. Lettuce and pears
    4. Oats and barley

48. The patient reports sensations of bloating, gas, and constipation after adding lots of fruits, vegetables, and whole grains to her diet. So she has decided to go back to her former dietary pattern and exclude these foods. What is the **best** advice that the nurse can give the patient? (528)
    1. "Resume former dietary patterns and contact your health care provider."
    2. "Slowly increase intake of fiber foods and drink at least 8 glasses of water each day."
    3. "Start with a fiber supplement instead of fruits, vegetables, and whole grains."
    4. "Excessive fiber intake can lead to osteoporosis and anemia in women."

49. The patient expresses a strong preference for beef that is marbled with fat at every meal, because of the flavor and the feeling of fullness and satisfaction. Nurse would advise that this eating habit is likely to increase risk for which health condition? (529)
    1. Osteoporosis
    2. Cirrhosis of the liver
    3. Diabetes mellitus
    4. Atherosclerosis

50. The patient tells the nurse that he has problems with his cholesterol so a friend told him to eat avocadoes. What is the **best** response? *(529)*
    1. "Avocadoes are very high in fat so the total cholesterol will increase."
    2. "Avocadoes are a source of monounsaturated fats, which are thought to lower bad cholesterol."
    3. "Avocadoes are yellow fruits, and fruits generally do not affect cholesterol levels."
    4. "Avocadoes are a source of trans-fatty acids, which will increase the good cholesterol."

51. The patient was advised by the provider to "watch intake of cholesterol." Which question is the **most** useful in assessing the likelihood of the patient's adherence to the provider's advice? *(547)*
    1. "Do you understand what 'watch your intake of cholesterol' means?"
    2. "How do you plan to manage your intake of cholesterol?"
    3. "Would you like a list of foods that contain high amounts of cholesterol?"
    4. "What do you normally eat in a 24-hour period?"

52. Which laboratory value would the nurse check to evaluate the protein status of a patient who has been receiving medical nutrition therapy? *(564)*
    1. Hemoglobin
    2. Albumin
    3. White blood cell count
    4. Electrolyte values

53. A patient has symptoms of steatorrhea and flatulence. Which diet is the provider **most** likely to recommend? *(554)*
    1. Carbohydrate-modified diet
    2. Protein-restricted diet
    3. Sodium-restricted diet
    4. Fat-controlled diet

54. The nurse is talking to a 17-year-old female whose parents have reluctantly allowed her to start a vegan diet if she agrees to talk to a health care provider before beginning the diet. The provider is **most** likely to monitor her for which nutrition-related condition? *(539)*
    1. Anorexia nervosa
    2. Rickets
    3. Iron deficiency anemia
    4. Marasmus

55. Which patient is at the **greatest** risk for a negative nitrogen balance that will lead to atrophy of muscles? *(531)*
    1. The patient gets nothing by mouth for several days due to intractable nausea and vomiting.
    2. The patient is in the first trimester of a normal pregnancy.
    3. The patient sustained severe burns to 50% of the body surface.
    4. The patient has been fasting for several days for a religious ritual.

56. During a trip to a developing country, the nurse observes that many of the toddlers appear very fat with enlarged abdomens and swollen extremities. Which nutritional deficiency is associated with these symptoms? *(532)*
    1. Carbohydrates
    2. Fats
    3. Vitamins
    4. Protein

57. The patient reports a habit of smoking at least one pack of cigarettes every day. Which foods would the nurse encourage the patient to eat, because of the heavy smoking habit? *(534)*
    1. Fish and poultry
    2. Milk products
    3. Citrus fruits
    4. Whole grains

58. A 69-year-old patient reports frequently taking antacids. Why does this patient have an increased risk for developing pernicious anemia? *(539)*
    1. Low stomach acidity blocks the absorption of vitamin B_{12} from foods.
    2. Antacids interfere with the body's ability to use heme iron.
    3. Older people who take antacids are less likely to produce intrinsic factor.
    4. Antacids inhibit the digestion of foods that supply vitamin C.

59. The mother reports that her child took a few extra chewable vitamins, because he thought they were gummy candies. Which question is the **most** important to assess for potential toxicity? *(539)*
    1. "Does the product contain vitamin C?"
    2. "How much does the child weigh?"
    3. "Is iron listed as one of the ingredients?"
    4. "Did you induce vomiting?"

60. Which patient should not be offered low-fat milk? *(543)*
    1. 15-year-old female with type 1 diabetes
    2. 26-year-old female who is in the third trimester of pregnancy
    3. 68-year-old female who has hip fracture related to osteoporosis
    4. 18-month-old female who is transitioning to cow's milk

61. Which parental action encourages good dietary habits in the child? *(544)*
    1. Allow the child to eat whenever he is hungry and skip meals if he is not hungry.
    2. Give the child whatever the rest of the family is eating; do not cater to special requests.
    3. Encourage the child to help with food preparation and create a positive environment.
    4. Give everyone the same serving size and quietly remove leftover food.

62. The nurse is talking to an adolescent girl about nutrition, but the girl seems bored, uninterested, and unlikely to try any of the nurse's suggestions. What should the nurse do? *(544)*
    1. Delay the discussion until the girl initiates interest.
    2. Explain the science of physiology and nutrition.
    3. Assess the girl's interest in other health topics.
    4. Describe how nutrition improves skin and facial appearance.

63. The UAP brings holiday cupcakes to the long-term care center and passes them out to all of the residents before checking with the nurse. What should the nurse do **first**? *(546)*
    1. Ask the UAP to collect the cupcakes and then determine who is allowed to have one.
    2. Praise the UAP for bringing seasonally appropriate good cheer to the residents.
    3. Remind the UAP that not all residents should have too much sugar, so next time, ask first.
    4. Sit with the residents, enjoy the cupcakes, and make the food into a social occasion.

64. A patient is on fluid restrictions because of renal failure. Which interventions would the nurse use? **Select all that apply.** *(557)*
    1. Encourage the patient to drink most of the fluid allowance in the morning.
    2. Explain the various sources of fluid such as IV fluids, gelatin, and fluids taken with medications.
    3. Suggest chewing gum and sucking on breath mints.
    4. Explain the rationale for fluid restrictions.
    5. Show the volume of fluid that is allowed for the shift.
    6. Post a sign in the room so that visitors are aware of fluid restrictions.

65. The patient is trying to lose weight because he is obese and has been told that he has a high risk for diabetes, coronary heart disease, and stroke. What is the **most** important point that the nurse should emphasize? *(549)*
    1. Strictly adhere to 1500 kcal/day, but eat a variety of foods.
    2. Take a multivitamin and mineral supplement while dieting.
    3. Exercise 60-90 minutes most days of the week.
    4. A weight loss of 5% to 15% can reduce health-related risks.

66. Which patient is **most** likely to be a candidate for bariatric surgery? *(551)*
    1. Body mass index of 40 or higher
    2. Body mass index of 35 or higher
    3. Body mass index of 23 with severe cardiovascular disease
    4. Body mass index of 17 with diabetes

67. The patient is newly diagnosed with type 2 diabetes. In talking to the patient about diet management, what would the nurse suggest? *(551)*
    1. Suggest the patient follow a standardized preprinted menu for each meal.
    2. Indicate that two or more servings of fried fish would be beneficial.
    3. Closely monitor and control intake of table sugar and desserts.
    4. Emphasize consistent mealtimes; approximately every 4-5 hours.

68. A patient who is a known diabetic presents with weakness, diaphoresis, and disorientation. What should the nurse do **first**? *(527, 552)*
    1. Encourage the patient to drink a lot of water.
    2. Give the patient a glass of milk.
    3. Establish intravenous access and give glucose.
    4. Have the patient suck on a hard candy.

CRITICAL THINKING ACTIVITIES

69. The nurse is working on a medical-surgical unit and has identified several patients who may need enteral feeding.

   a. What are the indications for the use of enteral feeding? *(557)* _____

   _____

   _____

   b. Identify the nursing assessments and interventions for enteral feeding in the following situations.

      i. Patient assessment before feeding: *(561)*_____

      _____

      ii. Assessment of gastric aspirate: *(561)* _____

      _____

      iii. Gastric residual based on provider's parameters: *(561)*_____

      _____

      iv. Formula is cold: *(559, 562)*_____

      _____

      v. Occlusion of the tubing is suspected: *(561)*_____

      _____

      vi. After feeding is given: *(563)* _____

      _____

      vii. Documentation: *(563)*_____

      _____

   c. What are the possible complications or problems associated with enteral feeding? *(559)*_____

   _____

   _____

   _____

70. The nurse is talking to a 25-year-old woman who is approximately 10 pounds underweight for her age and height, but is otherwise in good health. She would like some information about healthy diet and lifestyle, because she and her husband are thinking about trying to have a baby.

   a. Explain to this young woman why there is an increased need for nutrients during pregnancy. *(540)*

   _____

   _____

   b. Which vitamins would be recommended for the pregnant patient and what is the function of these vitamin supplements? What are the food sources for each vitamin? *(541)*

   _____

   _____

   _____

c. What can the nurse tell the patient about her current weight in relation to getting pregnant? *(540)*

_____

_____

_____

d. What can the nurse tell the patient about foods and lifestyle activities that should be avoided? *(542)*

_____

_____

71. In your own words, explain what you would tell a patient about "bad" cholesterol and "good" cholesterol. *(530)*

_____

_____

_____

Complementary and Alternative Therapies

MULTIPLE CHOICE

Directions: Select the best answer(s) for each of the following questions.

1. All patients should be advised to discuss use of complementary and alternative therapies with their health care provider; however, which patient needs extra encouragement to check with the provider before trying reflexology? *(575)*
   1. Has type 2 diabetes
   2. Is in the first trimester of pregnancy
   3. Has chronic pulmonary disease
   4. Had fractured ankle in childhood

2. The patient says, "I take an anticoagulant because I have atrial fibrillation and I like to use ginseng because I heard it can prevent diabetes." Based on the patient's comments, what is the **most** important data set for the nurse to follow up? *(572)*
   1. Look at the patient's current and previous blood glucose levels.
   2. Put the patient on the cardiac monitor and compare to previous tracings.
   3. Check the patient's current and previous clotting times.
   4. Take a full set of vital signs and compare current values to previous.

3. Which outcome statement indicates that valerian is being used appropriately and is a successful therapy for the patient? *(574)*
   1. The patient reports that his upper respiratory infection resolved much faster than expected.
   2. The patient states he feels more alert and has better mental concentration after several doses.
   3. The patient reports that the nausea is relieved, and the abdominal pain has subsided.
   4. The patient feels that he is sleeping more soundly, and quality of sleep seems much better.

4. The patient has a bone infection in the lower leg. Which patient education brochure is the nurse **most** likely to prepare for the patient? *(577)*
   1. Antibiotic Therapy and Surgery for Osteomyelitis
   2. How to Effectively Use Tea Tree Oil for Infections
   3. Risks and Benefits of Chiropractic Therapy
   4. Advantages and Disadvantages of Energy Field Therapy

5. Which nurse is correctly using a complementary and alternative therapy to assist older residents in a long-term care center to evoke memories of past Christmas holidays? *(580)*
    1. Nurse A puts up strings of red, white, and green lights to create a positive energy field.
    2. Nurse B uses biofeedback and monitors respiratory rate as people listen to Christmas music.
    3. Nurse C applies animal-assisted therapy by showing a movie about Santa's reindeer.
    4. Nurse D uses an aromatic infuser filled with pine scent and the residents decorate a tree.

6. For most patients, magnet therapy has neither beneficial nor detrimental effects; however, for which patient would magnet therapy be contraindicated? *(581)*
    1. The patient has rheumatoid arthritis.
    2. The patient has a pacemaker.
    3. The patient had knee replacement surgery.
    4. The patient has terminal ovarian cancer.

7. Currently, which patients are **most** likely to be prescribed and benefit from tetrahydrocannabinol (THC)? *(585)*
    1. Patients with fibromyalgia or chronic fatigue syndrome
    2. Patients with clinical depression or anxiety disorders
    3. Patients with addictions to alcohol or opioid analgesics
    4. Patients with cancer or acquired immunodeficiency syndrome

8. Which outcome statement indicates that the prescribed dronabinol is a successful therapy for a patient with cancer? *(585)*
    1. The tumor is reduced in size and pressure on surrounding tissues is reduced.
    2. The patient reports decreased nausea and an improvement in appetite.
    3. The patient reports sleeping longer and resting more comfortably.
    4. Fever and pain are reduced, and white cell count is improving.

9. What is the **most** common element of relaxation strategies? *(582)*
    1. Rhythmic breathing
    2. Control of muscle groups
    3. Awareness of environment
    4. Meditation

10. The patient suffered a traumatic event as a child; however, the event is not something the patient ever thinks or talks about. Which therapy would be **most** likely to trigger a memory that would require psychological intervention? *(584)*
    1. Biofeedback
    2. Reflexology
    3. Yoga
    4. Accupressure

11. The nurse is collecting data for the health history of a new patient. What is the **best** rationale for directly asking the patient about the use of complementary and alternative medicine therapies? *(571)*
    1. About 50% of patients use herbal supplements but usage is rarely reported.
    2. A complete health history is essential for every patient.
    3. Alternative therapies must be listed for insurance coverage.
    4. Nurses should be advocates for holistic care for patients.

12. The nurse is seeking evidence-based practice information related to complementary and alternative medicine (CAM) therapies for cancer patients. What would be the **best** source of this information? *(571)*
    1. Consult an updated comprehensive medical-surgical nursing textbook.
    2. Use the Internet to search for "cancer" and "CAM therapies."
    3. Access National Center for Complementary and Integrative Health website.
    4. Talk to the local chapter of the American Cancer Society.

13. Why do herbal products have the potential to cause problems for consumers? **Select all that apply.** *(572)*
    1. Do not have the same rigorous study as pharmaceuticals
    2. Reduced level of accountability for the manufacturers
    3. Not required by law to demonstrate safety, efficacy, or quality of products
    4. Wide variations in potency, quality, and chemical content
    5. No standardized dosages have been established for most herbs
    6. More potent than pharmaceuticals because the whole plant is used

14. Which patient statement indicates a correct understanding of the patient teaching information about using herbal preparations? *(575)*
    1. "Herbal preparations are made from plants and are natural and safe."
    2. "These are over-the-counter products so they don't have dangerous side effects."
    3. "If I follow the package instructions on dosage, I'll be okay."
    4. "The herbs should be discontinued at least 2 weeks before any surgery."

15. The patient has heart failure and takes digoxin. He tells the nurse that he is thinking about taking *Ginkgo biloba* because it is supposed to improve memory by increasing circulation to the brain. What is the **best** response? *(575)*
    1. "You sound like you might be worried about memory loss."
    2. "Digoxin has a lot of herb-drug and drug-drug interactions."
    3. "Let me contact your provider so you can discuss this with him."
    4. "I will get you some additional information about *Ginkgo biloba*."

16. A 42-year-old female patient has a family history of osteoporosis and would like advice about the use of CAM for prevention of osteoporosis. Which therapy would the nurse provide information about? *(584)*
    1. Acupuncture
    2. Chiropractic therapy
    3. Reflexology
    4. T'ai chi

17. Which patient statement indicates understanding of a therapy that could help with smoking cessation? *(577)*
    1. "I could consult an herbalist and smoke herbal leaf instead of tobacco."
    2. "Acupuncture stimulates acupoints and has been used to treat addictions."
    3. "Inhalation of lavender oil relieves stress and decreases craving for a cigarette."
    4. "Biofeedback would increase my awareness about my physiologic cravings."

18. Which patient would **not** be a candidate for therapeutic massage? *(579)*
    1. A pregnant woman who would like to have a foot massage
    2. A postsurgical patient who wants the legs massaged to relieve cramping
    3. An older patient who has an ache in the upper back after prolonged sitting
    4. A school-aged child who has been confined to bed for several days

19. The older patient disrobes to take a shower. The young nursing student who is assigned to assist with hygiene is shocked and repulsed by the appearance and condition of the patient's skin. What should the student do? *(580)*
    1. Quickly excuse herself and step out into the hall to recover composure.
    2. Smile and avoid looking at the patient directly, but continue to assist with care.
    3. Apologize to the patient and then seek out the instructor for advice.
    4. Make eye contact, smile, and assist the patient to maintain safety in the shower.

20. The nurse is working in a long-term care center and recognizes that older residents are at risk for "skin hunger." What would the nurse do to address this problem? *(580)*
    1. Ensure that herbal lotion enriched with vitamins and protein is applied after bathing.
    2. Identify residents who are comfortable with hugging and touching by staff members.
    3. Consult with a holistic nutritionist to design meals that supply nutrition for the skin.
    4. Apply herbal sunscreens to protect the skin and take residents into the sun.

21. Which patient should be cautioned that inhalation of essential oils could exacerbate symptoms? *(580)*
    1. Takes as-needed (PRN) medication for asthma
    2. Recently diagnosed with major depression
    3. Currently experiences excessive stress related to work
    4. Underwent chiropractic treatments for back pain

22. The nursing student has severe test anxiety. She is using guided imagery to help reduce anxiety just before the beginning of each test. What is the desired outcome of this type of therapy? *(581)*
    1. Controls response to stimuli by regulating expectations and perceptions
    2. Learns to deep-breathe and include all senses during times of stress
    3. Visualizes warmth entering the body on inspiration and tension leaving on expiration
    4. Creates an image of self successfully passing the exam

23. What are the advantages of animal-assisted therapy? **Select all that apply.** (583)
    1. Research indicates that animals have a calming effect.
    2. Animals can stimulate mental activity through interaction.
    3. Most families have a pet that will be familiar to the patients.
    4. Everyone likes animals because they decrease loneliness.
    5. Patients who like animals are usually not allergic to them.
    6. Being around an animal can reduce blood pressure and anxiety.

CRITICAL THINKING ACTIVITIES

24. The nurse is caring for a patient who is from a different culture than the nurse. The patient requests some ginseng tea and there is a vial of tea tree oil on the bedside table. Identify cultural considerations that arise in relation to complementary and alternative therapies. (588)

    _____

    _____

    _____

    _____

25. Consider the cognitive skills of focusing, passivity, and receptivity and discuss the use of relaxation therapy with the following patients. (581, 582)

    a. A 77-year-old woman with advanced dementia is frequently restless. She will pace and demonstrate non-purposeful movements. Her family has asked the nurse to help her to be calmer and relax.

    _____

    _____

    _____

    b. A 23-year-old college student is extremely anxious about doing well. At times, he has studied to the point of exhaustion. He reports taking "uppers" so that he can stay awake and study. Currently, it appears that he is under the influence of stimulants because he is talking very fast about a math problem that he is working on and he appears jittery and nervous.

    _____

    _____

    _____

    c. A 62-year-old retired military officer appears very tense, but he tells the nurse that he doesn't have any problems with anxiety, tension, or stress. Furthermore, he informs the nurse that if he did have any problems, he would control them on his own. His wife tries to tell the nurse that he does need some help to relax, but he cuts her off abruptly.

    _____

    _____

    _____

26. A neighbor tells the nurse that he is no longer seeing a health care provider and that he has discontinued his prescribed medications in favor of herbs and other types of complementary or alternative therapies for his health problems, which include diabetes, high blood pressure, and heart problems. What should the nurse do? (571)

    _____

    _____

    _____

Pain Management, Comfort, Rest, and Sleep

chapter
21

MULTIPLE CHOICE

Directions: Select the best answer(s) for each of the following questions.

1. Which nursing action empowers the patient to become an active partner in managing pain? *(592)*
   1. Administers prescribed pain medication in a timely fashion
   2. Acknowledges the patient as expert in his own experience of pain
   3. Advocates for therapies that provide sufficient relief of pain
   4. Assesses the pain before and after giving pain medication

2. The nurse identifies that the patient with coronary insufficiency is having referred pain. Which finding substantiates the nurse's interpretation? *(593)*
   1. Patient reports she is having pain in her left jaw.
   2. Patient demonstrates grimacing when pain starts.
   3. Patient reports that chest hurts during exercise.
   4. Patient reports that symptoms are relieved with rest.

3. The patient reports lower back pain that is dull and intermittent. Which description **most** strongly suggests that the patient is having chronic pain? *(593)*
   1. Sometimes the pain interferes with sleep or work.
   2. The pain has been off and on for about 11 months.
   3. Over-the-counter medications give temporary relief.
   4. Prolonged sitting seems to make the pain worse.

4. What is an expected assessment finding that demonstrates the action of epinephrine on the body during an episode of acute pain? *(593)*
   1. Blood glucose is lower than normal.
   2. Description of pain is disproportionate.
   3. Pain medication quickly relieves the pain.
   4. Pulse and respiratory rates are increased.

5. The patient reports that pain medication used to help, but now is less effective. The patient also reports fatigue, sleep disturbance, and depression. The nurse suspects a synergistic effect. Based on the nurse's interpretation of the data, which intervention would the nurse try **first**? *(593)*
   1. Advocate for a change of medication or an increase of dose.
   2. Tell the patient that this is an expected side effect that will pass.
   3. Assess sleep patterns and control environment to facilitate rest.
   4. Ask the provider to prescribe an antidepressant medication.

6. Although placebos are rarely used, what is the **best** physiologic explanation for how they relieve pain? *(593)*
   1. Action of a placebo mimics "fight or flight," which is triggered by epinephrine.
   2. Placebos partially close the "gate," so the passage of pain impulses is blocked.
   3. Chemically, placebos inhibit the synthesis of prostaglandins that mediate pain.
   4. Placebos cause the release of endorphins, which attach to opioid receptor sites.

7. For a patient who is having an acute myocardial infarction, the nurse anticipates that the provider will order morphine to relieve pain. Which harmful physical effect of unrelieved pain is the **greatest** concern for this patient? *(595)*
   1. Increased oxygen demand
   2. Decreased gastric motility
   3. Depressed immune response
   4. Increased mental confusion

8. It is now 2300 and the patient is requesting a PRN (as needed) dose of pain medication. The nurse checks the medication administration record and sees that the patient has received:

0400	2 tablets 500 mg acetaminophen
0900	2 tablets oxycodone 5 mg and 325 mg acetaminophen
1300	2 tablets 500 mg acetaminophen
1800	2 tablets 500 mg acetaminophen

   What should the nurse do **first**? *(596)*
   1. Give two tablets of oxycodone 5 mg and acetaminophen 325 mg.
   2. Wait 2 hours, and then give two tablets 500 mg of acetaminophen.
   3. Call the provider and report the overdose of acetaminophen.
   4. Use a drug reference to verify recommended dosage of acetaminophen/24 hours.

9. What is the **greatest** concern with patient-controlled analgesia (PCA) by proxy? *(600)*
   1. It's more difficult for the nurse to monitor dosage and assess response.
   2. There is a greater chance of oversedation and opioid toxicity.
   3. The patient becomes a passive recipient in the pain management process.
   4. The patient's pain is more likely to be unrelieved or undertreated.

10. A patient tells the nurse that he has been sleeping in a recliner chair for the past several months because "It is easier to fall asleep and stay asleep." What is the nurse **most** likely to suspect and assess for? *(607)*
    1. Back or spinal problems
    2. Problems with breathing
    3. Headaches with visual problems
    4. Restless leg syndrome

11. The patient had a surgical procedure this morning and is requesting pain medication. The nurse assesses the patient's vital signs and decides to withhold opioid medication. Which finding supports this decision? *(597)*
    1. Pulse = 90/min
    2. Respirations = 10/min
    3. Blood pressure = 130/80 mm Hg
    4. Temperature = 99° F rectally

12. The nurse is caring for a patient who has arthritis. Which medication does the nurse anticipate the provider will prescribe? *(602)*
    1. Naloxone
    2. Gabapentin
    3. Ibuprofen
    4. Morphine

13. The patient is receiving an epidural opioid. What is a complication of this treatment? *(601)*
    1. Diarrhea
    2. Hypertension
    3. Urinary retention
    4. Increased respiratory rate

14. An older adult patient diagnosed with osteoarthritis suffers from chronic pain. Based on the patient's age and condition, which pain medications will the provider **most** likely avoid? **Select all that apply.** *(598, 602)*
    1. Meperidine
    2. Acetaminophen
    3. Morphine sulfate
    4. Nonsteroidal antiinflammatory drugs
    5. Combinations of opioid drugs

15. Which nursing intervention demonstrates the application of the gate control theory of pain? *(593)*
    1. Performs a back massage using warmed lotion
    2. Administers acetaminophen as needed
    3. Elevates a patient's sprained ankle to prevent swelling
    4. Repositions the patient every 2 hours

16. Which nursing action demonstrates that the nurse is complying with the Joint Commission standards of pain management? *(594)*
    1. Documents that medication is given after the patient receives it
    2. Incorporates knowledge of the patient's culture in pain management
    3. Assesses the patient's pain and reassesses pain after interventions
    4. Stays current with the latest information about pain therapies

17. The nursing student reports to the nurse that a postoperative patient is asking for pain medication. What is the **most** important question that the nurse will ask the student to answer? *(594)*
    1. "Can you give the medication yourself?"
    2. "What did the patient tell you about his pain?"
    3. "Did you try any nonpharmacologic interventions?"
    4. "What do you know about the prescribed medication?"

18. The patient agrees to try guided imagery as a noninvasive method of pain relief. Before they begin the therapy, which instruction is the nurse **most** likely to give? *(595)*
    1. "I'll use a combination of firm and light strokes during the therapy."
    2. "The skin will be stimulated with a mild electric current that reduces pain."
    3. "Tell me about a place and time where you felt relaxed and peaceful."
    4. "We have to use specialized equipment to identify your biologic responses."

19. What is the **greatest** advantage of using non-pharmacologic pain management techniques as an adjunct to pain medication? *(595)*
    1. Inexpensive and easy to perform
    2. Based on the gate control theory
    3. Low risk and few side effects
    4. Gives patients some control over pain

20. The nurse is talking to a patient who wants to try transcutaneous electric nerve stimulation. Which condition is **most** important to bring to the attention of the provider? *(595)*
    1. The patient has a cardiac pacemaker device.
    2. The patient uses an older model of hearing aid.
    3. The patient has a metallic hip joint.
    4. The patient has a history of a broken back.

21. The provider prescribes 1000 mg acetaminophen every 4 hours as needed for pain. What should the nurse do? *(596)*
    1. Assess the patient every 4 hours and give the medication as needed.
    2. Give the medication as needed during the daytime hours only.
    3. Call the provider and ask for clarification of the order.
    4. Call the pharmacy and ask if the medication comes in 1000-mg tablets.

22. The nurse is caring for several patients who are receiving morphine. Which patient is **most** likely to have problems with respiratory depression? *(599)*
    1. A patient with a history of chronic back pain who is receiving epidural morphine for an acute exacerbation
    2. An older patient who is postoperative for a fractured hip and is receiving patient-controlled analgesia
    3. A child who received an intramuscular injection prior to having fracture reduction of the forearm
    4. An older patient with end-stage uterine cancer who is receiving an oral form of morphine

23. What is the physiologic rationale for avoiding use of meperidine for patients with sickle cell disease? *(598)*
    1. There is a direct action that causes sickling of blood cells.
    2. Renal insufficiency will be present to some degree.
    3. Underlying respiratory distress results in respiratory depression.
    4. Patients with sickle cell disease are more prone to seizures.

24. The home health nurse sees an order for meperidine for a 63-year-old patient with cancer who requires long-term opioid treatment. What is the **best** rationale for the nurse to question this medication order? *(598)*
    1. Meperidine is an older drug that is now rarely prescribed for any condition.
    2. The patient cannot be continuously monitored for adverse effects in the home setting.
    3. The patient is not young nor healthy and is therefore more likely to suffer side effects.
    4. Repeated administration of meperidine increases the risk of accumulation.

25. The nurse hears in report that the patient with diabetes has reported a tingling, burning sensation in the lower extremities. Which drug is the nurse **most** likely to administer for this type of discomfort? *(599)*
    1. Ketorolac tromethamine
    2. Tramadol
    3. Acetaminophen
    4. Duloxetine

26. The patient reports that the prescribed opioid dose does not seem to provide the same relief for his acute pain compared to 4 weeks ago. Based on the nurse's knowledge of pharmacology, what does the nurse recognize? *(598)*
    1. The patient has developed a physical tolerance.
    2. The patient has a psychological dependence.
    3. The patient probably has an addiction.
    4. The patient is experiencing chronic pain.

27. The nurse is talking to a patient who reports feeling tired and not getting enough sleep. Which question related to the patient's medication is **most** relevant to designing interventions for the patient's problem? *(608)*
    1. "Which antiinflammatory medication has the provider suggested?"
    2. "Has there been a recent increase in the dosage of your opioid medication?"
    3. "What time of the day do you usually take your diuretic medication?"
    4. "Are you taking your antiemetic medication before or after meals?"

28. The student nurse is looking at nursing jobs to consider after graduation. Which shift is **most** likely to cause sleep-wake cycle disruption? *(608)*
    1. Straight night shift
    2. Rotating day to night shift
    3. Weekends-only evening shift
    4. Monday to Friday day shift

29. The provider has ordered blood pressure, pulse, and respirations every 2 hours for 12 hours. It is currently 8:00 PM and the nurse knows that the patient has been having a lot of problems sleeping in the hospital. What strategy should the nurse try **first**? *(609)*
    1. Clarify the necessity of the order with the provider.
    2. Explain to the patient that vital signs will only be taken every 2 hours for 12 hours.
    3. Tell the unlicensed assistive personnel to quietly take vital signs every 2 hours.
    4. Apply an automatic blood pressure cuff that can programmed for every 2 hours.

30. The nurse enters the patient's room at 3:00 AM and finds that the patient is awake and sitting up in a chair. The patient tells the nurse that she is not able to sleep. What should the nurse do **first**? *(609)*
    1. Obtain a prescription for a hypnotic.
    2. Instruct the patient to return to bed.
    3. Provide a glass of warm milk with honey.
    4. Ask about methods that have helped her sleep.

CRITICAL THINKING ACTIVITIES

31. The patient is experiencing difficulty sleeping while in the hospital. She reports this is the first time she has been in the hospital and the sounds and smells seem very strange. In addition, she reports feeling mildly anxious because "so many people come in and out of the room at all hours of the day and night." She looks tired and seems mildly irritable. Identify nursing interventions that may be implemented to promote sleep. *(609, 610)*

32. a. Think about the patients whom you have cared for thus far during your clinical experiences and identify at least five possible causes for the discomfort that your patients were experiencing. *(591)*

b. Describe what you did to relieve your patient's discomfort. *(605, 606)* _____

_____

_____

_____

33. The "opioid epidemic" has been in the news. Discuss with your classmates and instructor how the opioid epidemic could affect your nursing practice. *(596, 598)*

_____

_____

_____

_____

_____

Surgical Wound Care

MULTIPLE CHOICE

Directions: Select the best answer(s) for each of the following questions.

1. What does the nurse observe during the first phase of healing if fibrin is functioning correctly? *(616)*
   1. Erythema, heat, edema, and pain occur.
   2. There is an overgrowth of whitish collagen.
   3. Wound looks irregular, raised, and purplish.
   4. Clot begins to form and bleeding subsides.

2. To address the signs and symptoms of the inflammatory phase, which action would the nurse perform? *(616)*
   1. Cover the wound with clean gauze and apply direct pressure.
   2. Elevate the injured part and apply an ice pack as ordered.
   3. Observe for purulent exudate and cleanse the wound.
   4. Observe for granulation tissue and keep the wound moist.

3. During the reconstruction phase of healing, what is the **most** serious complication? *(616)*
   1. Keloid formation
   2. Granulation tissue
   3. Wound dehiscence
   4. Phagocytosis

4. On the first day of surgery, how often does the nurse inspect the surgical dressings and what does he or she expect to see? *(619)*
   1. Inspects every hour for the first 24 hours and expects to see serous and serosanguineous fluid.
   2. Inspects every 2 to 4 hours for the first 24 hours and expects to see sanguineous and serosanguineous fluid.
   3. Inspects once every 8 hours for the first 24 and expects to see sanguineous and serosanguineous fluid.
   4. Inspects every 5 minutes for the first hour and expects to see serous and sanguineous fluid.

5. Which dressing requires that the nurse place tape strips on all sides of the dressing? *(621)*
   1. Wet-to-dry dressing
   2. Dry dressing
   3. Transparent dressing
   4. Occlusive dressing

6. The nurse observes that the dressing over the wound has exudate that has a strong, pungent odor. Which action is the **most** important? *(633)*
   1. Weigh the soiled dressing.
   2. Cleanse the wound with an antiseptic.
   3. Perform a wound culture.
   4. Circle and date the drainage on dressing.

7. What is an important nursing responsibility associated with a Penrose drain? *(633)*
   1. Drainage in bulb should be observed and measured, suction should be reestablished.
   2. Ensure that the irrigation pressure does not exceed 4 to 15 psi.
   3. Drain should be observed for patency and flushed as needed.
   4. Drainage on dressing should be observed, position of safety pin is noted.

8. With appropriate instruction and supervision, which tasks related to wound care can be delegated to unlicensed assistive personnel? **Select all that apply.** *(642)*
   1. Emptying a closed drainage container
   2. Removing sutures or staples
   3. Applying an abdominal binder
   4. Assessing breathing with a breast binder in place
   5. Measuring intake and output

9. The nurse sees that the patient takes steroids for a respiratory condition. What would be an expected affect of steroids on wound healing? *(618)*
   1. Decreased inflammatory response
   2. Prolonged bleeding times
   3. Decreased keloid formation
   4. Impaired formation of granulation tissue

10. The nurse is applying a dressing over the insertion site of a peripheral intravenous catheter. Which dressing is the **best** choice? *(625)*
    1. Sterile tape with dry gauze
    2. Steri-Strips and transparent dressing
    3. Transparent dressing
    4. Sterile pad with chevron taping

11. After abdominal surgery, a patient is at risk for wound stress related to coughing and moving. What equipment does the nurse need to teach the patient the self-care measure of splinting? *(617)*
    1. An abdominal binder
    2. A pillow or rolled blanket
    3. A large triangular bandage
    4. Several wide elastic bandages.

12. Which lunch tray is **best** for providing protein, vitamins A and C, and zinc, the nutrients required for wound healing? *(617)*
    1. A peanut butter sandwich with a glass of milk
    2. A bowl of bean soup with crackers and iced tea
    3. Broiled seafood with spinach salad and tomato juice
    4. Stir-fried mixed vegetables with rice and hot tea

13. The patient has no contraindications for fluid intake. Over a 24-hour period, he drank 16 ounces of decaffeinated coffee, 10 ounces of juice, 6 ounces of milk, and a half a liter of soda. What instructions does the nurse give the patient about fluid intake to promote wound healing? *(617)*
    1. Instructs the patient to continue drinking the same amount as he drank today
    2. Tells the patient that tomorrow he should try to drink twice as much as today
    3. Advises the patient that drinking excessive fluid is likely to decrease appetite for food
    4. Suggests that he drink 2-3 additional 8-ounce servings of his favorite fluid every day

14. The nurse is caring for a patient who has a large abdominal incision. The patient tells the nurse that she is afraid to sit up or even move because of the pain and the strain on the incision site. What instructions should the nurse give to the patient? *(617)*
    1. "Rest in bed until the incision site is less tender and healing has progressed."
    2. "Roll to one side, use your elbow as a lever, and push to a sitting position."
    3. "Hold a pillow next to your abdomen and roll forward into a sitting position."
    4. "Call for assistance whenever needed and someone will help you sit up."

15. A patient has just returned from surgery. What are the initial assessments that the nurse would make related to the surgical site? **Select all that apply.** *(620)*
    1. Inspect the protective dressing that was placed by the surgical team.
    2. Look at the area around the dressing and record observations.
    3. Check under the patient to make sure that exudate is not pooling.
    4. Carefully remove the dressing and inspect the suture line for intactness.
    5. Expect and note amount of serous drainage that is coming from the wound.

16. A patient had surgery 4 days ago and now reports an increase in pain and has a temperature of 101.6° (38.7° C). The incision site looks red compared to yesterday and a small amount of purulent drainage is seeping around the suture line. Which laboratory result will the nurse check before contacting the surgeon? *(619)*
    1. Hemoglobin and hematocrit
    2. White blood cell count
    3. Platelet count
    4. Blood glucose level

17. Which patient is **most** likely to benefit from the application of a triangular binder? *(639)*
    1. Has a chronic pressure injury on the sacral area
    2. Has a possible fracture in the forearm
    3. Has venous stasis ulcer on left ankle
    4. Has a surgical wound on the lateral chest area

18. The nurse is preparing to remove the patient's staples, but after assessment, the nurse decides that the staples should not be removed. The decision was based on which finding? *(630)*
    1. The wound edges were partially separated.
    2. Dried serous drainage was noted around the staples.
    3. The patient was anxious about staple removal.
    4. Early keloid formation was observed.

19. The nurse is preparing to change the patient's dry sterile dressing. Upon attempting the removal of the old dressing, it adheres to the site. What should the nurse do? *(621)*
    1. Notify the surgeon.
    2. Leave the dressing alone.
    3. Pull the dressing off quickly.
    4. Moisten the dressing with saline.

20. The patient returned to the unit 3 hours ago after having surgery on the abdomen, and the dressing is now saturated with red, watery drainage. What should the nurse do **first**? *(633)*
    1. Notify the charge nurse and the surgeon.
    2. Take the patient's vital signs and assess for pain.
    3. Securely reinforce the dressing with layers of gauze.
    4. Remove the dressing and observe the wound site.

21. After a total abdominal hysterectomy, a postoperative patient develops a wound evisceration. What should the nurse do **first**? *(629)*
    1. Check patency of the intravenous (IV) site for delivery of fluids.
    2. Place the patient in low Fowler's position to reduce strain on the wound.
    3. Prepare the patient for surgery and contact the surgeon.
    4. Cover the wound with a sterile dressing moistened with saline.

22. A postoperative patient who was happy and cheerful earlier now demonstrates restlessness and anxiety. He reports feeling "a little lightheaded." He is mildly diaphoretic and his pulse feels thready. What assessments does the nurse perform to identify a suspected complication? *(628, 629)*
    1. Checks the pulse rate, blood pressure, and assesses for pain
    2. Assesses for localized warmth or redness with tenderness
    3. Observes the incision site for wound edge approximation
    4. Takes the temperature and checks for purulent drainage

23. The patient has a T-tube in place following an abdominal cholecystectomy. What is the expected output of bile in the **first** 24 hours? *(635)*
    1. 30 mL per hour
    2. 250-500 mL
    3. 10-50 mL
    4. 1-2 L

24. The nurse is observing a new staff member perform a sterile dry dressing change. The nurse would intervene if the staff member performed which action? *(622)*
    1. Loosens tape and gently pulls towards the incision
    2. Uses sterile gloves to remove the old dressing
    3. Cleanses wound by starting at incision moving outward
    4. Allows antiseptic cleansing solution to air-dry

25. A nurse is supervising a nursing student who is doing a wet-to-dry dressing change. What does the nurse do when the student applies a dry dressing over the wet gauze? *(624)*
    1. Directs the student to moisten all of the layers.
    2. Hands the student an occlusive dressing.
    3. Tells the patient that the student is doing a great job.
    4. Suggests removal of all layers and starting over.

26. The nurse is assessing the amount of drainage that the patient has from a surgical wound and finds that 650 mL has drained from 9:00 AM until now, 11:40 PM. What should the nurse do **first**? *(628, 629)*
    1. Record the amount and appearance of the drainage and continue to observe.
    2. Take the patient's vital signs, assess for other symptoms, and inform the surgeon.
    3. Make sure that the patient's linens are clean and dry and empty the drainage receptacle.
    4. Apply a pressure dressing and place the patient in a supine position.

27. The patient needs a breast binder. What is the **most** important consideration for the nurse when implementing this application? *(642)*
    1. Respiratory function must not be restricted.
    2. Vomiting and nausea are a contraindication.
    3. Binders cannot be used for patients who are obese.
    4. Older patients have difficulty tolerating the binder.

CRITICAL THINKING ACTIVITIES

28. The nurse is caring for a 72-year-old patient who is being treated for a chronic ulcer on the right lower leg. The patient lives alone. He is diabetic and reports poor vision. The nurse notes that the patient has trouble with fine motor control. He reports that he does his own meal preparation, although he admits that he doesn't make the effort to prepare fresh produce. He is 15 pounds underweight and he has "cut down on his smoking."

    a. Identify factors that may impair wound healing for this patient. *(614)* _____

    _____

    _____

    b. Discuss how the nurse applies knowledge about older adults to help this patient achieve wound healing. *(644)*

    _____

    _____

    _____

    _____

    _____

29. The student nurse is preparing to implement wound irrigation for a patient. The nursing instructor asks the student to answer the following questions before starting the procedure. *(625, 627, 628)*

    a. What is the purpose of wound irrigation?_____

    b. What equipment is needed for irrigation at the patient's bedside?_____

    c. How is the syringe positioned for the irrigation?_____

    d. What is the direction of cleansing? _____

    e. What findings should be immediately reported to the provider? _____

30. Discuss some of the difficulties that a homeless patient could have performing wound care after being discharged from the hospital. What strategies could the nurse use to help a homeless patient achieve wound care and prevent complications? *(644)*

_____

_____

_____

_____

_____

Specimen Collection and Diagnostic Testing

MATCHING

Directions: Match the suffix on the left to the correct definition on the right and give an example for each. (667)

Suffix

_____ 1.   -oscopy
_____ 2.   -ogram
_____ 3.   -ography
_____ 4.   -centesis

Definition

a.   Procedure involving puncture of a body cavity

Example _____

b.   Procedure in which an image is produced

Example _____

c.   Actual image or results of a test

Example _____

d.   Procedure in which body structures are visualized

Example _____

FIGURE LABELING

5.   Directions: Label the veins of the arms and hands on the figure. *(683)*

Basilic vein
Cephalic vein
Median cubital vein
Radial vein
Median vein of forearm
Superficial dorsal vein
Dorsal venous arch

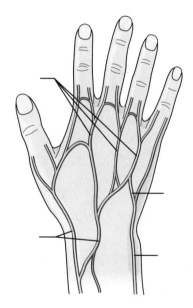
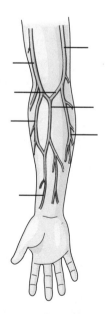

FIGURE LABELING

6. Directions: Label the placement of the chest (precordial) leads on the figure. *(689)*

    V_1—Fourth intercostal space (ICS) at right sternal border
    V_2—Fourth ICS at left sternal border
    V_3—Midway between V_2 and V_4
    V_4—Fifth ICS at midclavicular line
    V_5—Left anterior axillary line at level of V_4 horizontally
    V_6—Left midaxillary line at level of V_4 horizontally

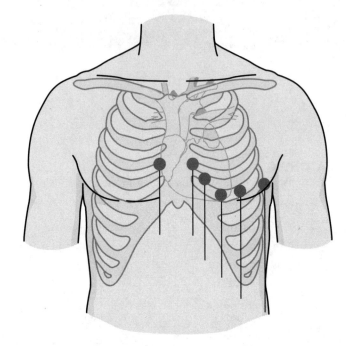

DELEGATION

7. Directions: Determine which specimen collections are usually possible to delegate to unlicensed assistive personnel (UAP) and indicate yes or no in the space provided. *(691)*

    _____ a. Urine by midstream collection
    _____ b. Gastric secretion from nasogastric tube
    _____ c. Blood sample by venipuncture
    _____ d. Sputum specimen by suctioning
    _____ e. Blood sample for glucose
    _____ f. Wound cultures
    _____ g. Stool for ova and parasites
    _____ h. Throat culture
    _____ i. Sputum specimen by expectoration
    _____ j. Nasal culture
    _____ k. Emesis
    _____ l. Nasopharyngeal culture
    _____ m. Cerebrospinal fluid
    _____ n. Stool for hemoccult
    _____ o. Stool from colostomy

MULTIPLE CHOICE

Directions: Select the best answer(s) for each of the following questions.

8. Which laboratory blood test is **more** likely to require written informed consent? *(649)*
   1. Complete blood count
   2. Human immunodeficiency virus test
   3. Platelet count
   4. Blood glucose testing

9. The patient reports seeing black, tarry stool. Which question is the nurse **most** likely to ask? *(673)*
   1. "Are you straining or noticing discomfort with bowel movements?"
   2. "Have you eaten a lot of red meat in the past few days?"
   3. "Are you having any pain or discomfort in the upper mid-abdomen?"
   4. "Have you ever had a problem with hemorrhoids?

10. The clinic nurse sees that the provider has ordered a sputum specimen for acid-fast bacillus. What is the nurse most likely to clarify with the provider? (673)
    1. "Shall I instruct the patient to collect the specimen in the early morning?"
    2. "If the patient cannot expectorate a specimen, is nasotracheal suction allowed?"
    3. "Is the patient allowed to smoke, drink, and eat after the sputum is collected?"
    4. "Should the patient be placed in a negative pressure isolation room?"

11. The postsurgical patient has chills, fever, and malaise. The provider has instructed the nurse to report the laboratory results as soon as they are available. Which laboratory result is definitive for confirmation of infection and effective treatment? *(673)*
    1. White blood cell count
    2. Wound culture and sensitivity
    3. Red blood cell count
    4. Electrolyte levels

12. According to the bloodborne pathogen standards of Occupational Safety and Health Administration, health care facilities are required to make a written exposure control plan. Which health care worker has sustained a major significant exposure? *(681)*
    1. Nursing student injures self while recapping a needle used to draw up the patient's insulin.
    2. UAP picks up blood-stained linen without donning gloves.
    3. Nurse sustains a deep cut with profuse bleeding while trying to raise a patient's side rails.
    4. Phlebotomist sustains a deep puncture caused by a needle used to collect blood.

13. What is the **best** rationale for drawing at least two blood cultures from two different sites? *(681)*
    1. This is the standard method used to detect bacteremia.
    2. If only one culture shows bacteria, technician error is assumed.
    3. If both cultures show an infecting agent, bacteremia is confirmed.
    4. If both cultures show different infecting agents, skin contamination is assumed.

14. The nurse is planning care for several patients who will need postprocedural care. Which patient will require serial neurovascular assessments on bilateral extremities? *(654)*
    1. Patient having cardiac catheterization
    2. Patient having a bone scan
    3. Patient having electrocardiography
    4. Patient having paracentesis

15. The nurse is interviewing a patient who needs to be scheduled for colonoscopy. Which patient comment would cause the nurse to contact the provider before giving instructions for the usual oral bowel preparation? *(655)*
    1. "I take insulin for my diabetes."
    2. "I have heard the bowel prep is awful."
    3. "I think I might have acute diverticulitis."
    4. "My father died of colon cancer."

16. The patient had a colonoscopy 2 hours ago and reports that abdominal pain seems to be increasing. What assessments would the nurse perform if colon perforation is suspected? **Select all that apply.** *(655)*
    1. Take vital signs and compare with baseline.
    2. Gently palpate abdomen for tenderness and distention.
    3. Perform digital rectal examination to check for blood.
    4. Observe for tolerance of clear oral fluids.
    5. Observe stools for bleeding and note color and amount.

17. Shortly after the patient returns from having a liver biopsy, he reports chest pain and trouble breathing. He seems restless and anxious. The RN says that he might have a pneumothorax. What will the nurses do before calling the provider? **Select all that apply.** *(660)*
    1. Assess rate, rhythm, and depth of respirations.
    2. Check pulse oximeter reading.
    3. Assess blood coagulation profile.
    4. Listen to breath sounds.
    5. Apply oxygen if needed.

18. The postoperative patient demonstrates some mild dizziness and mild shortness of breath when moving from sitting to standing position. Which laboratory value would the nurse check **first**? *(692)*
    1. Red blood cell count
    2. White blood cell count
    3. Blood urea nitrogen
    4. Creatinine level

19. Prior to a paracentesis, which assessments should be performed? **Select all that apply.** *(662)*
    1. Weight
    2. Height
    3. Abdominal girth
    4. Baseline vital signs
    5. Peripheral pulses

20. The nurse needs to perform venipuncture on an older patient whose veins are very fragile. What is the **best** strategy for the nurse to use? *(661)*
    1. Gently tap over the vein.
    2. Apply a warm compress.
    3. Use a vacutainer.
    4. Use a small-gauge needle.

21. The nurse is using a commercially prepared tube for the collection of an aerobic wound specimen for culture. After collecting the specimen with the swab, what should the nurse do? *(679)*
    1. Place the swab into the collection tube, close it tightly, and keep the specimen warm.
    2. Take the swab and mix it with the special color-changing reagent in the collection tube.
    3. Place the swab into the collection tube and add the liquid culture medium.
    4. Crush the ampule at the end of the tube and put the tip of the swab into the solution.

22. Following a lumbar puncture, what does the nurse do to prevent a postpuncture spinal headache? *(660)*
    1. Reduces the patient's fluid intake
    2. Places the patient in a high Fowler's position
    3. Informs the provider if a headache develops
    4. Instructs the patient to lie in the supine position

23. The patient is to have a thoracentesis performed. The nurse assists the patient to which position for this test? *(664)*
    1. Dorsal recumbent
    2. Supine with the arms held above the head
    3. Sitting up and leaning over a table
    4. Side-lying with the knees drawn up

24. The patient requests information about a scheduled magnetic resonance imaging study. What should the nurse tell the patient to expect? *(661)*
    1. "You shouldn't eat or drink for 4 hours before the test."
    2. "You will hear humming and loud thumping sounds."
    3. "You will have minor discomfort in the area being tested."
    4. "You will be assisted to make frequent position changes."

25. The nurse is teaching the patient how to collect a specimen for blood glucose monitoring. Which patient action demonstrates correct technique? *(671)*
    1. Allows the blood specimen to drop onto the test strip
    2. Uses the center of the finger for the puncture
    3. Holds the finger upright after puncture
    4. Vigorously squeezes the fingertip after puncture

26. What is included in the instructions to the patient for collection of a midstream urine sample? *(668)*
    1. Use a clean specimen cup and try not to touch the inside of the cup.
    2. Collect at least 200 mL of urine into the specimen cup.
    3. Void into the toilet, stop urinating, and then urinate into the cup.
    4. Bathe or shower the perineal area before collection.

27. The student nurse is obtaining a urine specimen from a patient with an existing indwelling catheter. When would the supervising nurse intervene? *(667)*
    1. Performs hand hygiene and applies clean gloves for the procedure.
    2. Clamps the drainage tubing for 30 minutes before specimen collection begins.
    3. Disconnects the catheter from the drainage tubing and collects the urine in a specimen cup.
    4. Unclamps the drainage tube after collection and observes for urine flow.

28. The patient will be catheterized for residual urine. What is the correct technique for this procedure? *(667)*
    1. Catheterize the patient when the bladder is full.
    2. Obtain an order for an indwelling catheter.
    3. Catheterize the patient within 10 minutes of voiding.
    4. Use clean technique to obtain the sample.

29. A patient requires venipuncture to obtain a blood sample for diagnostic testing. Which laboratory result is the **greatest** concern related to the venipuncture? *(680)*
    1. High blood glucose level
    2. Low platelet count
    3. Elevated blood urea nitrogen
    4. Low sodium level

30. How does the nurse properly use a tourniquet when performing a venipuncture? *(682)*
    1. Ties it into a single knot
    2. Leaves it in place for no more than 1-2 minutes
    3. Places it 6-8 inches above the selected site
    4. Ties it tight enough to occlude the distal pulse

31. The patient is suspected of having a urinary tract infection (UTI). The provider has ordered a urine specimen for culture and sensitivity testing. The patient asks, "Can't I just get a prescription for antibiotics?" What is the **best** response? *(673)*
    1. "This is just a routine test for any patient suspected of having a UTI."
    2. "Your provider feels this test is necessary in determining your diagnosis."
    3. "I can contact your provider if you would like to ask for a prescription."
    4. "Different bacteria can cause a UTI and the test results will indicate the best antibiotic."

32. When performing a Hemoccult slide test to determine the presence of occult blood in a stool specimen, the nurse would be correct in performing which action? *(674)*
    1. Use two separate areas of the stool when obtaining the specimen.
    2. Obtain the specimen from the toilet bowl.
    3. Perform the test control before obtaining the specimen.
    4. Take the specimen immediately to the laboratory to prevent hemolysis.

33. An older patient had a bronchoscopy several hours ago and now seems restless and confused compared to baseline behavior. Which assessment is the **most** important? *(654)*
    1. Orientation to person, place, and time
    2. Pulse oximeter reading and respiratory rate
    3. Use of antianxiety medications during procedure
    4. Time of last food and fluid ingestion

34. An older female patient is supposed to have diagnostic testing that requires nothing by mouth for 12 hours prior to the test and a bowel preparation. The test has been cancelled 2 days in a row; once for a large amount of retained stool and once because of equipment problems. Which intervention is the **priority**? *(652)*
    1. Explain the cancellations to the patient using terms that she can easily understand.
    2. Call the diagnostic technician to ensure that the test gets done.
    3. Assess the patient for dehydration and fluid and electrolyte imbalances.
    4. Call the provider and ask if the test can be postponed for a few days.

35. The nurse has just informed the patient that he should collect a sputum specimen in the morning. Which additional instruction will the nurse give? *(673)*
    1. "Brush your teeth and use mouthwash just prior to collecting the specimen."
    2. "Drink extra water the day before collection to decrease the thickness of mucus."
    3. "Inhale and cough deeply and then spit the clear saliva into the sterile cup."
    4. "Do not eat any red meat or drink any caffeinated beverages."

36. The nurse has just received laboratory results for an unfamiliar test, so he is unsure if the results are within normal limits. What should the nurse do **first**? *(650)*
    1. Call the provider and read the results exactly as they are shown.
    2. Ask the patient if he is having any unusual symptoms or complaints.
    3. Call the laboratory technician and ask for an explanation of the results.
    4. Check the facility's laboratory manual for information about the test.

37. The nurse has orders for voided midstream urine specimens for several patients. Which patient is **most** likely to require an order for a straight catheterized specimen rather than a voided midstream specimen? *(668)*
    1. A 25-year-old female who finished her menstrual period yesterday
    2. A 55-year-old female diabetic patient who is very overweight
    3. A 63-year-old male who has difficulty with urination due to prostate problems
    4. An 18-year-old male who has a Glasgow coma score of 4 after a head injury

38. The nurse sees that several patients require stool specimens for diagnostic testing. Which patient's stool specimen must be taken immediately to the laboratory after it has been obtained? *(669)*
    1. Patient traveled to a foreign country and reports abdominal cramping with diarrhea.
    2. Patient saw very dark black stool several days ago, but now stool seems normal.
    3. Patient (small child) is suspected of swallowing a plastic marble 3 days ago.
    4. Patient saw stool floating in toilet and there was an oily film in the water.

39. The nurse is suctioning the patient to obtain a sputum specimen. During the 10 seconds of suctioning, the cardiac monitor shows bradycardia and the patient becomes very diaphoretic. What is the **best** explanation for this occurrence? *(673)*
    1. Patient demonstrated anxiety due to the procedure.
    2. Nurse caused hypoxia by suctioning for a prolonged time.
    3. Cardiac changes are unrelated to the procedure.
    4. Catheter caused direct stimulation of vagal nerve fibers.

40. The nurse notes purulent drainage from a wound and decides to obtain an order for a wound culture. Prior to contacting the surgeon, what other data will the nurse obtain? **Select all that apply.** *(673)*
    1. Check oral temperature.
    2. Look at trends of white blood cell count.
    3. Ask about subjective symptoms such as chills or fatigue.
    4. Assess for pain at the wound site.
    5. Review the previous documentation about the wound.

41. A patient is newly admitted for pneumonia with possible early sepsis. The nurse is reviewing the admission orders. Which order should be done **first**? *(681)*
    1. Intravenous antibiotics
    2. Blood cultures from two sites
    3. Chest x-ray
    4. Blood chemistries

42. The nurse is supervising a nursing student who will perform venipuncture to obtain a blood sample for blood chemistries. The nurse will intervene if the student performs which action? *(682)*
    1. Applies a warm compress to the arm on the side of a mastectomy
    2. Obtains a vacutainer and different colors of collection tubes
    3. Applies a tourniquet 3 inches above elbow and palpates the antecubital space
    4. Releases the tourniquet after 2 minutes of trying to locate a vein

43. A patient had a diagnostic study with a contrast medium 4 hours ago. Now he has swelling and itching around the eyes, a rapid pulse, and mild dyspnea. What should the nurse do **first**? *(650)*
    1. Administer an as-needed (PRN) dose of diphenhydramine and call the provider.
    2. Call the Rapid Response Team and bring resuscitation equipment to the bedside.
    3. Contact the health care team member who administered the contrast medium.
    4. Apply a cool compress to reduce the swelling and instruct the patient to rest.

44. The UAP made two attempts to test a patient's blood glucose but was unable to get enough blood to adequately cover the test strip. What factors will nurse assess that could interfere with getting an adequate drop of blood? **Select all that apply.** *(665, 671)*
    1. Environmental temperature of the room
    2. Technique used to obtain the sample
    3. Position of the patient's arm
    4. Improper calibration of the glucometer
    5. Problems with peripheral circulation
    6. Condition of the skin on hands and fingers

45. The nurse is supervising a new nurse who must collect gastric secretions from a nasogastric (NG) tube. When would the supervising nurse intervene? *(675)*
    1. New nurse uses an alcohol swab to scrub the NG tube prior to inserting a sterile needle.
    2. New nurse assists the patient to a high Fowler's position and places a towel underneath the NG tube.
    3. New nurse disconnects the NG tube from the suction or the gravity drainage.
    4. New nurse verifies NG tube placement to ensure aspiration of gastric contents.

46. The nurse is suctioning a patient to obtain a sputum specimen. Which occurrence is expected? *(676)*
    1. As the suction catheter is inserted into the tracheostomy, there is resistance.
    2. As the suction catheter is inserted into the trachea, the patient begins to cough.
    3. As suction is applied, oxygen saturation drops below normal for several minutes.
    4. As the suction catheter is withdrawn, the patient begins to exhale very deeply.

47. The nurse has tried several times to obtain a throat culture on a patient, but the patient has gagged, moved, and contaminated the tip of the swab during each attempt. What should the nurse do **first**? *(679)*
    1. Have the patient look in the mirror, give him the swab, and coach him through the procedure.
    2. Inform the provider that several unsuccessful attempts have been made.
    3. Instruct the patient to open mouth and say a very long "ahhhhh" and avoid using a tongue blade.
    4. Obtain an order for a mild local anesthetic that will temporarily suppress the gag reflex.

48. The nurse needs to perform venipuncture to obtain a blood sample for blood chemistries. What factors influences the nurse's choice of sterile needles? **Select all that apply.** *(685)*
    1. Age of patient
    2. Condition of veins
    3. Nurse's familiarity with product
    4. Syringe method versus vacuum tube method
    5. Type of blood chemistry test ordered
    6. Color of the collection tube

49. Nurse A is aware that Nurse B, who is not very skilled at venipuncture, is sticking her patients more than the recommended two times as stated by hospital policy. What should Nurse A do **first**? *(686)*
    1. Report Nurse B to the nurse manager for violating hospital policy.
    2. Watch Nurse B and offer to perform venipunctures after two attempts.
    3. Assess Nurse B's understanding and skill in performing venipuncture.
    4. Ask the charge nurse to assess Nurse B's understanding of hospital policy.

50. As the nurse is performing an electrocardiogram (ECG), the patient reports very mild left anterior chest pain. What should the nurse do **first**? *(656)*
    1. Stop the procedure and obtain the crash cart and other emergency equipment.
    2. Continue the procedure, and tell the patient to relax and not to worry.
    3. Stop the procedure and obtain an order for pain medication.
    4. Continue procedure and make notation of pain on the request slip or ECG strip.

CRITICAL THINKING ACTIVITIES

51. The nurse is caring for a patient who is scheduled to have a thoracentesis.

    a. What assessments should be performed prior to the procedure? *(664)* _____

    _____

    _____

    _____

    b. Why would it be particularly important to assess this patient's lung sounds and presence of cough before the procedure? *(664)*

    _____

    _____

    _____

    _____

    c. Describe the nursing responsibilities related to the care of the patient before and during the thoracentesis. *(649, 664)*

    _____

    _____

    _____

    d. Describe the assessments and care that the nurse should perform after the thoracentesis procedure. *(664, 690)*

    _____

    _____

    _____

52. The nurse is caring for a 68-year-old woman who is scheduled to have a urinalysis, blood chemistries, and an intravenous pyelogram (IVP). The patient is alert and cooperative. She is thin and reports a poor appetite and fluid intake. The patient demonstrates some trouble with fine motor movements of the hands and some mobility issues related to arthritis, but she is able to independently perform most activities of daily living. Identify considerations for this older patient with regards to the urinalysis, blood chemistries, and IVP. *(665)*

    _____

    _____

    _____

    _____

    _____

    _____

Lifespan Development

chapter

24

SHORT ANSWER

Directions: Using your own words, answer each question in the space provided.

1. Identify factors that have contributed to the changes that families today have undergone and are still undergoing. *(698)*

    _____

    _____

2. Discuss the qualities of functional families. *(700)* _____

    _____

    _____

3. Three common causes of family stress are: *(702)* _____

    _____

TABLE ACTIVITY

4. Directions: Insert the expected values of vital signs for different age groups.

Age Group	Temperature	Pulse	Respirations (at Rest)	Blood Pressure
Infants at 12 months *(704)*				
Toddler 1-3 years *(708)*				
School age 6-12 years *(715)*				
Adolescent 12-19 years *(718)*				

MULTIPLE CHOICE
Directions: Select the best answer(s) for each of the following questions.

5. Which nursing actions contribute to accomplishing the *Healthy People 2020* Health Indicators? **Select all that apply.** (696)
   1. Administers medication on time using the six rights
   2. Reinforces the need for preventive dental care
   3. Encourages patients to routinely exercise
   4. Assists patients to locate smoking cessation literature
   5. Shows respect and courtesy to older patients
   6. Teaches patients how to limit fats and sugar in the diet

6. The nurse is interviewing a woman who is from a different culture than the nurse's. The nurse directs the questions to the woman, but the woman consistently looks toward her husband and he gives all of the answers. What should the nurse do **first**? (698)
   1. Ask the husband to leave the room and continue the interview with the wife.
   2. Continue the interview and observe for additional nonverbal behaviors.
   3. Direct the questions to the husband, because the wife is deferring to him.
   4. Discontinue the interview and seek advice about how to interact with this couple.

7. The nurse determines that the family is primarily autocratic. Which observation supports the nurse's analysis? (700)
   1. Mother assumes dominance in decision-making.
   2. Parents implement strict rules and expectations.
   3. Uncle controls the finances.
   4. Children participate in negotiations.

8. Which patient needs to get both pneumococcal and influenza vaccines? (730)
   1. 68-year-old resident in an assisted-living facility
   2. 3-year-old who goes to daycare every weekday
   3. 21-year-old who lives in a college dorm
   4. 30-year-old pregnant woman in the first trimester

9. Which patient group is the nurse **most** likely to assess for possible exposure to teratogens? (697)
   1. A group of preschoolers who attend a day-care setting
   2. Residents who live at a long-term care center
   3. A group of young women who are planning pregnancy
   4. A group of adolescents who are at risk for substance abuse

10. The nurse is assessing a 6-month-old infant, who was 21 inches long at birth. Based on expected growth patterns, what height would the nurse expect on measuring this healthy baby? (704)
    1. 22 inches
    2. 27 inches
    3. 30 inches
    4. 31 inches

11. The nurse is assessing a 1-year-old child who weighed 9 lbs at birth. Based on expected growth patterns, how much should this healthy child weigh? (704) _____ lbs

12. Most of the weight gain in the first months of life is in the form of fat. What is the **best** physiologic explanation for this gain of fat? (704)
    1. Fat provides insulation and a source of nourishment if teething or other problems decrease food intake for a few days.
    2. In cephalocaudal growth, fat must be deposited in areas of the trunk and abdomen before growth in extremities can occur.
    3. Breast milk or prepared formulas are high in nutrients that are more readily converted to fat than to muscle or bone tissue.
    4. Muscle and bone require more protein and calcium, so development of these tissues is concurrent with intake of solid foods.

13. The mother of a 5-month-old infant reports the child is irritable; gums are red and edematous, and he demonstrates excessive drooling. What would the nurse recommend? (705)
    1. Advise the mother to contact the provider for treatment of infection.
    2. Suggest the mother wipe and massage the gums and offer sips of clear water.
    3. Teach the mother to brush the gums with a soft brush and fluoride toothpaste.
    4. Advise the mother to give an infant dose of acetaminophen for discomfort.

14. Under what circumstance would the nurse advise the parents to contact the provider about their 1-year-old infant? *(707)*
    1. Child seems restless and makes little noises during short naplike periods.
    2. Baby cries persistently during usual sleep periods and is inconsolable.
    3. Infant sleeps 12 hours a night and takes one nap during the day.
    4. Child frequently kicks and stretches when in the supine position.

15. Which infant behavior is consistent with Piaget's theory that infants are in the sensorimotor stage of cognitive development? *(708)*
    1. Clings to the parent and protests any separation
    2. Reaches for objects and puts them into mouth
    3. Demonstrates shoulder control prior to hand control
    4. Frequently says, "me" and "no"

16. The working mother has an 8-month-old child who has to go to daycare while she works. How can the nurse **best** help the mother prepare for the first day of daycare? *(706)*
    1. Explain the likelihood of separation anxiety as a normal behavior.
    2. Emphasize that the child is likely to sleep most of the day, so he won't miss her.
    3. Describe the benefits of parallel play for cognitive development.
    4. Validate the mother's feelings of guilt and reassure that daycare is beneficial.

17. The nurse is teaching the parents of an infant the principles of introducing new foods. Which information should be provided? **Select all that apply.** *(707)*
    1. Citrus fruits may be given before the infant is 6 months of age.
    2. Foods should be mixed together to improve intake of nutrients.
    3. Cereals should be started before vegetables and meats.
    4. New foods should be introduced one at a time.
    5. Several days should pass between introducing new foods.

18. The nurse is watching a group of mothers interact with their young children. Which behavior by a mother would **most** strongly suggest that additional assessment for potential child abuse might be required? *(703)*
    1. Retrieves toddler whenever he tries to run or jump or perform active movements
    2. Allows toddler to climb on a table space that is meant for snacks and drinks
    3. Berates and shames her toddler for refusing to share toys with other children
    4. Talks to other mothers and allows the toddler to fuss without comforting him

19. The nurse is interviewing the parents of a toddler who must be admitted for 23-hour observation for a febrile illness. What would be the **most** important question to ask about the child's bedtime? *(710)*
    1. "Would you prefer that he gets milk or juice in a night bottle?"
    2. "What do you usually do when you put him to bed?"
    3. "How many hours does he usually sleep?"
    4. "What would you like me to tell him about sleeping away from home?"

20. The mother is ordering lunch for her toddler. The nurse would intervene if the mother selected which food for the toddler? *(709)*
    1. Milk
    2. Peanut butter sandwich
    3. Carrot sticks
    4. Small banana

21. The parents report that their 3-year-old child has not started talking, but he seems happy and active and very interactive with the world in nonverbal ways. What should the nurse advise the parents to do? *(713)*
    1. Advise the parents to read to the child and ask him to name familiar objects.
    2. Suggest expanding opportunities for parallel play, such as at daycare or play groups.
    3. Reassure parents that children grow and develop at their own individual pace.
    4. Suggest consultation with the provider for possible hearing or speech problems.

22. The provider asks the nurse to please watch the 4-year-old child because she needs to talk privately to the mother. What would be the **best** way for the nurse to interact with the child? *(714)*
    1. Take the child to the cafeteria and buy him a snack.
    2. Give him some crayons and paper and ask him to draw a picture.
    3. Ask him to "help" by sorting a bag of rubber bands by size and color.
    4. Explain why he has to wait and give him a book to read.

23. The school nurse notices that an 8-year-old boy comes to her office during recess for a "tummy ache" which seems to disappear as soon as recess is over. What should the nurse do **first**? *(715)*
    1. Call the parents and review symptoms that warrant an appointment with the provider.
    2. Ask the teachers if there are any unusual classroom behaviors going on.
    3. Alert the principal that there may be some bullying or rough play during recess.
    4. Contact the parents and discuss the pattern of stomachache and recess time.

24. A mother reports that her child occasionally complains of pain in the legs particularly at night. Which question would the nurse ask to determine if this is an expected symptom? *(714)*
    1. "Has the child been running?"
    2. "How old is your child?"
    3. "Has your child appeared anxious?"
    4. "How much does your child weigh?"

25. The nurse must give the school-age child an immunization. Based on the nurse's awareness that the child is in the concrete operational stage, what would the nurse do prior to giving the child the injection? *(715)*
    1. Ask a helper to hold the child to prevent movement.
    2. Suggest that the child pretend that she is getting a fairy's kiss.
    3. Tell the child that it hurts a bit, but prevents sickness.
    4. Make extra efforts to protect modesty and privacy.

26. Which routine check-ups or screenings are recommended for school-age children? **Select all that apply.** *(714, 715)*
    1. Vision testing
    2. Dental examination every 6 months
    3. Hearing testing
    4. Scoliosis screening
    5. Cancer screening
    6. Human immunodeficiency virus testing

27. The nurse must perform a dressing change on a 7-year-old child. The nurse explains that the procedure will not be painful, but the child appears apprehensive. What is the **best** approach for the nurse to use? *(715)*
    1. Demonstrate the procedure on a doll and answer questions.
    2. Ask the child to hold the tape strips and praise her.
    3. Premedicate with a mild anxiolytic medication and explain.
    4. Coach the parent through the procedure and stand back.

28. The school nurse is talking to a child who sustained an abrasion and bruise during recess. When the nurse asks the child what happened, he begins to cry, shakes his head, and refuses to answer. What should the nurse do **first**? *(715)*
    1. Tell him that all information is confidential, so he doesn't have to feel embarrassed or afraid.
    2. Call the parents and inform them that the child is emotionally overwhelmed and can't talk.
    3. Consult the school principal to see if something unusual happened on the playground.
    4. Talk to him while treating the wounds and give encouragement to establish rapport.

29. A parent expresses concern because her healthy, active 11-year-old son seems very short. She reports that all men on both sides of the family are tall. What is the **best** information that the nurse can give to the mother about growth and development? **Select all that apply.** *(714)*
    1. During the school-age period, the growth pattern is usually gradual and subtle.
    2. A second period of rapid growth is expected during adolescence.
    3. From ages 6-12, height increases by about 2 inches.
    4. He is probably lacking essential nutrients that contribute to height and weight.
    5. Distant genetic factors are likely to predispose him to a shorter height.

30. Which parent is doing the **best** job of using good parenting tips in dealing with an adolescent child? *(719)*
    1. Parent permits 17-year-old son to set own curfew time on weekends.
    2. Parent gives up smoking cigarettes and encourages 18-year-old to quit too.
    3. Parent respects 15-year-old daughter's privacy by not asking questions about friends.
    4. Parent allows 13-year-old unlimited computer time if grades are maintained.

31. The parent reports that her 15-year-old daughter seems more moody than usual and she is concerned because there was a teenager in the neighborhood who recently committed suicide. What is the **most** important question that the nurse should ask to determine if the daughter has a high risk for suicide? *(720)*
    1. "Has she had a change in appetite?"
    2. "Does she seem to have an inability to concentrate?"
    3. "Is she preoccupied with thoughts of death?"
    4. "Has she talked about ways to commit suicide?"

32. The nurse is working with a group of parents of high school students. During the discussion, the following statements are made by the parents. Based on an understanding of the needs of adolescents, which statement requires follow-up by the nurse? *(720)*
    1. "We try to set reasonable limits on dating and are encouraging group activities."
    2. "The car has to be back home by 9:00 PM on school nights."
    3. "We are generally not in favor of allowing sex education to be taught at school."
    4. "The number of after-school activities are tremendous, so we suggest finding a focus."

33. Which behaviors indicate that the young adult is achieving the developmental tasks of early adulthood? **Select all that apply.** *(720)*
    1. Lives at home with parents, but is saving for an apartment deposit.
    2. Accepts that sister's decision to have a big family is okay.
    3. Establishes a permanent relationship with a same-sex partner.
    4. Decides to postpone marriage and focus on career.
    5. Identifies with and seeks out gay and lesbian peer groups.

34. Which behavior demonstrates that a 60-year-old adult is meeting his developmental task of generativity? *(724)*
    1. Ruminates over fears and lifetime failures
    2. Reorganizes personal belongings and assets
    3. Gives advice to nephew about succeeding in life
    4. Reviews will for distribution of worldly goods

35. A 53-year-old woman tells the nurse that she has been experiencing flushing, mood swings, night sweats, and breast tenderness for the past several months. Based on knowledge of lifespan development, which question is the nurse **most** likely to ask? *(723)*
    1. "Do you have a personal or family history of breast cancer?"
    2. "When was your last normal menstrual period?"
    3. "Have you experienced a change in libido?"
    4. "Have you ever been told that you have osteoporosis?"

36. The nurse is assessing the vision of an older adult patient. Which finding is **not** associated with the aging process? *(727)*
    1. Presbyopia
    2. Visualization of half of the field
    3. Decreased depth perception
    4. Slowed accommodation

37. The nurse is working in a long-term care facility. Which activity will help the residents to meet the developmental task of ego integrity as described by Erikson? *(727)*
    1. Taking the residents out to lunch at a restaurant
    2. Reminiscing about past important events
    3. Assisting residents to maintain personal hygiene
    4. Leading the residents in an arts and crafts project

38. The home health nurse is interviewing an older patient who lives alone. The patient is underweight and the kitchen is so cluttered that it appears impossible to do any cooking or cleaning. What should the nurse do **first**? *(730)*
    1. Contact a local organization that will deliver meals to the house.
    2. Start an investigation to determine if elder neglect is an issue.
    3. Assess for additional factors that are contributing to the malnutrition.
    4. Weigh the patient and calculate the body mass index.

39. Based on knowledge of normal changes of the cardiovascular system, which recommendation would the nurse make to an older adult? *(721)*
    1. Maintain a low-fat, low-sodium diet.
    2. Obtain streptococcal pneumonia vaccine.
    3. Encourage coughing and deep-breathing.
    4. Change position frequently.

40. Which behavior **most** strongly indicates that the older adult is successfully aging? *(726)*
    1. Spends a lot of time with adult children trying to make up for lost time
    2. Studies Latin and combines subject matter with previous interest in literature
    3. Tries various complementary and alternative therapies to improve appearance
    4. Works through his "bucket list" with an uncharacteristic enthusiasm

41. Which health care worker is demonstrating ageism? *(725)*
    1. Unlicensed assistive personnel helps a resident who lives in a long-term care facility to go outside for a walk
    2. Phlebotomist examines an older patient's veins and tells the nurse that successful blood draw is unlikely
    3. Provider tells an older woman that it would be best if her husband was in hospice care
    4. Nurse continuously smiles and nods as an older patient makes a complaint about the nursing care

CRITICAL THINKING ACTIVITIES

42. Visit the home of friend, family member, or classmate who has an infant or very young child or visit a daycare center that cares for infants or very young children. Observe the setting, the way that the child interacts with the environment and other family members/people, and then review the safety rules for infants and children. Identify which rules that the family/daycare center already has in place and identify areas where safety could be improved. *(709)*

_____

_____

_____

43. A young mother expresses frustration because she is having trouble toilet training her 18-month-old child. She reports that the child shows no interest in learning to use the "potty chair." She tells you that she has tried to sit the child on the potty chair and instructed the child to "urinate." She says that her child frequently has temper tantrums when she places him on the chair.

    a. What can you tell the mother about physiologic development related to toilet training? *(709)*

    _____

    _____

    _____

    b. Use Erikson's stages of psychosocial development to explain how the mother can respond to the child during toilet training. *(710)*

    _____

    _____

    c. What can you tell the mother about the child's temper tantrums? *(710)* _____

    _____

    _____

    _____

    _____

44. The nurse is working in an assisted-living facility. The majority of the residents are older and have some chronic health problems; however, many of the residents are active and only manifest changes associated with aging. Describe the physical changes that the nurse might observe in each of the following systems as a result of the aging process. *(727)*

    a. Sensory: _____

    _____

    b. Integumentary:_____

    _____

    c. Cardiovascular: _____

    _____

    d. Respiratory: _____

    _____

    e. Gastrointestinal:_____

    _____

    f. Genitourinary: _____

    _____

    g. Musculoskeletal: _____

    _____

    h. Neurologic:_____

    _____

45. What influence does the aging process have on the following? *(724, 729)*

    a. Ability to cope:_____

    _____

    b. Intelligence and learning:_____

    _____

    c. Memory: _____

    _____

46. Recall a recent interaction with an older person (patient, family member, neighbor, friend) and select one of the theories of aging that helps you understand an aspect of aging for that person. Describe what you saw and then explain how the selected theory supports your understanding. *(725, 726)*

    _____

    _____

    _____

    _____

    _____

    _____

    _____

    _____

Loss, Grief, Dying, and Death

chapter
25

MULTIPLE CHOICE

Directions: Select the best answer(s) for each of the following questions.

1. Which nursing action supports the structure and process of care and represents one of the eight domains established by the National Consensus Project for Quality Palliative Care? *(735)*
   1. Assists the provider to intubate a patient who is in respiratory arrest
   2. Teaches the patient self-care measures to resume independent life at home
   3. Helps the patient to identify previously used coping strategies and develop new ones
   4. Assists the patient to maintain hope for a successful recovery and return to function

2. Which action is the **best** indicator that an older widow is moving through grief towards closure? *(737)*
   1. Shuts the door of her husband's study so that his belongings are out of sight
   2. Tells her son to throw out all of her husband's belongings so that she won't have to look at them
   3. Sorts through husband's belongings and saves some items for grandchildren and donates the rest
   4. Sits in the study every evening and handles items that represent shared memories

3. For which patient should the nurse design and implement interventions to facilitate anticipatory grief? *(737)*
   1. Woman reports fatigue and depression after death of a child and subsequent divorce.
   2. Young athlete is informed that he needs a below-the-knee amputation due to osteosarcoma.
   3. Reluctant older adult is brought by daughter-in-law to live in an assisted-living center.
   4. Young woman who never knew her father continues to grieve over the missing relationship.

4. The nurse has a good relationship with an older man who was recently placed on hospice care. He speaks fondly about his adult children but admits to being very rough on them while they were growing up. What should the nurse do **first** to facilitate anticipatory grieving for the man and his family? *(737)*
   1. Call the children and suggest that their father would like to see them.
   2. Ask the provider if the circumstances and prognosis was explained to the family.
   3. Invite the family in and observe the interaction and relationship between the members.
   4. Talk to the man about his perception of his current relationship with his children.

5. The home health nurse is visiting an older patient who had an exacerbation of chronic obstructive pulmonary disease (COPD). Which finding **best** supports the nurse's analysis of dysfunctional grieving? *(739)*
   1. In addition to COPD, the patient has multiple other chronic health problems.
   2. Patient ruminates over loss of health and vigor that started years ago.
   3. Nurse observes pictures of family and friends and fun times from past years.
   4. Patient lives alone and appears to have limited social or familial support.

6. The nurse is caring for a hospice patient who is frequently experiencing episodes of pain and dyspnea. The family is devoted and frequently visits, but today the patient is difficult to arouse, and they accuse the nurse of overmedicating the patient. What should the nurse do **first**? *(740)*
   1. Listen to their concerns and clarify their goals for the patient.
   2. Explain that the medication was administered as prescribed.
   3. Call the provider and ask that the medication be discontinued.
   4. Contact the RN so that the care plan can be adjusted.

7. The nurse enters the room and the family is standing around the dying patient loudly praying and chanting. The wife invites the nurse to join in. What should the nurse do **first**? *(743)*
   1. Instruct them to quietly pray and chant.
   2. Decline to join but allow them to continue.
   3. Politely set a time limit on the chanting.
   4. Assess effects of the activity on the patient.

8. The nurse is teaching the entire family, which includes a preschooler and a school-aged child, about how to care and interact with an older member of the family who is dying and being cared for at home. Which activities would be **best** to suggest to the preschooler and school-aged child, respectively? *(740, 748)*
   1. Listen to music with grandma and help her brush her teeth.
   2. Eat breakfast with grandma and help her swallow liquids.
   3. Watch television with grandma and help her to the bathroom.
   4. Draw a picture for grandma and organize her photo album.

9. Which outcome statement **best** indicates that one of the primary goals of palliative care has been met? *(752)*
   1. Patient reports relief from pain and nausea.
   2. Patient verbalizes a wish to die as soon as possible.
   3. Patient was not alone at the time of death.
   4. Patient had personal affairs arranged before death.

10. In the care of the dying patient, which tasks can be delegated to the unlicensed assistive personnel (UAP)? **Select all that apply.** *(753)*
    1. Recognize grief and communicate therapeutically.
    2. Assist the patient into a position of comfort.
    3. Assist the patient with taking oral fluids.
    4. Ensure that patient is clean and dry, and linens are changed as needed.
    5. Support the family when patient's condition changes.

11. Which person is **most** likely to suffer from a maturational loss? *(736)*
    1. A woman married to a police officer is informed that he has been shot and killed.
    2. A college student who has never been away from home goes to Europe to study.
    3. A school-aged child witnesses the family pet being killed by a speeding car.
    4. A middle-aged woman who was married for 30 years is divorced by her husband.

12. A student who normally gets "As" receives a "C" on her project and experiences a loss of confidence. Which behavior **best** indicates that the student is achieving growth because of this situational loss? *(736)*
    1. Does the project over and over again until the teacher gives her an "A."
    2. Tells her parents to go to see the teacher and advocate for a grade change.
    3. Asks another teacher to look at the project and give an opinion about the grade.
    4. Requests a review of the project's strengths and weaknesses against the criteria.

13. Following the death of her husband, a wife feels that he is still with her. She also reports having dreams and vivid memories of him. Which question should the nurse ask to assess the sense of presence that the wife has described? *(737)*
    1. "Do you think he is trying to tell you something?"
    2. "What are your religious beliefs about life after death?"
    3. "How do you feel about these dreams and experiences?"
    4. "Would you like to see a doctor about these symptoms?"

14. On seeing the body of his little brother who just died from cancer, a 10-year-old sibling screams, "I won't go to the funeral! I won't go!" The mother is sobbing and the father begins to yell. What should the nurse do **first**? *(737)*
    1. Take the child aside and quietly talk to him about his feelings about death.
    2. Encourage the father to stop yelling because it is not helpful.
    3. Ask the mother to hold her child so that he can be supported and comforted.
    4. Calmly close the door and stay with the family while they express themselves.

15. A nurse is talking to a 63-year-old woman who underwent grief therapy for unresolved grief related to the death of her husband. Which behavior **best** indicates that the therapy is helping? *(735)*
    1. She frequently visits his grave site.
    2. She invites his old friends to dinner.
    3. She talks about things they used to enjoy.
    4. She cooks and serves his favorite foods.

16. As the nurse is performing medication teaching, the older woman begins to cry. "My grandson got into my pills and overdosed. He didn't die, but my daughter won't even speak to me." What is the **most** therapeutic response? *(734)*
    1. "Well, thank goodness he is okay. She should be happy about that."
    2. "I'm sure everything will work out. She'll get over it; give her time."
    3. "You feel like you were to blame for this, but accidents do happen."
    4. "Every time you look at your medicine, you think about your family."

17. The hospice nurse is visiting a family of a deceased patient. During the visit, the son displays symptoms of a grief attack. Which intervention would the nurse use? *(738)*
    1. Ensure that other members of the household do not get attacked.
    2. Reassure the son that he is safe and that no one will attack him.
    3. Help the son recognize that the attack is a type of grief response.
    4. Report the symptoms of the attack to the provider.

18. The UAP tells the nurse that the dying patient's family keeps calling for assistance with minor tasks that they could easily do for the patient. What should the nurse do? *(743)*
    1. Tell the UAP to do whatever the family or patient wants him/her to do.
    2. Encourage the family to participate in care to increase feelings of control.
    3. Ask the UAP to clarify what he/she means by "assistance with minor tasks."
    4. Assess the family's desire and ability to participate in the care of the patient.

19. Which statement by the family member of a dying patient **best** indicates a healthy retention of hope? *(744)*
    1. "We are planning to take our father on one last trip to Europe next year."
    2. "My sister is coming from California next week; I know he wants to see her."
    3. "He really loves to golf and is looking forward to playing again this summer."
    4. "We know a man from our church who beat his cancer; Dad can do the same."

20. The patient is sobbing. When the nurse tries to find out what is wrong, the patient angrily says, "I'm dying! I have pain! My children are losing their mother! We are in debt up to our eyeballs! And God seems to be on a coffee break!" What does the nurse do **first** to identify and prioritize the patient's problems? *(744, 745)*
    1. Use Maslow's Hierarchy and first address the physical issue of pain.
    2. Ask the RN to assume care because of multiple complex problems.
    3. Collect additional data about each concern and consult with the RN.
    4. Review the plan of care and determine if these are old or new issues.

21. What signs and symptoms would the nurse expect to observe in the patient who is nearing death? **Select all that apply.** (754)
    1. Lowered blood pressure
    2. Rapid, bounding pulse
    3. Irregular respiratory pattern
    4. Mouth-breathing with dry mucous membranes
    5. Rapid, anxious eye movements

22. The terminally ill patient has been experiencing severe pain and has requested that the physician assist her to end her suffering. What should the nurse do if the physician prescribes a morphine dosage that could cause respiratory depression and respiratory arrest? (749)
    1. Administer the medication as prescribed.
    2. Refuse to give the prescribed dose.
    3. Tell the physician to administer the dose.
    4. Consult the nursing supervisor for advice.

23. On assessing the dying patient, the nurse notes that the pulse rate is 30/min, the respiratory rate is 8/min, and the systolic blood pressure is palpated at 60. The patient has a Do Not Resuscitate (DNR) order. What should the nurse do **first**? (750)
    1. Call the family to the bedside.
    2. Make the patient comfortable.
    3. Call for help and get the crash cart.
    4. Start an IV and give a fluid bolus.

24. Which nursing action demonstrates that the nurse is performing his/her responsibilities according to the National Organ Transplantation Act (Public Law 98-507, 10-14, 1984) and the Uniform Anatomical Gift Act? (750)
    1. Assists the physician who certified death to remove suitable organs.
    2. Ensures that the clinical signs of death are present before death is certified.
    3. Explains the process of organ donation and transplant to the family.
    4. Contacts a qualified health care professional to ask family about organ donation.

25. Which actions indicate that the health care team is fulfilling the Dying Person's Bill of Rights? **Select all that apply.** (751)
    1. Nurse assesses pain and administers pain medication accordingly.
    2. Patient's choice of spiritual leader is contacted and rituals are allowed.
    3. Family is allowed to decide how much information is given to patient.
    4. Health care team creates a living will and advance directives for the patient.
    5. Nurse gives comfort measures and talks to a patient who is in a coma.
    6. Patient is allowed to make decisions, even though she seems indecisive.

26. Which nursing action is **most** likely to be affected by the patient's advance directives? (750)
    1. Instructing UAP on how to perform postmortem care
    2. Advising the provider that the pain medication is not working
    3. Assisting the provider to intubate for respiratory arrest
    4. Contacting the family if the patient dies unexpectedly during the night

27. The nurse is working in a pediatric outpatient clinic. There is an 8-year-old child whose grandfather has just died. Based on the developmental level of the child, what type of response would the nurse anticipate? (740)
    1. "Grandpa will come back soon. He just went to see Grandma."
    2. "Grandpa was old and supposed to die. My cat was old; he died too."
    3. "I was bad at school and talked back to Mom. That's why Grandpa died."
    4. "It was better that Grandpa died quickly and didn't have to suffer a long time."

28. The patient tells the nurse that he has a durable power of attorney for health care and medical treatment. What is the **most** important information to obtain from the patient? (750)
    1. The name and phone number of the person who will make health care decisions
    2. The name and phone numbers of the family member who is next of kin
    3. The patient's written permission to disclose information to the attorney
    4. The patient's wishes about his or her care when death is near

29. What is **most** likely to be included in postmortem care? **Select all that apply.** (754, 756)
    1. Remove all tubings, dressings, and drains.
    2. Wash hands and don gloves.
    3. Care for valuables and personal belongings.
    4. Close patient's eyes and mouth if needed.
    5. Place patient supine with arms at the sides.

CRITICAL THINKING ACTIVITIES

30. The patient's husband died in an automobile accident a year ago. She is still experiencing insomnia and feelings of worthlessness and anger, and she continues to avoid family and social functions.

    a. What physical assessments will the nurse perform on this patient? *(740)* _____

    _____

    _____

    _____

    _____

    b. Discuss how physical and social aspects of human functioning influence the grieving process. *(740)*

    _____

    _____

31. Nurse A is a new nurse who recently started working on the unit. Nurse A likes and respects Nurse B, an experienced nurse who has been caring for terminal patients for a long time. Nurse A notices that Nurse B is efficiently caring for patients, but seems progressively cold, uncaring, and indifferent about everyone's feelings. Nurse B is particularly critical of one family because of how they act toward the staff and the dying family member.

    a. Discuss what could be happening to Nurse B. *(738)* _____

    _____

    _____

    _____

    _____

    _____

    b. What can Nurse A do to help Nurse B? *(738)* _____

    _____

    _____

    _____

    _____

    _____

32. The older patient who is receiving palliative care verbalizes the "wish to die." What would the nurse do to differentiate whether the patient is experiencing acceptance or depression? *(746, 751)*

_____

_____

_____

_____

_____

_____

Health Promotion and Pregnancy

TABLE ACTIVITY

1. Directions: For the parameters on the left, enter the expected change on the right. *(785)*

Cardiovascular Changes in Pregnancy

Parameter	Change
Heart rate	
Blood pressure	
Blood volume	
Red blood cell mass	
Hemoglobin	
Hematocrit	
White blood cell count	
Cardiac output	

MULTIPLE CHOICE

Directions: Select the best answer(s) for each of the following questions.

2. What would the nurse expect the patient to report as presumptive signs of pregnancy? **Select all that apply.** *(778)*
   1. Amenorrhea
   2. Nausea and vomiting
   3. Breast changes
   4. Positive home pregnancy test
   5. Urinary frequency

3. The woman is in the first trimester of pregnancy and tells the nurse that she has morning sickness almost every day. Which intervention would the nurse suggest **first**? *(783)*
   1. Taking an over-the-counter antacid
   2. Keeping a daily symptom diary
   3. Drinking a tea made of ginger root
   4. Nibbling a few soda crackers before rising

4. While there are many variations that the nurse might see, what would be the **most** likely behaviors that a man would demonstrate during paternal adaptation? *(789)*
   1. Establishes a relationship with the unborn child, and prepares for the birth experience
   2. Prepares for the parental role accompanied by fantasy, pleasure, and intense learning
   3. Experiences the *couvade syndrome* with nausea, other gastrointestinal issues, and fatigue
   4. Views pregnancy as proof of masculinity and dominant role within the family

5. The woman is in the third trimester of pregnancy and the nurse observes that the woman's feet and ankles are unusually swollen. What is the **most** important assessment for the nurse to make? *(782)*
   1. Ask the woman if she has been resting and elevating her legs.
   2. Assess the peripheral pulses and movement of the ankle joints.
   3. Assess for edema of the face, presacral area, or fingers.
   4. Ask the woman how much fluid she typical drinks in a day.

6. The provider tells the nurse that a couple expecting their first child is considering diagnostic testing to detect chromosomal abnormalities. Which informational pamphlets is the nurse **most** likely to prepare? **Select all that apply.** *(772, 773, 774)*
   1. "Amniocentesis Can Reveal Information About Genetic Factors"
   2. "What an Ultrasound Shows About the Health of Your Baby"
   3. "Chorionic Villus Sampling to Detect Genetic Disorders of the Fetus"
   4. "Maternal Serum Alpha-Fetoprotein Screening: A Low-Risk Test"
   5. "The Biophysical Profile of You and Your Baby"
   6. "Nuchal Translucency Screening to Assess for Potential Down Syndrome"

7. The pregnant woman reports blurring and double vision. Which assessment should the nurse **immediately** perform? *(788, 789)*
   1. Check the patient's blood pressure.
   2. Assess the patient's visual acuity.
   3. Auscultate the lungs and count respirations.
   4. Assess balance and coordination.

8. The woman has entered her 16th week of pregnancy and asks the nurse, "How is the baby growing?" What does the nurse tell the mother? *(765)*
   1. "Your baby has developed head hair."
   2. "Your baby weighs about 27 ounces."
   3. "Your baby has settled into a favorite position."
   4. "Your baby has formed all organs and structures."

9. The nurse notices that the patient has facial swelling. What is the nurse's **best** response? *(782)*
   1. "This is a temporary condition caused by increased blood flow resulting from high estrogen levels."
   2. "An increased blood volume results in increased water retention, but the swelling should go away."
   3. "Facial swelling is something that has to be reported to your provider for follow-up care and evaluation."
   4. "This should be reported to your provider because swelling signals an increased amount of melanocyte-stimulating hormone."

10. The nurse notes in the provider's documentation that the patient is experiencing ptyalism. What should the nurse instruct the patient to do? *(783)*
    1. Eat small, frequent meals.
    2. Suck on hard candy.
    3. Sit up after eating.
    4. Avoid eating spicy foods.

11. The patient in the first trimester is advised to avoid exercising for more than 35 minutes in hot, humid weather. What is the **best** rationale for this advice? *(787)*
    1. An altered calcium and phosphorus balance could cause leg cramps.
    2. Maintaining balance and posture is more difficult during this time period.
    3. Prolonged or repeated fetal temperature elevation may result in birth defects.
    4. Stretching of the ligaments causes pain or tenderness in the lower abdomen.

12. The pregnant patient has been instructed to count fetal movements (kick count). Which statement demonstrates that the patient understands the procedure? *(772)*
    1. "I should count all movements during a 24-hour period."
    2. "I should choose a time of day after I have done my own exercises."
    3. "My baby should move at least 10 times in a 1- to 2-hour period."
    4. "I should feel the baby move at least four times after I have eaten a meal."

13. Which patient response indicates that she understands how to perform Kegel exercises? *(786)*
    1. "The exercises are most beneficial if they are done 10 times in a row, at least three times a day."
    2. "If I could perform the exercises 100 times in a row, I will only have to do them once a day."
    3. "I will perform the exercises whenever I have time to sit and concentrate for at least 20 minutes."
    4. "The exercises are most beneficial if I start performing them right after I deliver my baby."

14. After delivery, the nurse is examining the placenta. What is the **most** important observation that the nurse should note and document? *(763)*
    1. Weight of the placenta
    2. Presence of the placental barrier
    3. Appearance of the "Shiny Schultz"
    4. Intactness of the placenta

15. The nurse is examining the umbilical cord immediately after delivery. Which finding should be reported to the provider for further investigation of fetal anomalies? *(763, 770)*
    1. The cord has two vessels, one artery and one vein.
    2. The cord contains a significant amount of Wharton's jelly.
    3. The cord is 50 cm long and 2.5 cm in diameter.
    4. The cord has a pale white, ropelike appearance.

16. The nurse is assessing fetal heart tones on a woman who is 12 weeks pregnant. What is the correct method for this procedure? *(771)*
    1. Use an amplified stethoscope and listen at the midline of the abdomen.
    2. Place the Doppler just above the symphysis pubis and apply firm pressure.
    3. Instruct the patient to drink a quart of water prior to abdominal ultrasound.
    4. Insert the transvaginal ultrasound probe into the vagina.

17. The nursing student is preparing to measure fundal height. At which step would the supervising nurse intervene? *(771)*
    1. Reviews the established protocol to measure this specific patient
    2. Verifies the patient's identity by asking name and birthdate
    3. Obtains a disposable paper tape measuring device
    4. Instructs the patient to lie supine on the examination table

18. The nurse is comparing today's fundal height measurement with the previous recording taken 5 weeks ago. What is the significance of a stable or decreased measurement? *(771)*
    1. Possible intrauterine growth restriction
    2. Possible multifetal gestation
    3. Possible excessive amniotic fluid
    4. Expected normal finding

19. The patient is at risk for a miscarriage. Which diagnostic test result is consistent with a miscarriage? *(773)*
    1. Elevated levels of maternal serum alpha-fetoprotein
    2. Declining levels of quantitative human chorionic gonadotropin
    3. Increasing levels of amniotic fluid
    4. Positive findings for chorionic villus sampling

20. The nurse is helping the woman prepare for an abdominal ultrasound. Which information is correct? *(774)*
    1. "You will have to drink several cups of water after the procedure to flush the bladder."
    2. "We will help you assume the lithotomy position for the examination."
    3. "The procedure is a little uncomfortable; just signal if you need to take a break."
    4. "You and your partner can watch the images on the screen if you would like to."

21. The mother has diabetes and is at risk for placental insufficiency. The results of the nonstress test shows three fetal movements accompanied by two increases of 15 bpm in a 20-minute period. On hearing the results, she starts crying. What should the nurse be prepared to do for the patient? *(775)*
    1. Encourage the mother to express feelings of anxiety or uncertainty.
    2. Prepare the mother for additional testing, such as the contraction stress test.
    3. Reassure the mother that crying with relief and joy is an understandable response.
    4. Support the mother through a repeat of the nonstress test for validation.

22. The mother is in her second trimester and reports "premilk" is leaking from her breasts. What should the nurse tell the mother? *(777)*
    1. "Any discharge from the nipples should be considered abnormal and evaluated by the provider."
    2. "Premilk or colostrum is not supposed to start until immediately after delivery."
    3. "Premilk will be pumped and discarded in order to stimulate the true breast milk."
    4. "If excessive leakage is a problem, breast pads can be useful."

23. The nurse is interviewing a woman who has just found out that she is pregnant. From a nursing standpoint, what is the **best** rationale for asking about insurance coverage for maternity and newborn care? *(777)*
    1. Information is used to determine the frequency of the prenatal visits.
    2. Admission to the hospital is based on the type of insurance coverage.
    3. Family will have additional stress related to finances if there is no insurance coverage.
    4. Number and frequency of diagnostic tests can be altered if there is no coverage.

24. The nurse is taking a health history and the information is likely to be used later during genetic counseling. Which question is the **most** appropriate in the initial data collection? *(777)*
    1. "How do you feel about undergoing genetic testing?"
    2. "What would you do if an abnormality is detected?"
    3. "Have you ever had rubella or have you had the vaccination?"
    4. "Would you like information about genetic defects?"

25. The patient had her last menstrual period (LMP) on August 18, 2018. Using Nägele's rule, when is the estimated date of birth (EDB)? _____ *(780)*

26. Define the parity of the pregnant woman using the GTPAL system: She has been pregnant four times, delivered three full-term infants, had no abortions or preterm deliveries, and has three living children. _____ *(780)*

27. The pregnant woman reports frequently feeling ill in the morning with bouts of nausea throughout the day. Which question is **most** important to differentiate between morning sickness and the more serious condition of hyperemesis gravidarum? *(783)*
    1. "How much and how frequently are you eating meals?"
    2. "Do you notice that you are salivating more than usual?"
    3. "Have you been vomiting? If yes, how frequently?"
    4. "Are you experiencing heartburn? If yes, when does it occur?"

28. The pregnant woman is a heavy smoker and she feels that it is unlikely that she will be able to quit. Because of the oxygen deprivation in utero, which outcome should the health care team be prepared to deal with? *(781)*
    1. Fetal respiratory distress requiring resuscitation
    2. Preterm delivery with low birth weight
    3. Intrauterine infection and fetal distress
    4. No change in fetal heart rate during contraction

29. The pregnant patient phones the clinic and reports having some symptoms that are causing discomfort and worry. Which symptom is the **most** serious and warrants immediate evaluation by the provider? *(782)*
    1. Shortness of breath when climbing the stairs
    2. Perineal discomfort and pressure with standing
    3. Muscle aches and difficulty walking
    4. Pain and burning sensation with urination

30. Which laboratory result should be reported to the provider because pregnancy increases the risk for blood clots? *(783)*
    1. Increased platelet count
    2. Decreased hematocrit
    3. Presence of protein and glucose in the urine
    4. Increased cholesterol level

31. The woman with a low-risk pregnancy tells the nurse that she frequently has to travel for her job. Which questions are **most** relevant? **Select all that apply.** *(793)*
    1. "Will you have to travel to areas where the water is untreated?"
    2. "Will you be terminated if you refuse to travel?"
    3. "Have you checked the policies of the airline that you usually fly?"
    4. "Are you aware that magnetometers at airports are harmful to the fetus?"
    5. "Are you planning to travel to a foreign country?"
    6. "When you drive, do you use the lap belt and shoulder harness?"

CRITICAL THINKING ACTIVITIES

32. The nurse is working at an OB-GYN clinic and is aware that pregnancy is usually a time when women want to improve health habits and that expectant mothers are likely to want and welcome information about how to have a healthy baby.

    a. What counseling should the nurse give patients about self-care according to the trimester checklist? *(781)*

    b. Identify five drugs that the mother should avoid during pregnancy. *(764-770)*

    c. In addition to selected medications, what are other activities or substances that the nurse will instruct the woman to avoid during pregnancy? *(781, 785, 786)*

33. The nurse is talking with a woman who is in the first trimester of pregnancy. The patient reports feeling "fat, sluggish, and bloated." She begins to cry and expresses feelings of guilt because she resents the pregnancy for making her feel this way and dreads what is coming because "I'm just going to get bigger; then I'll start waddling like a duck and my skin will get all stretched out." The nurse recognizes that the patient has low self-esteem related to perceived loss of control over lifestyle and a distorted body image related to physiologic changes of pregnancy. What can the nurse do to assist the patient? *(788, 793)*

_____

_____

_____

_____

_____

34. While it is not the nurse's responsibility to perform genetic counseling, the nurse may be involved in the care of couples who undergo testing for genetic counseling and may have to support families who get bad news or those are conflicted about what to do with the information. Discuss the scenarios with your classmates or instructor.

   a. The nurse is caring for a couple who has just been told that it is likely that their unborn child has Down syndrome. The wife is crying, and the husband is very withdrawn. The nurse has a younger brother who has Down syndrome and he is happy and healthy and active in the community. What should the nurse do? *(777, 778)*

_____

_____

_____

_____

   b. The nurse is caring for a couple who have several children with severe congenital and genetic abnormalities. The children are frequently seen in the pediatric clinic and are generally undernourished and not well cared for. The parents are currently expecting another child but they have no money for genetic testing and they seem unconcerned about the current or any future pregnancies. What is the best way for the nurse to help and support this family? *(771, 791)*

_____

_____

_____

_____

Labor and Delivery

chapter 27

MATCHING
Directions: Match the term/phrase on the left to the correct definition on the right.

Term

_____ 1. bloody show *(799)*
_____ 2. effacement *(799)*
_____ 3. primary powers *(805)*
_____ 4. cardinal movements of labor *(807)*
_____ 5. second stage of labor *(811)*

Definition

a. Begins with complete dilation at 10 cm and ends with the birth of the baby
b. Involuntary uterine contractions that signal the beginning of labor
c. Turns and adjustments that occur as the fetus moves through the maternal pelvis
d. Vaginal drainage and blood-tinged mucus typically increase as term approaches
e. Thinning and shortening or obliteration of the cervix that occurs during late pregnancy, labor, or both

SHORT ANSWER
Directions: Using your own words, answer each question in the space provided.

6. What are the five Ps of the complex process of labor and delivery? *(800)*

   a. _____
   b. _____
   c. _____
   d. _____
   e. _____

7. Briefly define the four qualities of uterine contractions that are important to assess. *(827)*

   a. _____
   b. _____
   c. _____
   d. _____

FIGURE LABELING

8. Directions: Label the figure to indicate the fetal position in relation to the quadrant of the maternal pelvis. *(803)*

Right occipitoposterior (ROP)
Right occipitotransverse (ROT)
Right occipitoanterior (ROA)

Left occipitoposterior (LOP)
Left occipitotransverse (LOT)
Left occipitoanterior (LOA)

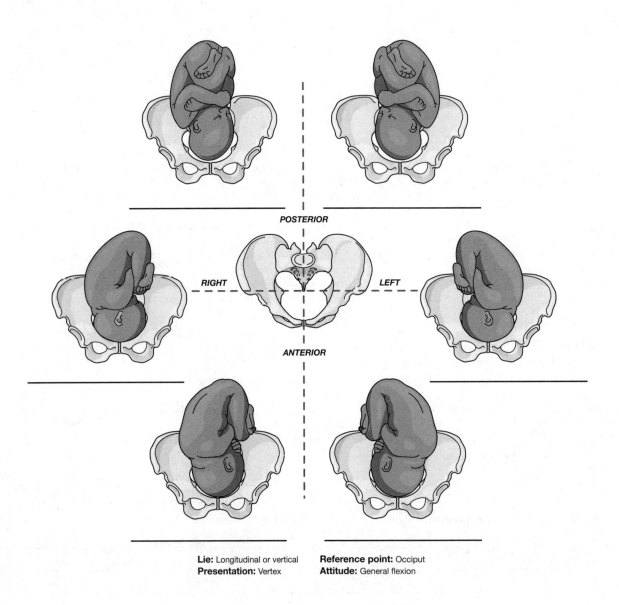

Lie: Longitudinal or vertical
Presentation: Vertex

Reference point: Occiput
Attitude: General flexion

MULTIPLE CHOICE
Directions: Select the best answer(s) for each of the following questions.

9. What topics would be included in a discussion about the birth plan? **Select all that apply.** *(797)*
   1. When to get pregnant
   2. Labor
   3. Delivery
   4. Postpartum period
   5. Fetal development
   6. Genetic counseling

10. Which factor would negate the woman's personal preference to use a birthing center? *(798)*
    1. Low-risk pregnancy
    2. Unavailability of doula
    3. Need for cesarean section
    4. Limited insurance coverage

11. About 2 weeks before the due date, a nullipara patient reports that the "lightening" that was described in the prenatal classes has occurred. Which physical change is likely to occur because of the lightening? *(798)*
    1. Urinary frequency
    2. Decreased fetal movement
    3. Shortness of breath
    4. Leakage of amniotic fluid

12. The nurse informs the mother that the results of the nitrazine test are blue-green, pH 6.5. What additional information should the nurse give to the mother? *(799)*
    1. Advise her that precipitous labor is likely.
    2. Instruct her to go home and resume usual activity.
    3. Inform her that delivery should occur within 24 hours.
    4. Tell her that the test is nonreactive and that urine leakage is normal.

13. The patient in the first trimester reports an irregular tightening of the uterus and the provider informs her that these are Braxton Hicks contractions. What additional information should the nurse give the patient? *(799)*
    1. Call the provider whenever these occur.
    2. Expect Braxton Hicks to increase in frequency as pregnancy progresses.
    3. Anticipate that a headache and backache will accompany these contractions.
    4. Monitor these contractions for a few hours and then call the provider.

14. The provider tells the mother that it is likely that she is having a vaginal discharge called *bloody show.* Which action is the nurse **most** likely to perform? *(799)*
    1. Prepare the mother for an emergency cesarean section.
    2. Assist the provider to perform a vaginal examination.
    3. Prepare the internal transducer to assess fetal heart rate.
    4. Place in side-lying position to reduce pressure on the vena cava.

15. Premature rupture of membranes increases the risk for which complication? *(799)*
    1. Infection for mother and fetus
    2. Failure to progress
    3. Uterine hemorrhage
    4. Precipitous labor

16. Which behaviors/symptoms would be considered normal and expected a few days before onset of true labor? *(799)*
    1. Depression and fatigue
    2. Vomiting and loss of appetite
    3. A loss of 5-10 pounds
    4. Renewed energy for cooking and cleaning

17. The nurse is assisting the provider to measure the pelvis of several patients. Which patient is **most** likely to undergo pelvimetry? *(801)*
    1. Patient is relatively thin and is in the early part of the first trimester.
    2. Patient is not currently pregnant but has a history of pelvic fracture.
    3. Patient is in the second trimester and multiple fetuses are suspected.
    4. Patient is in the third trimester and placental location is questionable.

18. The patient gives a history of multiple pregnancies. What is the potential clinical significance for the fetus' attitude and lie within the womb? *(802)*
    1. A weakened abdominal wall increases the risk for a transverse lie.
    2. The fetus is more likely to be small and change positions frequently.
    3. The spine of the fetus will be parallel to the spine of the mother.
    4. The presentation is likely to be a complete breech.

19. The provider informs the nurse that the patient will have trial labor as a candidate for vaginal birth after cesarean (VBAC). The nurse would closely monitor the patient and alert the health care team. If complications occur, which procedure would be performed? *(831)*
    1. Forceps-assisted or vacuum-assisted delivery
    2. Amniotomy for induction of labor
    3. Epidural analgesia early in labor
    4. Emergency cesarean section

20. What is an acceptable practice in labor and delivery? *(821)*
    1. Maintenance of a full bladder
    2. Maintenance of supine position
    3. Ambulation before membrane rupture
    4. Administration of enemas in the presence of vaginal bleeding

21. For which patient would the nurse anticipate that the uterine contractions may temporarily become less frequent and intense? *(806)*
    1. Woman who received an epidural analgesia early in labor
    2. Woman who has been paraplegic for past several years
    3. Adolescent who is nullipara
    4. Older woman who is multipara

22. Which patients may be candidates for induction of labor? **Select all that apply.** *(828)*
    1. Patient had rupture of membranes 2 hours ago and labor has not started.
    2. Patient has high blood pressure with symptoms of headache and dizziness.
    3. Patient has a history of one stillbirth and one fetal demise.
    4. Patient has a history of diabetes mellitus.
    5. Patient has documented placenta previa.
    6. Patient has active herpes simplex infection.

23. Which patients may be candidates for cesarean delivery? **Select all that apply.** *(830, 831)*
    1. Cephalopelvic disproportion is present.
    2. Mother is a nullipara.
    3. Mother has a cardiac condition.
    4. Prolapse of cord is present.
    5. Presentation is breech.
    6. Fetus has a heart rate of 140 bpm.

24. Put the following steps (1-7) in the mechanism of labor in the order in which they occur for vertex positions. *(811)*
    _____ a. Extension and restitution
    _____ b. Flexion
    _____ c. Descent
    _____ d. Internal rotation
    _____ e. Expulsion
    _____ f. Engagement
    _____ g. External rotation

25. The provider informs the nurse that there is a prolapsed umbilical cord. What should the nurse do **first**? *(804)*
    1. Assist the mother into a high Fowler's position.
    2. Apply a fetal monitoring device and count heart rate.
    3. Prepare the mother for a cesarean birth.
    4. Ensure that the provider has sterile gloves.

26. The nurse is caring for a patient who has completed the third stage of labor. What is the purpose and goal of massaging the fundus? *(805)*
    1. To achieve uterine atony
    2. To facilitate separation of the placenta
    3. To regain uterine muscle tone
    4. To determine the number and size of clots

27. The nurse is encouraging the mother to make frequent position changes during the first stage of labor. Which position promotes maternal cardiac output and placental perfusion? *(807)*
    1. Lateral side-lying
    2. Squatting
    3. Knee-chest
    4. Lithotomy

28. Assessment of the amniotic fluid reveals yellow staining. What is the significance of this finding? *(820)*
    1. This is associated with hydramnios.
    2. Fetal hemolytic disease is likely.
    3. Woman has sustained abruptio placentae.
    4. Meconium passage occurs with a breech birth.

29. On examination, the patient is found to be 8 cm dilated with contractions every 3 minutes that last for 70 seconds. Which behavior is likely to occur in this transitional phase? *(811)*
    1. Alert and talkative
    2. Confused and disoriented
    3. Less talkative and focused on breathing
    4. Irritable and deeply focused

30. What is an expected finding for a woman who is in the mid- to active phase of labor? *(809)*
    1. Cervical dilation of 2 cm
    2. Contractions every 3 to 5 minutes
    3. A desire to ambulate
    4. Very mild, easily controlled pain

31. When coaching the patient through the early or latent phase of labor, which breathing technique is the nurse **most** likely to encourage? *(829)*
    1. Shallow panting
    2. Slow, deep chest or abdominal breathing
    3. Acceleration through contractions
    4. Holding the breath for 5 seconds and exhaling

32. All members of the health care team have performed hand hygiene. Which members are appropriately using personal protective equipment while caring for the mother and infant during childbirth? **Select all that apply.** *(800)*
    1. Unlicensed assistive personnel wears clean gloves when cleaning the perineal area after a bowel movement.
    2. Obstetrician wears a sterile waterproof gown and gloves, a mask with shield, cap and shoe covers when delivering infant.
    3. Nurse wears a sterile gown and sterile gloves when handling the newborn immediately after birth.
    4. Nurse wears clean gloves and gown when inserting an internal scalp electrode.
    5. Nurse wears sterile gloves when inserting a urinary catheter.

33. The patient is receiving intravenous (IV) oxytocin for uterine inertia. The nurse notes that the fetal heart rate (FHR) is dropping below 100 bpm. What should the nurse do? *(829)*
    1. Stop the infusion.
    2. Slow down the infusion.
    3. Monitor the FHR for 5-10 full cycles of contractions.
    4. Do nothing, as this is an expected response.

34. The baby is assessed after birth and the following are noted: heart rate 124 bpm; respiratory effort good, crying; some flexion of the extremities; grimacing; body pink, extremities bluish. Based on this information, what is the Apgar score?_____ *(820)*

35. What is the **first** intervention that the nurse would perform in the care of an infant who has just been delivered? *(812)*
    1. Place the infant in contact with the mother's skin.
    2. Use a bulb syringe to remove fluid from mouth and nasopharynx.
    3. Place identification bracelets on both mother and infant.
    4. Immediately dry the infant to help reduce heat loss from evaporation.

36. The neonate has just been delivered. What is an indication that placental separation is occurring? *(804)*
    1. Uterus is relaxed and flaccid.
    2. Sudden gush of bright-red blood with large clots.
    3. Contractions are progressively weaker.
    4. The umbilical cord is obviously lengthening.

37. A new nurse is performing fundal massage. When would the supervising nurse intervene? *(805)*
    1. Massages to produce uterine fatigue and atonia
    2. Supports uterus from below with one hand
    3. Uses upper hand to apply firm downward pressure
    4. Observes perineum for number and size of clots

38. The woman received general anesthesia by inhalation. Because the mother has increased risk for uterine relaxation, which action will the nurse perform? *(825)*
    1. Administer glycopyrrolate as prescribed.
    2. Monitor for increased abdominal pain.
    3. Monitor for postpartum hemorrhage.
    4. Administer magnesium sulfate.

39. Following a precipitous labor and emergency birth, what is likely to be the **greatest** concern? *(826)*
    1. Grief and loss due to fetal demise
    2. Prolonged contractions and abdominal pain
    3. Severe hypertension and seizures
    4. Postpartum hemorrhage and hypovolemia

CRITICAL THINKING ACTIVITIES

40. a. The admission assessment to the labor area includes: *(821)* _____

_____

_____

b. Nursing assessment of a patient's status throughout labor includes: *(827)* _____

_____

_____

c. For the fourth stage of labor, what are the nursing assessments and how often are they done? *(812)*

_____

_____

41. Discuss how the fetus is monitored and circumstances that would warrant notification of the provider. *(815, 816)*

_____

_____

42. Discuss the use of Standard Precautions during childbirth. *(800)* _____

_____

_____

43. The nurse is caring for a pregnant woman who is in the latent phase of labor. The woman becomes very agitated and panicky during the initial vaginal examination. She begins to cry and apologize after the provider leaves the room and confides in the nurse that she is a survivor of sexual abuse. She says, "I don't know how I am going to get through this. I feel so vulnerable and exposed."

a. Discuss how history of sexual abuse may affect patients. *(824)* _____

_____

_____

b. What can the nurse do to help this patient? *(824)* _____

_____

_____

Care of the Mother and Newborn

TABLE ACTIVITY

1. Directions: Complete the table below with the expected values for the newborn. *(860)*

Assessment of Newborn	Normal Value
Head circumference	
Relationship of head to chest circumference	
Temperature	
Pulse	
Respirations	
Blood pressure	

CLINICAL APPLICATION OF MATH AND CONVERSION

Directions: Calculate or make the necessary conversions for math problems encountered in performing skills for patients.

2. The breastfeeding mother has an intake as indicated in the flow sheet. What should the nurse tell the mother? *(846)*

24-Hour Fluid Intake	
Time	Amount
7:00	6 oz juice, 8 oz water, 16 oz of low-fat milk
10:00	8 oz juice
12:00	350 mL water
14:00	16 oz of low-fat milk
17:00	250 mL water
20:00	16 oz of low-fat milk

1. Encourage the mother to drink an additional 2-3 servings of liquid each day.
2. Tell the mother that she is drinking more than required, but that's not a problem.
3. Advise the mother that there is a potential for fluid overload; then assess for edema.
4. Reinforce need for fluids and tell her that she is drinking the recommended amount.

3. The healthy neonate weighs 6.8 lbs. How much fluid does the neonate need every day? _____ mL/day *(867)*

4. The healthy newborn weighs 3.5 kg. How many kilocalories does the newborn need each day? _____ kcal/day *(867)*

MULTIPLE CHOICE
Directions: Select the best answer(s) for each of the following questions.

5. When the let-down reflex occurs, what action will the nurse perform? *(834)*
   1. Offer the mother oral fluids to prevent dehydration.
   2. Assess the color change and consistency of the lochia.
   3. Assist the mother with breastfeeding as needed.
   4. Observe for frequency of saturation of perineal pads.

6. After an uncomplicated vaginal delivery, the mother reports that her appetite has returned; however, the nurse recognizes that gastric motility may continue to decline. Which action is the nurse likely to perform **first**? *(839)*
   1. Assess for abdominal discomfort and possible paralytic ileus.
   2. Encourage activity, fluid intake, and increased fiber in the diet.
   3. Obtain an order for antacids as needed and encourage small meals.
   4. Administer an enema or suppository to promote bowel evacuation.

7. The nurse is monitoring the flow of lochia for several postpartum patients. Which condition is cause for the **greatest** concern? *(835)*
   1. There is a gush of dark lochia as the patient gets out of bed.
   2. Lochia alba changes back to lochia rubra.
   3. Pad with scant lochia serosa has a fleshy smell.
   4. One pad is saturated in 20 minutes with lochia rubra.

8. What instructions would the nurse give to a mother who has elected to use bottle-feeding rather than breastfeeding? *(854)*
   1. Pump the breasts regularly to prevent engorgement.
   2. Apply warm, moist packs or shower breasts with hot water.
   3. Wear a supportive bra within a few hours of delivery.
   4. Decrease fluid intake to suppress milk production.

9. The nurse hears in report that the woman had a cesarean birth with general anesthesia. The combination of general anesthesia and lost abdominal tone prompts the nurse to be watchful for which potential complication? *(847)*
   1. Paralytic ileus
   2. Hyperemesis
   3. Loss of sensation in legs
   4. Urinary incontinence

10. The woman is in the later postpartum period. The urinary output is noted below. What should the nurse do **first**? *(846)*

Urine Output	
Time	**Amount**
7:00	50 mL
7:30	75 mL
8:15	30 mL
8:45	60 mL
9:00	30 mL

   1. Continue to observe output and then record the total at the end of the shift.
   2. Assess the patient for urgency, dysuria, or bladder distention.
   3. Obtain an order for urinalysis and culture and sensitivity.
   4. Obtain an order for straight catheterization to check for residual.

11. The mother has lost a large volume of blood and appears to be in hypovolemic shock following the delivery. What should the nurse do **first**? *(836)*
   1. Raise the head of the bed to 80 degrees.
   2. Discontinue the oxytocic agent in the intravenous infusion.
   3. Massage the fundus firmly and continuously.
   4. Provide oxygen by facemask at 8-10 L/min.

12. Which action by the mother indicates a need for additional teaching about the care of the infant's umbilicus? *(844)*
    1. Gives a tub bath in the first 3 days after delivery
    2. Uses alcohol on the stump daily
    3. Folds the diaper down from the umbilicus
    4. Reports a foul odor or redness from the stump

13. What is included in the care of the circumcision? *(844)*
    1. Removing the yellow crusting right away.
    2. Applying the diaper loosely.
    3. Assessing for bleeding every hour for 4 hours.
    4. Using petroleum gauze under the Plastibell.

14. What is an appropriate technique to teach the new mother about the baby's bath? *(868)*
    1. Vigorous removal of the vernix caseosa
    2. Use of plain water on the perineal area
    3. Washing the baby twice daily
    4. Having the bathwater at 100° F (37.7° C)

15. The nurse is discussing sexuality with the new mother. What information should the nurse provide? *(842)*
    1. Menses usually returns in 3-5 months.
    2. Breastfeeding acts as an effective contraceptive.
    3. Discomfort and bleeding are expected with sexual activity.
    4. Avoid sexual activity until after the first postpartum office visit.

16. In teaching the new mother about breastfeeding, what should the nurse tell her? *(853)*
    1. Use one breast for two consecutive feedings.
    2. Have the baby nurse for 5 minutes at each breast.
    3. Put as much of the areolar tissue into the baby's mouth as possible.
    4. Pull the breast straight away from the baby's mouth to break the suction seal.

17. The nurse is teaching the patient about the signs and symptoms that should be reported to the provider. After 5 days from the delivery date, which sign/symptom warrants contacting the provider? *(843)*
    1. Temperature is 99° F.
    2. Lochia is light pink-brown in color.
    3. Breast is tender and red.
    4. Fundus feels like a softball.

18. The patient has opted to bottle-feed her newborn. Which the patient statement indicates that she understood discharge teaching related to breast engorgement? *(852)*
    1. "I will most likely not experience breast engorgement if I manually express the milk."
    2. "If I experience engorgement, I should use a covered ice pack for relief."
    3. "Engorgement will most likely occur about 10 days from my delivery date."
    4. "Breast engorgement is unlikely since I am not breastfeeding my baby."

19. The nurse is assessing a newborn infant who was born at 30 weeks gestation. Which findings would be considered normal? **Select all that apply.** *(861)*
    1. Vernix caseosa
    2. Lanugo
    3. Desquamation
    4. Good skin turgor
    5. Good tissue elasticity

20. The mother reports that the new infant is making a weak, high-pitched crying sound. She has tried feeding, changing, rocking, and ignoring the baby, but the crying continues. What should the nurse do **first**? *(871)*
    1. Assess the mother-child interaction to see if there are problems with bonding.
    2. Try swaddling or bundling the baby to make him feel secure.
    3. Ask the mother to hold the baby while vital signs are obtained.
    4. Contact the pediatrician, because the crying is excessive.

21. What are normal variations in the physical characteristics of a newborn? **Select all that apply.** *(860, 861)*
    1. Acrocyanosis in a 5-day-old infant
    2. The harlequin sign in a 2-day-old infant
    3. Jaundice during the first 24 hours after delivery
    4. Epstein's pearls on the hard palate of a 2-week-old infant
    5. Lacy mottling on pale skin immediately at birth

22. The home health nurse is assessing the mother's peripads 6 days after delivery. What is the expected finding? *(835)*
    1. Bright-red blood with tissue
    2. Thin pinkish-brown drainage
    3. Slightly yellow to white drainage
    4. Small clots with a fleshy odor

23. After delivery, which patient has the **greatest** risk for life-threatening postpartum hemorrhage? *(836)*
    1. Has a vaginal hematoma secondary to forceps-assisted delivery
    2. Has a vulvar hematoma associated with vulvar varicosity
    3. Has a vaginal hematoma related to primigravidity
    4. Has a retroperitoneal hematoma due to rupture of cesarean scar

24. Which treatment related to bowel function would the nurse question for a woman with a fourth-degree laceration of the perineum? *(837)*
    1. Administer stool softener for constipation as needed.
    2. Assist with ambulation in hall 3 or 4 times/day.
    3. Administer enema for constipation as needed.
    4. Encourage fluid intake of at least 3 L/day.

25. The nurse is explaining to a mother who had an episiotomy how to use a Peri bottle to clean herself after urination or a bowel movement. Which information is correct? *(839)*
    1. "First, clean perineal area front to back with toilet tissue."
    2. "Use the whole Peri bottle of water to cleanse the perineum."
    3. "Fill the Peri bottle with sterile water warmed to approximately 98° F (37.7° C)."
    4. "Flush the perineal area twice a day for 20 minutes."

26. The nurse sees that the postpartum patient has a platelet count that is on the high end of the normal range. Based on this observation, which action will the nurse perform? *(848)*
    1. Observe the patient for fatigue, particularly after exertion.
    2. Monitor temperature and watch for signs of infection.
    3. Encourage the patient to get out of bed and walk around.
    4. Watch for signs and symptoms of hemorrhage.

27. In the postpartum period, the patient has no urge to void, but the nurse notes that the patient's bladder is distended. What complications are **most** associated with bladder distention in postpartum patients? *(849)*
    1. Uterine hemorrhage and urinary tract infections
    2. Rectocele and uterine prolapse
    3. Kidney dysfunction and painful sexual intercourse
    4. Urinary incontinence and perineal lacerations

28. The postpartum patient complains of a persistent headache. Which action would the nurse perform **first**? *(839)*
    1. Obtain an order for a mild analgesic, such as acetaminophen.
    2. Reassure that pregnancy-induced headaches will abate.
    3. Check the blood pressure and compare it to baseline measurements.
    4. Check the record for history of epidural or spinal anesthesia.

29. The nurse notes that the patient is profusely diaphoretic during the first night after delivery. Based on the nurse's knowledge of what is expected for the healthy mother in the immediate postpartum period, which action is the nurse **most** likely to take? *(840)*
    1. Assist the patient to change clothes and explain that diaphoresis is normal.
    2. Monitor the patient's temperature, because diaphoresis suggests a fever.
    3. Check the patient's blood sugar to validate that the patient is not hypoglycemic.
    4. Assist the patient to sit upright, to facilitate respiratory effort and oxygenation.

30. The nurse is trying to teach a 15-year-old mother how to swaddle the baby, but the young mother seems more interested in fixing her hair and makeup. She states, "My boyfriend is coming in a little while." How should the nurse respond? *(841)*
    1. "Let's focus on the swaddling, then you can show him when he gets here."
    2. "You look very pretty. He will be delighted to see you and the baby."
    3. "Don't you want to spend some time holding and snuggling your baby?"
    4. "Well, you finish with your makeup and I'll take the baby back to the nursery."

31. The nurse hears in report that a patient who had a cesarean section should receive liquids for the first day with a gradual reintroduction to a regular diet. How does the nurse know when to offer solid foods? *(845)*
    1. Follow the protocol or clinical pathway for cesarean section patients.
    2. Give solid food when the dietary kitchen includes it on the meal tray.
    3. Call the provider to clarify specific parameters.
    4. Assess the abdomen and auscultate for bowel sounds.

32. The woman is interested in returning to her prepregnant weight as soon as possible. She has decided to breastfeed because "it's better for the baby and it will also help me lose weight." What information should the nurse give to the mother about nutrition and diet? *(845)*
    1. During breastfeeding, continue the diet recommended during pregnancy.
    2. For gradual weight loss, follow MyPlate suggestions and drink 3 L of fluid each day.
    3. Eliminate approximately 300-500 kcal/day for 6-8 weeks for weight loss.
    4. Breastfeeding does require extra calories, so weight loss is expected.

33. What is the **most** important nursing action to perform before assisting the woman to stand up and ambulate for the first time after the delivery of the baby? *(848)*
    1. Obtain a wheelchair and place it close to the bedside.
    2. Assist the patient to slowly sit and dangle legs while seated.
    3. Compare the blood pressure in the supine and upright positions.
    4. Assist the patient to apply a pair of slippers with a nonslip sole.

34. The patient received an epidural block. In the early recovery stage, what would be considered a normal finding? *(848)*
    1. Decreased sensation in both legs
    2. Altered level of consciousness
    3. Elevated blood pressure compared to baseline
    4. Low-grade fever

35. The woman's temperature is slightly elevated 12 hours after delivery of the baby. What additional assessment would the nurse perform **first**? *(847)*
    1. Check the appearance and odor of the lochia.
    2. Assess skin turgor and condition of mucous membranes.
    3. Palpate the fundus for height and firmness.
    4. Check a urine specimen for foul odor and cloudiness.

36. The unlicensed assistive personnel (UAP) tells the nurse that there was a gush of brownish vaginal drainage when the patient got out of bed and stood up. What should the nurse do **first**? *(848)*
    1. Inform the UAP that secretions pool in the supine position and flow is expected.
    2. Ask the UAP to describe the amount and color of the drainage and the patient's response.
    3. Check on the patient and assess for pain, dizziness, or continued vaginal flow.
    4. Tell the patient that there is nothing to worry about and help her clean up.

37. The mother reports to the nurse that the baby doesn't seem to be getting enough breast milk. What should the nurse do **first**? *(853)*
    1. Suggest that the mother supplement with formula feedings.
    2. Teach the mother how to manually pump the breasts.
    3. Assess the axillary region for engorgement of milk supply.
    4. Assess how the mother places the areola in the baby's mouth.

38. The nurse notices that the grandmother seems to be dominating the care of her own daughter and the new infant to the point of excluding the new father. What should the nurse do? *(855)*
    1. Gently suggest that the grandmother leave so that the new family can bond.
    2. Refer the family to counseling so that parental roles can be clarified.
    3. Assess the father's feelings about his role and his knowledge of child care.
    4. Wait until the grandmother leaves and then teach the father how to hold the baby.

39. The mother reports a mild cramping during the postpartum period. The nurse anticipates that the provider will write an as-needed (PRN) order for which medication? *(856)*
    1. Morphine
    2. Acetaminophen
    3. Aspirin
    4. Codeine

40. When is infant abduction **most** likely to occur? *(858)*
    1. During visiting hours
    2. In the middle of the night
    3. During the discharge process
    4. Upon admission to the nursery

41. Which assessment finding in a new infant should be reported to the provider for additional investigation? *(862)*
    1. Molding
    2. Strabismus
    3. Low-set ears
    4. Nystagmus

42. The nurse notes on assessing the newborn that there is a small tuft of hair at the base of the spine. What is the clinical significance of this finding? *(863)*
    1. This is the lanugo that frequently covers the newborn's body.
    2. This is part of the vernix caseosa that is usually left in place for 48 hours.
    3. Different skin colorations and hair patterns are related to genetic factors.
    4. Hair tufts indicate possible abnormalities of spinal column development.

43. Newborns are at risk for bleeding because of the lack of intestinal flora that synthesizes blood clotting factors. Which action would the nurse take? *(851)*
    1. Administer vitamin and mineral supplements as prescribed.
    2. Administer an injection of vitamin K as prescribed.
    3. Administer an injection of $Rh_o(D)$ immune globulin as prescribed.
    4. Monitor the color, frequency, and consistency of bowel movements.

44. Parents of a newborn have limited funds, but they want to provide something to stimulate their newborn. What is the **best** response? *(862)*
    1. "Your baby would like an object that makes happy sounds."
    2. "Your baby prefers to look at your face and eyes."
    3. "Many babies like intricate black and white images."
    4. "Most parents like to get something soft and snugly."

45. In the first few hours after birth, the neonate has a blood glucose level of 40 mg/dL. The nurse prepares for which intervention? *(867)*
    1. Oral feeding of sterile glucose water
    2. Oral feeding of prepared formula
    3. Oral feeding of 15-30 mL of sterile water
    4. Administration of intravenous dextrose

46. Which nursing observation of the newborn's bowel function should be reported to the provider? *(869)*
    1. Initial stool is black-green with a sticky consistency.
    2. Stool contains strands of lanugo, mucus, and vernix.
    3. No stool is passed 24 hours after birth.
    4. Newborn appears to be straining when passing stool.

CRITICAL THINKING ACTIVITIES

47. What information would the postpartum nurse expect to get in a transfer report on a new patient who has delivered her baby and is being moved from the recovery area to the postpartum unit? *(840)*

    _____

    _____

    _____

48. Identify the changes that occur in the mother's body systems after delivery. *(837, 839, 840)*

    a. Cardiovascular: _____

    _____

    b. Urinary: _____

    _____

    c. Gastrointestinal: _____

    _____

    d. Endocrine: _____

    _____

    e. Integumentary: _____

    _____

Care of the High-Risk Mother, Newborn, and Family With Special Needs

chapter
29

CROSSWORD PUZZLE

1. Directions: Use the clues on the next page to complete the crossword puzzle.

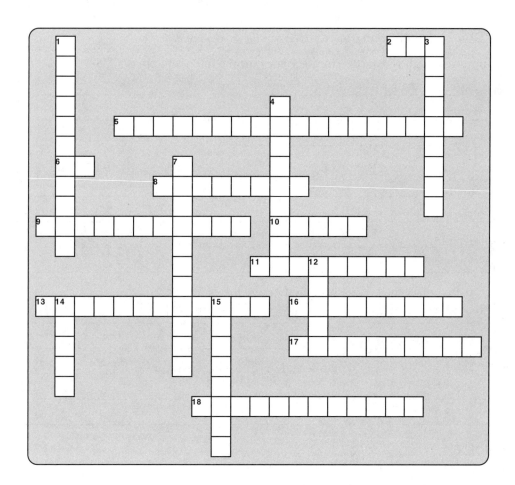

Across

2. Abbreviation for gestational diabetes mellitus *(875)*
5. Excess of bilirubin in the blood of the newborn *(912)*
6. Abbreviation for gestational hypertension *(875)*
8. Uses suture material to constrict the internal os of the cervix *(883)*
9. Phototherapy at home *(913)*
10. Organisms capable of crossing the placenta: toxoplasmosis, other infections, rubella virus, cytomegalovirus, and herpes simplex viruses *(895)*
11. Increased blood pressure after 20 weeks gestation with seizure activity *(890)*

13. Exposing the skin to fluorescent lights *(912)*
16. Number of deaths in a given population *(875)*
17. Excessive amount of amniotic fluid *(888)*
18. Increase in blood pressure *(890)*

Down

1. Twins begin with one fertilized ovum *(879)*
3. State of having disease *(877)*
4. Fertilization of two separate ova *(879)*
7. Abnormal toxic accumulation of bilirubin in central nervous system tissues *(912)*
12. Lack of normal tone or strength *(888)*
14. H, hemolysis; EL, elevated liver enzymes; LP, low platelet count *(893)*
15. Massive, generalized edema *(890)*

SHORT ANSWER
Directions: Using your own words, answer each question in the space provided.

2. Identify examples of high-risk factors in pregnancy for the following areas. *(876)*

    a. Biophysical:_____

    _____

    b. Psychosocial:_____

    _____

    c. Sociodemographic: _____

    _____

    d. Environmental:_____

    _____

3. Identify factors that place the postpartum mother and infant at risk. *(877)* _____

    _____

    _____

4. What are the characteristic physical manifestations of a preterm infant? *(910)* _____

    _____

    _____

MULTIPLE CHOICE
Directions: Select the best answer(s) for each of the following questions.

5. For a patient with hyperemesis gravidarum, which laboratory value is the **most** important to monitor for the prevention of cardiac arrhythmias? *(878)*
    1. White blood cell count
    2. Human chorionic gonadotropin level
    3. Potassium level
    4. Clotting factors

6. Which high-risk patient is **most** likely to need support and encouragement for follow-up because of the risk for developing cancer? *(880)*
    1. Woman has had two multifetal pregnancies.
    2. Woman's first pregnancy was ectopic.
    3. Woman had severe hyperemesis gravidarum.
    4. Woman was diagnosed with hydatidiform mole.

7. A woman comes to the emergency department. She recently had a positive home pregnancy test and is now having severe lower abdominal pain. She is pale, diaphoretic, and reports feeling lightheaded and dizzy. What should the nurse do **first**? *(881)*
   1. Take vital signs and assess abdominal pain.
   2. Put her on a stretcher and alert the provider.
   3. Obtain an order for a pregnancy test.
   4. Provide privacy and check for vaginal bleeding.

8. What teaching points should be included for a patient who had a spontaneous abortion? **Select all that apply.** *(883)*
   1. Report any heavy, profuse, or bright-red bleeding to the provider.
   2. Do not to use tampons until bleeding has stopped.
   3. Avoid sexual intercourse until bleeding has stopped.
   4. Be aware that scant, dark discharge may persist for 1 to 2 weeks.
   5. Postpone attempts to get pregnant for at least 1 year.

9. The nurse hears in report that the patient needs assessment for 1-2 hours after placement of prophylactic cerclage. What assessments does the nurse plan to make for this patient? *(883)*
   1. Monitor for dyspnea and abnormal lung sounds.
   2. Assess for headache and hyperreflexia.
   3. Check the fetal heart tones and the vital signs.
   4. Observe perineal pad count and signs of pooling.

10. Under which circumstance would the nurse anticipate a double setup? *(885)*
    1. Patient has undiagnosed vaginal bleeding and provider needs to do a vaginal examination.
    2. Patient has sudden onset of chest pain, dyspnea, cyanosis, and frothy blood-tinged sputum.
    3. Patient has a complete abortion and all products of conception are expelled from the uterus.
    4. Patient with no prenatal care and history of substance abuse arrives at hospital in active labor.

11. The nurse hears in report that the patient is at risk for disseminated intravascular coagulation (DIC), but so far the patient has showed no signs/symptoms. What is an assessment finding that alerts the nurse that DIC may be in progress? *(888)*
    1. Urinary frequency
    2. Elevated blood pressure
    3. Bleeding gums
    4. Low-grade fever

12. What are signs of cold stress in the neonate? **Select all that apply.** *(910)*
    1. Decreased temperature
    2. Shivering
    3. Pallor
    4. Lethargy
    5. Inconsolable crying

13. The preterm infant's greatest potential problem is respiratory distress syndrome. What is an **early** sign? *(910)*
    1. Nasal flaring
    2. Substernal retractions
    3. Circumoral cyanosis
    4. Grunting on expiration

14. Which patient may be a candidate for methotrexate therapy? *(882)*
    1. Patient has unruptured ectopic pregnancy.
    2. Patient has incompetent cervix.
    3. Patient has gestational hypertension.
    4. Patient has a vaginal infection.

15. The patient is diagnosed with a missed abortion. Which signs and symptoms does the nurse expect to find during assessment of the patient? *(882)*
    1. Malodorous bleeding, increased temperature, and cramping
    2. Some, but not all, products of conception are expelled
    3. Amenorrhea continues, but no uterine growth is measurable
    4. Bleeding increases and membranes rupture

16. What is the target outcome for a woman experiencing hyperemesis gravidarum? *(915)*
    1. Relief of painful uterine contractions
    2. Absence of fetal withdrawal symptoms
    3. Normalization of partial thromboplastin time
    4. Adequate caloric intake for maternal and fetal health

17. In the care of a patient who has just been admitted for hyperemesis gravidarum, which tasks can be delegated to the unlicensed assistive personnel? **Select all that apply.** *(878)*
    1. Assist with breakfast tray and encourage liquids.
    2. Measure and report frequency and amount of emesis.
    3. Assess for and report signs of dehydration.
    4. Assist with oral hygiene after episodes of vomiting.
    5. Assist the patient to maintain bedrest.
    6. Weigh the patient every day.

18. A patient is diagnosed with placenta previa. The provider indicates to the patient that she is stable enough to manage the condition at home. What instructions will the nurse give? *(886)*
    1. Take small amounts of clear fluid until vomiting subsides.
    2. Maintain bedrest, but getting up to the bathroom is allowed.
    3. Painless, bright-red bleeding is expected to continue.
    4. The prescribed tocolytic drug is used to relax the uterus.

19. The nurse's assignment on the postpartum unit includes patients with the following assessment data. Which patient should the nurse see **first**? *(890)*
    1. The patient has saturated one peripad within the last 2 hours.
    2. The patient has a blood glucose of 160 mg/dL.
    3. The patient had a spontaneous abortion and is experiencing moderate dark bleeding.
    4. The patient has had a continuous headache, upset stomach, and blurred vision.

20. The patient has a fasting blood glucose of 130 mg/dL. What sign/symptom would the nurse expect to find in conjunction with this laboratory result? *(897)*
    1. Cool, pale skin
    2. Increased appetite
    3. Frequent urination
    4. Irritability and tremors

21. The nurse is assisting an inexperienced provider who is in training to examine a patient with abruptio placentae. When would the nurse intervene? *(886)*
    1. The provider measures the fetal heart rate with a fetoscope.
    2. The provider sets up for a vaginal examination.
    3. The provider places the patient in a side-lying position.
    4. The provider orders an ultrasound scan.

22. Which patient is **most** likely to need vital signs every 15 minutes until stable and then every hour as indicated? *(886)*
    1. Has probable hydatidiform mole
    2. Had placement of prophylactic cerclage
    3. Has low-implantation placenta previa
    4. Has abruptio placentae requiring cesarean section

23. The nurse recognizes that the chance of hemolytic disease in the newborn is very low if which findings are present? *(911)*
    1. Mother blood type O, infant blood type A
    2. Mother Rh negative, father Rh negative
    3. Mother Rh negative, infant Rh positive
    4. Mother blood type B, infant blood type A

24. What are significant signs of gestational hypertension that should be immediately reported? *(890)*
    1. Weight gain with edema
    2. Vomiting and low potassium
    3. Tachycardia and fever
    4. Hyperglycemia and polyuria

25. Which medication does the nurse anticipate for the patient who is experiencing severe gestational preeclampsia? *(891)*
    1. Mcperidine
    2. Heparin
    3. Oxytocin
    4. Magnesium sulfate

26. The nurse is working with an adolescent mother who has just delivered her first child. What is the **most** likely problem for this patient? *(903)*
    1. Insufficient knowledge
    2. Inadequate fluid volume
    3. Poor health maintenance
    4. Insufficient cardiac output

27. The nurse is teaching the pregnant woman about prevention of infection. What is the **most** important teaching point related to toxoplasmosis? *(895)*
    1. Hand hygiene after using the bathroom
    2. Vaccination with an attenuated virus
    3. Delay of sexual relations
    4. Avoidance of cat litter

28. The nurse suspects that a postpartum patient being seen for her 6-week postdelivery check-up is experiencing postpartum depression (PPD). Which patient behavior is evidence of PPD? *(915)*
    1. Demonstrates little interest in her baby
    2. Talks extensively about her labor experience
    3. Reports fatigue due to infant's feeding schedule
    4. Admits to having some problems with breastfeeding

29. A woman who had an incomplete abortion several days ago reports sudden onset of chest pain and dyspnea. The nurse notes bleeding gums, petechiae, and ecchymoses. To support suspicion of DIC, which laboratory results will be immediately investigated and reported to the provider? *(887)*
    1. Cardiac enzymes
    2. Electrolyte levels
    3. Clotting factor studies
    4. Type, screen, and crossmatch

30. In the early postpartum period, the nurse notes a boggy uterus and the flow of lochia is heavy. What should the nurse do **first**? *(889)*
    1. Report suspected hemorrhage.
    2. Start intravenous oxytocin.
    3. Perform fundal massage.
    4. Continue routine assessments.

31. In the early postpartum period, the mother complains of severe, deep rectal pain. She has an increased pulse and respiratory rate and her skin is pale and cool. There are no obvious signs of hemorrhage that the nurse can see. What assessment should the nurse make to detect a possible hematoma? *(889)*
    1. Take the patient's blood pressure and compare it to baseline.
    2. Examine the vulva for a bulging mass or skin discoloration.
    3. Palpate the suprapubic area and listen for bowel sounds.
    4. Save all pads, linen savers, and linen to estimate blood loss.

32. The patient is diagnosed with gestational hypertension that is severe enough to warrant a prescribed antihypertensive medication. The morning blood pressure is 150/95 mm Hg. What should the nurse do **first**? *(891)*
    1. Administer the medication as ordered.
    2. Call the provider and clarify parameters for holding the medication.
    3. Compare blood pressure to baseline; then administer medication.
    4. Call the pharmacy and ask for contraindications.

33. The pregnant patient with HELLP (*H,* hemolysis; *EL,* elevated liver enzymes; *LP,* low platelet count) syndrome reports right upper quadrant and lower right chest pain, with nausea and vomiting. Which assessment technique should **not** be performed on this patient? *(893)*
    1. Auscultation of lung sounds
    2. Abdominal palpation
    3. Inspecting for hemorrhage
    4. Monitoring fetal status

34. To prevent mastitis, which teaching point would the nurse emphasize? *(894)*
    1. Take prophylactic antibiotics as ordered.
    2. Increase fluid intake to flush organisms from breasts.
    3. Empty both breasts regularly by feeding or pumping.
    4. Apply cold packs between feedings to reduce edema.

35. Which outcome statement **best** indicates that the plan of care for the patient with gestational diabetes is successful? *(898)*
    1. Patient continues in euglycemic state.
    2. Patient reports dietary compliance.
    3. Patient shows weight gain as expected.
    4. Patient is able to self-administer insulin.

36. The nurse is caring for a postpartum mother who was diagnosed and managed for peripartum cardiomyopathy. During labor, the mother required oxygen and demonstrated some transient arrhythmias, but otherwise had a normal delivery. What will the nurse plan to do in the care of this patient? *(902)*
    1. Routine care and assessment, because labor was the critical time for cardiac problems to occur.
    2. Obtain an order for oxygen as needed and continuous telemetry monitoring.
    3. Increase frequency of assessment for cardiac decompensation during the 48 hours after birth.
    4. Consult the provider to see if transfer to the coronary care unit is warranted.

37. In caring for the postpartum patient during the hospital stay, which intervention would the nurse use to prevent thromboembolic disease? *(907)*
    1. Assist to elevate both legs.
    2. Gently massage the legs.
    3. Administer oral anticoagulant.
    4. Encourage early ambulation.

38. The nurse is reviewing the laboratory results for a woman who comes to the clinic for routine prenatal visits. The nurse sees that the mother is Rh negative. Which question is the **most** important to ask the mother? *(911)*
    1. "How many children do you have?"
    2. "Do you know the blood type of the father?"
    3. "Have you ever received Rh$_O$(D) immune globulin ?"
    4. "Do you plan on having an amniocentesis?"

39. For a pregnant patient who is having a convulsion, place the nurse's responsibilities in the correct order (1-6). *(892)*

    _____ Provide oxygen by mask at 8-10 L/min.

    _____ Notify the provider that a convulsion has occurred.

    _____ Insert an airway after the convulsion, and suction mouth and nose.

    _____ Remain with the woman and press the emergency bell for assistance.

    _____ Observe fetal monitor patterns for bradycardia, tachycardia, or decreased variability.

    _____ If she is not on her side already, turn the woman onto her side when the tonic phase begins.

CRITICAL THINKING ACTIVITIES

40. During a routine prenatal appointment, the patient's blood pressure is 140/90 mm Hg. The nurse sees that this is an elevated reading compared to the past several appointments. The patient is currently at 22 weeks gestation.

    a. Describe the additional assessments that the nurse will make that will assist the provider in determining if the patient is developing gestational hypertension. *(890)*

    _____

    _____

    _____

    _____

    _____

    _____

    b. What is the treatment for mild preeclampsia? *(891)*_____

    _____

    _____

41. The nurse is interviewing a woman who comes into the clinic for prenatal care. She reports feeling thirstier than before with frequent urination and excessive hunger. When the nurse performs urine testing, the results indicate the presence of glucose. The provider recommends testing for gestational diabetes.

    a. Which diagnostic tests may be performed for gestational diabetes? *(898)* _____

    _____

    _____

    b. What complications for mother and infant are related to gestational diabetes? *(901)* _____

    _____

    _____

    _____

Health Promotion for the Infant, Child, and Adolescent

chapter

30

SHORT ANSWER

Directions: Using your own words, answer each question in the space provided.

1. Identify strategies to promote dental health for the following age groups. *(927)*

    a. Infant: _____

    _____

    b. Preschooler: _____

    _____

    c. Adolescent: _____

    _____

2. Identify at least one nutritional consideration for the following age groups. *(921)*

    a. Infant: _____

    b. Preschooler: _____

    c. Adolescent: _____

3. Identify three barriers to immunization for children. *(926)*

    a. _____

    b. _____

    c. _____

MULTIPLE CHOICE

Directions: Select the best answer(s) for each of the following questions.

4. Which lunch tray reflects a review of the top three caloric sources for children ages 2 to 17 years? *(920)*
    1. Fruit juice, granola bar, and ham sandwich
    2. Pizza, garlic bread, and a chocolate chip cookie
    3. Hamburger with French fries and a soda
    4. Chicken nuggets, potato chips, and ice cream

5. Which lunch tray for a school-aged child **best** reflects the Dietary Guidelines for Americans (USDA)? *(921)*
    1. Low-fat milk, vegetable soup, and orange slices
    2. Orange juice, whole wheat crackers and jelly
    3. Chocolate milk, plain pasta, and a cookie
    4. Skim milk, nachos with queso and sour cream

6. A group of adolescents decides to experiment with a hookah. Which adolescent is **most** likely to experience an immediate adverse effect? *(922)*
   1. Has a significant family history for throat and stomach cancer
   2. Has a significant family history for stroke and heart problems
   3. Has recently started taking antidepressant medication
   4. Had a recent episode of bronchitis with underlying asthma

7. The nurse is talking to an adolescent about responsible sexual behavior. Which question **best** demonstrates use of the principle of anticipatory guidance? *(924)*
   1. "What kind of precautions do you plan to use for protection during sexual intercourse?"
   2. "Are you sexually active now or thinking about having sex in the near future?"
   3. "Would you like to have information about sexually transmitted infections?"
   4. "Abstinence is 100% effective; is this consistent with your beliefs and behavior?"

8. What would be the **best** way for the nurse to contribute to the overall achievement of the *Healthy People 2020* goals? *(919)*
   1. Administer immunizations to infants during routine well-baby visits.
   2. Teach health promotion classes for parents/children at a community center.
   3. Pass out healthy snack samples in the waiting room at a local children's hospital.
   4. Give burn prevention brochures to parents when children are treated for minor burns.

9. A young couple is seeking advice about how to help their toddler develop good lifelong health habits. What would the nurse recommend as the **best** method? *(919)*
   1. Schedule the child for regular medical and dental check-ups.
   2. Encourage the parents to obtain the recommended immunizations.
   3. Enroll the child in a daycare program that includes exercise.
   4. Role-model a lifestyle that includes exercise and healthy foods.

10. Which male child has the **greatest** risk for developing obesity? *(920, 921)*
    1. A 3-year-old whose mother must work full-time
    2. A 9-year-old who eats at a fast-food restaurant every day
    3. A 13-year-old who spends 2-4 hours/day at the computer
    4. A 17-year-old who eats 5 meals a day with large portions

11. When an infant begins to transition from breastfeeding or formula to solid foods, which is recommended as the introductory food? *(921)*
    1. Strained applesauce
    2. Farina with whole milk
    3. Thinned rice cereal
    4. Strained bananas

12. The nurse is assisting a toddler to eat a healthy diet tray. Based on the child's developmental age, what would the nurse say? *(921)*
    1. "Drink your milk, then you can continue to play."
    2. "Let's have a race to see who can eat the most."
    3. "Would you like cheese or peanut butter on your bread?"
    4. "If you eat your vegetables, you will be strong like Daddy."

13. The nurse has a 14-year-old daughter who is refusing to wear sunscreen because "I want a tan just like my best friend." Using knowledge of growth and development for adolescents, what is the nurse's **best** response? *(921)*
    1. Tell the daughter that she can't go out unless she wears sunscreen.
    2. Review the dangers of skin cancer that are linked to sun exposure.
    3. Suggest that the best friend has heredity for naturally darker skin.
    4. Point out that red, peeling skin takes away from summer fashions.

14. Which age group is **most** at risk for foreign-body aspiration? *(928)*
    1. 1-5 months
    2. 6-12 months
    3. 1-2 years
    4. 2-4 years

15. The nurse is developing a nutrition plan with the parents of an overweight 12-year-old child. Which statement(s) by the parents demonstrate(s) an understanding of the plan? **Select all that apply.** *(920)*
    1. "Our child's calories from saturated fats should be no more than 7% daily."
    2. "We should not allow our child to drink milk that is less than 2% milk fat."
    3. "Our child should participate in physical activity for at least 60 minutes a day."
    4. "We should give our child foods from all the food groups except for grains."
    5. "Children outgrow obesity and complications when they reach adolescence."

16. Which statement by the child indicates an understanding of safety principles to reduce injury caused by motor vehicle accidents? *(925)*
    1. "I won't play outside anymore unless somebody goes with me."
    2. "I will wear my helmet if I am going a long ways on my bike."
    3. "I will 'stop, look, and listen' if I have to run to get my ball."
    4. "I won't play behind parked cars or at the curbside of the street."

17. Which child has the **highest** risk for accidental ingestion of a poisonous substance? *(928)*
    1. Infant who is just learning to crawl
    2. A toddler who is visiting grandma
    3. A school-aged child who is cleaning paint brushes
    4. An adolescent who is studying chemistry

18. The health care team seeks to reduce or eliminate substance abuse among all persons; however, which child represents the group that is currently of particular concern? *(923)*
    1. 15-year-old girl who admits to smoking cigarettes to impress older boys
    2. 17-year-old reports his parents allow him to drink beer whenever they do
    3. 12-year-old reports he and his friends experiment with any drugs they can get
    4. 9-year-old admits to watching her older brother smoke marijuana in the park

19. A nursing student is interested in a career in pediatrics and asks several pediatric nurses about common pediatric disorders and conditions. Which response **best** matches the health concerns for the current pediatric population in the United States? *(924)*
    1. "Childhood obesity is a problem and we are now treating kids for hypertension and heart problems."
    2. "We see a lot of physically abused or neglected children who are usually from low-income single-parent homes."
    3. "We see children with chronic illnesses or physical limitations and they are usually bullied at school."
    4. "Mental health issues that we see in pediatrics include depression, suicide, eating disorders, and substance abuse."

CRITICAL THINKING ACTIVITIES

20. Discuss benefits of physical activity and suggest ways that the nurse can promote physical activity for children. *(919)*

_____

_____

_____

_____

_____

_____

_____

21. The nurse is preparing a discussion for a community group about how to prevent accidental poisoning. What strategies will the nurse share that will help participants prevent accidental poisoning? *(928)*

_____

_____

_____

_____

_____

22. Explain the factors that contribute to tobacco use among adolescents and suggest interventions that the nurse can use to help teens stop or never start using tobacco. *(921, 922)*

_____

_____

_____

_____

_____

_____

_____

Basic Pediatric Nursing Care

chapter

31

SHORT ANSWER

Directions: Using your own words, answer each question in the space provided.

1. According to the Social Policy Task Force of the American Nurses Association, what are four essential features of nursing practice? *(935)*

   a. _____

   b. _____

   c. _____

   d. _____

2. Identify six stress points that are common for children undergoing surgery. *(957)*

   a. _____

   b. _____

   c. _____

   d. _____

   e. _____

   f. _____

3. Identify five things that the nurse can do to gain the trust of the pediatric patient's parents. *(957)*

   a. _____

   b. _____

   c. _____

   d. _____

   e. _____

FIGURE LABELING

4. Directions: Look at the Wong-Baker FACES Pain Rating Scale below and label each face with the appropriate description, then write an explanation that the nurse would give to a child about the scale so he or she could assess the child's pain. *(956)*

_____

_____

_____

_____

_____

TABLE ACTIVITY

5. Directions: Complete the table below with the average vital signs for each age. *(942)*

Vital Signs (Averages)

Age	Heart Rate/Min	Respirations/Min	Blood Pressure
Newborn			
1-11 months			
2 years			
4 years			
6 years			
10 years			
12 years			
16 years			

CLINICAL APPLICATION OF MATH AND EQUIVALENTS

Directions: Calculate or make the necessary conversions for math problems encountered in pediatrics.

6. The mother reports that her 4-year-old has grown 3 inches (1 inch = 2.54 cm) in the last year. How many centimeters has he grown? _____ cm   Is this growth within the normal range? _____ *(940)*

7. A 12-year-old is voiding 35 mL/hr. Over a period of 8 hours, how many mL of urine will he void? _____ mL *(946)*

8. The mother tells the nurse that she gave the child 4 cc (cubic centimeters) of liquid acetaminophen according to the instructions on the package. How many mL did the mother administer? _____ mL *(967)*

9. The nurse is measuring the urine output for an infant. The wet diaper weighs 20 g more than the dry diaper. How many mL does the nurse record as urine output? _____ mL *(964)*

10. A 6-year-old proudly hands the nurse an 8-ounce plastic cup full of urine, because he knows that "nurses like you to pee in a cup." Convert this to mL, so that the total can be added to the intake and output for the day. _____ mL *(964)*

11. A 16-year-old male weighs 161 lbs. He tells the nurse that he intentionally eats around 1,500 kcal/day to lose weight to secure his position on the wrestling team. What is the deficit of kcal/day according to daily caloric needs for his age and weight? _____ kcal/day. What should the nurse do? *(948)*

_____

12. A 15-year-old girl tells the nurse that obesity runs in her family and she would like to avoid gaining weight. She currently weighs 105 lbs. How many kilocalories per day does she need? _____ kcal/day *(948)*

13. A child has a temperature of 98.3° F. The nurse needs to record the temperature in Fahrenheit and Centigrade. Convert Fahrenheit to Centigrade. _____ ° C *(941)*

14. Determine the expected systolic blood pressure of a 5-year-old using the quick formula to calculate normal systolic blood pressure. What is the calculated systolic blood pressure? _____ mm Hg *(942)*

15. Determine the expected diastolic blood pressure of a 6-year-old using the quick formula to calculate normal diastolic blood pressure. What is the calculated diastolic blood pressure? _____ mm Hg *(942)*

MULTIPLE CHOICE
Directions: Select the best answer(s) for each of the following questions

16. Which family is **most** likely to be eligible for and benefit from a referral to the Women, Infants, and Children (WIC) program? *(934)*
    1. 22-year-old mother who needs emotional support to cope with a child who sustained a serious head injury
    2. 53-year-old mother of a 13-year-old child who is developmentally disabled and needs a new wheelchair
    3. 35-year-old single working mother of a toddler and preschooler, who is currently expecting her third child
    4. 15- and 16-year-old sisters who need counseling for prevention of pregnancy and sexually transmitted infections

17. Which nurse is **best** demonstrating the family-centered concept of enabling? *(936)*
    1. Nurse A tells the parents that the adolescent needs privacy and independence.
    2. Nurse B encourages the mother to show her partner how to burp the infant.
    3. Nurse C gives the child a small reward after a painful procedure is completed.
    4. Nurse D is truthful with the child and the family and follows up on promises.

18. The nurse reads in the provider's notes that the toddler is having physiologic anorexia. Which intervention is the nurse **most** likely to use? *(938)*
    1. Suggest three meals/day with planned snacks so the child eats every 2-3 hours.
    2. Obtain an order from the provider for a referral to a registered dietitian.
    3. Teach the parents how to do calorie counts and measure intake and output.
    4. Tell the mother that this is normal and that the child will eat when he gets hungry.

19. The nurse is working at a health fair performing growth measurements on children. Which children need follow-up for further investigation? **Select all that apply.** *(940)*
    1. 9-year-old male with height in the 10th percentile and weight in the 90th percentile
    2. 10-year-old male who had a sudden increase in height putting him in the 90th percentile
    3. 17-year-old male who has had no increase in height or weight since age 13
    4. 11-year-old male who continues in the 50th percentile for weight and height
    5. 13-year-old male with height in the 90th percentile and weight in the 10th percentile

20. A student nurse is performing routine measurements on an 18-month-old child. When would the supervising nurse intervene? *(940)*
    1. Student positions the child recumbent and extends the child's legs to measure length.
    2. Student uses a paper measuring tape to measure arm circumference
    3. Student asks the nurse if the child's clothes should be removed prior to weighing.
    4. Student puts the tape under the chin and over the top of the head for head circumference.

21. Which child is **most** likely to benefit from the en face position? *(941)*
    1. Toddler falls down and looks up at mother to gage her response.
    2. School-age child wants parent to look at a completed school project.
    3. Newborn infant shows quiet alertness after breastfeeding.
    4. Adolescent wants privacy while talking to friends on the phone.

22. A 4-year-old child comes to the clinic because of a sore throat and cough. The child is holding a doll and standing behind her mother and peering out around the mother's leg. The nurse needs to take a history, do the child's vital signs, and then do a focused assessment on the throat and upper airway. What action should the nurse perform **first**? *(953)*
    1. Say hello to the child and ask what her doll's name is.
    2. Stand at eye level of the child and welcome her.
    3. Talk to the doll and show the stethoscope to the doll.
    4. Ask the mother to sit and hold her child on her lap.

23. The mother tells the nurse that her 9-year-old daughter has pain on urination with frequency, and some brown spotting in her underpants. The mother also says the child seems more anxious than usual. What should the nurse do **first**? *(951)*
    1. Ask the mother to elaborate on symptoms and behavior.
    2. Ask the child about the discomfort and the brown spots.
    3. Alert the provider about possibility of sexual abuse.
    4. Help the child obtain a midstream urine specimen.

24. There is a cry for help; a child is having a grand mal seizure and the mother is cradling his head and sobbing. The child recovers quickly, but the mother repeatedly sobs, "I didn't know what to do." What can the nurse do to empower the mother? *(936)*
    1. Stay with the family and observe for complications.
    2. Reinforce the fact that the child is going to be fine.
    3. Tell her that managing the head was the correct action.
    4. Ask her if this was the first time she witnessed a seizure.

25. Which nursing action **best** exemplifies partnering with the parent of a toddler who has been admitted for an exacerbation of asthma? *(936)*
    1. Suggests that the mother take the toddler to the play area
    2. Instructs the mother on how to hold the nebulizer
    3. Asks the mother for advice about the child's preferred rituals
    4. Maintains a cheerful and warm attitude toward the toddler

26. What factors does the nurse consider when deciding which method to use to take a temperature measurement on a pediatric patient? **Select all that apply.** *(941, 942)*
    1. Child's ability to cooperate
    2. Parent's preference for route
    3. Child's developmental age
    4. Parent's familiarity with route
    5. Child's need for precise temperature
    6. Child's psychological response to method

27. Which set of vital signs is closest to the average findings for a 2-year-old child? *(942)*
    1. P 110, R 25, BP 94/66
    2. P 100, R 20, BP 110/80
    3. P 90, R 22, BP 108/70
    4. P 70, R 24, BP 120/76

28. Which vocalization exemplifies the vocabulary of a typical 1-year-old child? *(949)*
    1. "Mama, me; dada, me"
    2. "Burrr, ahhh, eeeehhhh"
    3. "Give me cookie cup."
    4. "When is daddy coming?"

29. Which set of vital signs for a 12-year-old child requires a follow-up intervention? *(942)*
    1. P 124, R 32, BP 126/66
    2. P 90, R 20, BP 100/80
    3. P 88, R 20, BP 110/70
    4. P 74, R 22, BP 110/76

30. The nurse is reviewing infant development. What is an expected finding? *(938)*
    1. Having a visual acuity of 20/100 at birth
    2. Enjoying "peek-a-boo" games throughout infancy
    3. Controlling bladder elimination by 18 months
    4. Tripling of birth weight by 6 months

31. The nurse is preparing to administer an immunization to a 4-year-old child in the pediatric clinic. What is the **best** way to communicate this event to the child? *(949)*
    1. "This may feel like a pinch."
    2. "Don't move when I give you this."
    3. "Do you want to take this medicine now?"
    4. "I will be coming back to give you a shot."

32. The nurse has to administer a liquid medicine that has a bitter taste to a 5-year-old. Which strategy would be the **best** to use? *(966)*
    1. Use a syringe to squirt the liquid along the side of the mouth.
    2. Give the child an ice pop to suck on beforehand to numb the tongue.
    3. Give the child a glass of sweetened juice immediately after the medicine.
    4. Hand the child the medication cup and allow independent sipping.

33. The nurse is evaluating the bath given to the infant by the adult caregiver. Identify what actions indicate a need for additional teaching. **Select all that apply.** *(959)*
    1. Using soap around the eyes
    2. Using a cotton-tipped swab to clean the ear canal
    3. Supporting the head while bathing the infant in a tub
    4. Washing the extremities after washing the face
    5. Washing the perineum in an anterior to posterior direction
    6. Retracting the foreskin of the male infant

34. An older school-age child will be having surgery with anesthesia. What would the nurse do to reduce anxiety? *(957)*
    1. Show the child the mask that will be used for the anesthesia.
    2. Introduce the child to a peer so they can talk about the experience.
    3. Reassure the child that the procedure is safe and necessary for health.
    4. Explain the special type of sleep that will occur with the anesthetic.

35. The mother of a toddler asks the nurse how to get him to eat right. What advice should the nurse give? *(960)*
    1. "Food should be left out, so the child can eat when he feels like it."
    2. "The child should be restrained in the high chair for meals."
    3. "The child should sit at the table for scheduled meals."
    4. "Meals should be arranged about every 5 hours for the child."

36. Which statements by the mother of a 3-month-old indicate that health promotion teaching has been successful? **Select all that apply.** *(938)*
    1. "My baby's birth weight should be doubled at the age of 6 months."
    2. "My baby should be actively exploring his environment."
    3. "My baby should enjoy parallel play by the age of 8 months."
    4. "My baby should enjoy toys that bang, shake, or can be pulled."
    5. "My baby should start eating rice cereals just before bedtime."

37. The nurse prepares to give an injection to an infant in the vastus lateralis muscle. Why does the nurse select this site? *(967)*
    1. This is the easiest area to expose on the baby.
    2. No blood vessels or nerves are near this site.
    3. This site is the least painful site for injections.
    4. The leg muscle is the least developed in an infant.

38. Which child is exhibiting behavior that warrants additional assessment? *(951)*
    1. 6-month-old infant coos and babbles to himself
    2. 2-year-old refuses to eat as much as he used to
    3. 10-year-old exhibits apprehension when another child cries
    4. 17-year-old is resistant to any parental suggestions

39. Which question **best** demonstrates the nurse's use of anticipatory guidance in helping the parents of an 8-month-old child? *(969, 971)*
    1. "Has your child been eating and drinking like he should?"
    2. "Have you looked at floor space from his perspective?"
    3. "Would you like to have a brochure on infant growth?"
    4. "Have you talked to the provider about immunizations?"

40. The nurse is trying to auscultate the bowel sounds of a 4-year-old child, but the child is resisting the placement of the stethoscope. What should the nurse do **first**? *(939)*
    1. Document the attempt as "deferred by patient."
    2. Let the child handle the stethoscope.
    3. Obtain the assistance of a helper.
    4. Ask the parent if the child has been eating.

41. Which vital sign should be performed **first** on an infant? *(941)*
    1. Temperature
    2. Pulse
    3. Respirations
    4. Blood pressure

42. Which assessment findings would be reported to the provider for follow-up? **Select all that apply.** *(944, 949)*
    1. Two palmar flexion creases in a newborn
    2. Tufts of hair along the spine of a newborn
    3. Preference for en face position in newborn
    4. Bumping into obstacles by 1-year-old
    5. Lack of babbling by a 9-month-old
    6. Tongue protrusion by a toddler

43. The mother who is breastfeeding her infant tells the nurse that the infant's bowel movements "look terrible." What should the nurse say to the mother? *(946)*
    1. "Infant stool is supposed to look different from ours because of immaturity."
    2. "The stool of breastfed babies is a light mustard color with seedlike particles."
    3. "The stool should be soft and formed with a pale greenish-yellow color."
    4. "As long as the baby does not have runny diarrhea, you should not worry."

44. What is the **best** rationale for advising the parent to withhold whole cow's milk until the child passes the 12-month mark? *(947)*
    1. Breast milk is cheaper and a better source of high-quality protein.
    2. The child is more likely to develop allergies to milk later in life.
    3. The protein and minerals in whole milk place stress on immature kidneys.
    4. Whole milk is more likely to cause vomiting, diarrhea, and flatus.

45. The aunt of an 11-month-old infant is making homemade baby food using materials that she has on hand. When would the mother intervene? *(947)*
    1. Aunt adds white sugar.
    2. Aunt uses a blender.
    3. Aunt mixes in honey.
    4. Aunt uses frozen peaches.

46. What is the **best** indicator of readiness to wean in a 9-month-old breastfed infant? *(947)*
    1. The provider says that most children wean around 9 or 10 months.
    2. The infant reaches for his siblings' or parents' cup or drinking glass.
    3. The father remembers that the sibling was weaned at 8 months.
    4. The mother has to return to work, so breastfeeding is increasingly difficult.

47. Which child needs cholesterol testing somewhere between the age of 2 and 10 years? *(948)*
    1. Mother has a total cholesterol level of 200 mg/dL.
    2. Father has a total cholesterol level of 300 mg/dL.
    3. Grandparent died of a heart attack at age 65.
    4. Grandmother had a coronary bypass at age 70.

48. While examining a child, the nurse finds human bite marks, linear ecchymosis patterns, and round red sores. According to the parent, "he frequently gets into fights at school." What should the nurse do **first**? *(951, 952)*
    1. Assist the provider to examine for occult injuries.
    2. Contact Child Protective Services and report suspected abuse.
    3. Ask the child to give details about how he sustained specific injuries.
    4. Assess the parent for signs of hostility toward the child.

49. How does the nurse use knowledge of body position and space to engage the preschooler and begin the nurse-patient relationship? *(953)*
    1. Stands in the doorway and greets the child by making a funny face.
    2. Directs the child to sit on mother's lap; then nurse holds child's hand.
    3. Puts chairs in a small circle and invites everyone to sit down.
    4. Allows the child to get comfortable; then nurse gets to child's eye level.

50. The nurse is placing electrodes on the chest of a 4-year-old child. What should the nurse say to the child? *(949)*
    1. "Feel this; like little round band-aids with a bit of cold jelly."
    2. "These snaps will hook you to the machine, so we can watch you."
    3. "The electrodes allow us to watch your heart beat all the time."
    4. "This won't hurt. It's just a way for us to see your heart."

CRITICAL THINKING ACTIVITIES

51. A 9-year-old child is being admitted to the hospital for surgical repair of a hernia. The nurse knows that the procedure should have an uncomplicated outcome, but the parents appear very nervous. The child is carefully watching his parents' reactions and the nurse sees that he is also fearful and distrustful of this new experience.

   a. What should the nurse do to reduce anxiety for the child and the parents? *(952)* _____

   _____

   _____

   _____

   _____

   b. What strategies can the nurse use when communicating with the child? *(953)* _____

   _____

   _____

   _____

52. a. Identify the guidelines for performing a physical assessment on a child. *(939)* _____

   _____

   _____

   _____

   _____

   b. Describe methods that can be used to have the child assist while you auscultate his/her lungs. *(945)*

   _____

   _____

   _____

   _____

53. Identify characteristics in yourself that would make you a good pediatric nurse. *(935)* _____

   _____

   _____

   _____

   _____

   _____

   _____

Care of the Child With a Physical and Mental or Cognitive Disorder

MATCHING

Directions: Match the disorder with the clinical manifestations. Indicate your answer in the space provided.

Physical Disorder

_____ 1. hypertrophic pyloric stenosis *(1008)*

_____ 2. nephrotic syndrome *(1013)*

_____ 3. pneumonia *(994)*

_____ 4. septic arthritis *(1024)*

_____ 5. cerebral palsy *(1029)*

_____ 6. hyperthyroidism *(1017)*

_____ 7. severe diarrhea *(1006)*

_____ 8. otitis media *(1042)*

_____ 9. hypothyroidism *(1015)*

_____ 10. Duchenne's muscular dystrophy *(1024)*

Clinical Manifestations

a. Cough, wheeze or crackles, respiratory distress, chest pain, fever, malaise, myalgia, nasal discharge

b. Cool, pale skin; sunken eyes and fontanelles; poor skin turgor; lethargy; rapid pulse and respirations; weight loss

c. Projectile vomiting, hungry, weight loss, peristaltic waves from left to right, palpable olive-shaped mass

d. Delayed growth, dry skin, constipation, lethargy, mental slowness, cold intolerance

e. Nervous, irritable, hyperactivity, tremors, excessive appetite, exophthalmos, palpable thyroid gland, tachycardia

f. Involuntary movement, hypertonic movements, arching of back, delayed gross motor development, drooling

g. Increased body weight, decreased urine output, ascites, periorbital edema, vomiting, anorexia, diarrhea, irritability

h. Clumsy, frequent falls, a waddling gait, difficulty running or climbing, Gowers' sign

i. Limited ROM to affected joint with erythema, edema, warmth, and exquisite pain; fever; limps or refuses to walk

j. Pulling, tugging, or rubbing the affected ear; fever; rhinitis; fussiness; irritability; decreased appetite

SHORT ANSWER

Directions: Using your own words, answer each question in the space provided.

11. The most current congenital heart disease categories are related to which four physiologic characteristics? *(977)*

   a. _____

   b. _____

   c. _____

   d. _____

12. Tetralogy of Fallot (TOF) involves a combination of which four defects? *(982)*

   a. _____

   b. _____

   c. _____

   d. _____

13. What are three pathophysiologic changes of blood components and the associated effects that develop as a result of leukemia? *(988)*

   a. _____

   b. _____

   c. _____

14. Identify the four classifications by causative agent for pneumonia. *(994)*

   a. _____

   b. _____

   c. _____

   d. _____

15. The ESSR feeding technique works especially well for infants with cleft lip/palate prior to corrective surgery. What does ESSR stand for? *(1004)*

   E _____

   S _____

   S _____

   R _____

TABLE ACTIVITY

16. Directions: Complete the table below by filling in the signs and symptoms for each assessment that indicates the clinical manifestations of dehydration. *(1005)*

Clinical Manifestations of Dehydration

Assessment	Signs and Symptoms
Skin	
Mucous membranes	
Eyes	
Fontanelles	
Behavior	
Pulse	
Blood pressure	
Respirations	

FIGURE LABELING

17. Directions: On the figure below, identify the assessment findings for the infant. *(1021)*

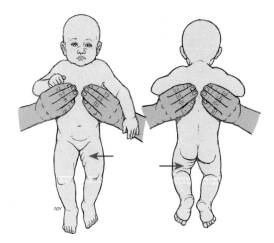

CLINICAL APPLICATION OF MATH AND CONVERSIONS

Directions: Calculate or make the necessary conversions for math problems encountered in pediatrics.

18. The nurse is performing a physical examination on a 6-month-old infant. At birth, the infant weighed 7 lbs. The current weight is 14 lbs. How much weight has the child gained in kilograms? _____ kg *(983)*

19. Toddlers require 7 mg/day of iron. The mother has purchased a bottle of liquid iron and the label indicates that there are 40 mg/15 mL. The mother is unable to determine how much to give. How many mL does the nurse tell her to give the child to achieve the correct dose? _____ mL *(983)*

20. The nurse must calculate an infant's urine output by weighing the wet diaper. The wet diaper weighs 35 g more than the dry diaper. What does the nurse record for urine output? _____ mL *(1005)*

MULTIPLE CHOICE

Directions: Select the best answer(s) for each of the following questions.

21. Which assessment is the provider **most** likely to ask the nurse to perform to assist in the diagnosis of possible coarctation of the aorta? *(983)*
    1. Take the blood pressure (BP) in the arms and the legs.
    2. Take manual BP in both arms, rather than using the automatic cuff.
    3. Take orthostatic BP: lying to sitting to standing positions.
    4. Take BP every 15 minutes for 1 hour; then every 30 minutes for 2 hours.

22. Which lunch tray provides the **best** food sources to help a toddler get the required 7 mg/day of iron? *(984)*
    1. Milk, chicken fingers, and biscuit
    2. Fruit punch, cheese and crackers
    3. Orange juice, and beef and bean burrito
    4. Low-fat milk and egg salad sandwich

23. An 11-month-old infant presents at the walk-in clinic with fever, vomiting, and irritability. He has a bulging fontanelle and demonstrates a high-pitched cry. The nurse also observes generalized petechiae over the trunk area. What is the **best** rationale for immediately notifying the provider about the infant's symptoms? *(1026)*
    1. Infant shows signs/symptoms of meningococcal meningitis.
    2. It is likely that infant has something contagious and requires isolation.
    3. Age of the infant creates an increased risk for sepsis and septic shock.
    4. Signs/symptoms suggest an illness that requires immediate attention.

24. For a child in sickle cell crisis, what are the **priority** interventions? **Select all that apply.** *(986)*
    1. Analgesics
    2. Comfort measures
    3. Sickle-turbidity test
    4. Oxygenation
    5. Hydration

25. Which child and family are **most** likely to need emotional support for anticipatory grief and loss immediately after being told about the medical diagnosis of their child? *(1024)*
    1. 3-year-old boy is diagnosed with acute bronchitis
    2. 4-year-old boy is diagnosed with Legg-Calvé-Perthes disease
    3. 2-year-old girl is diagnosed with Duchenne's muscular dystrophy
    4. 3-year-old girl is diagnosed with idiopathic thrombocytopenia purpura

26. The nurse is reviewing the child's medication list and sees that etanercept is prescribed. Based on the nurse's knowledge of pharmacologic therapy for juvenile rheumatoid arthritis, which intervention is the nurse likely to use **first**? *(992)*
    1. Encourage normal routines, such as homework and playing with friends.
    2. Plan a time for physical therapy to review range-of-motion exercises.
    3. Discuss how to use heat and cold to reduce swelling.
    4. Ask the parent and child about strategies they use to reduce pain.

27. Which nurse is **most** likely to encounter a child who needs care for respiratory distress syndrome? *(993)*
    1. Nurse A works in an after-school drop-in center.
    2. Nurse B works in a newborn intensive care unit.
    3. Nurse C works in a general pediatric hospital unit.
    4. Nurse D works in an allergy and asthma clinic.

28. The nurse is sitting at the front desk of a walk-in clinic. Simultaneously, several children come in with their parents. Which child should the nurse attend to **first**? *(997)*
    1. 12-year-old has no symptoms, but parents report that a sibling was recently diagnosed with tuberculosis
    2. 5-year-old has low-grade fever, malaise, anorexia, pharyngeal erythema, and sore throat
    3. 2-year-old demonstrates hoarseness, nasal flaring, intercostal retractions, and a barking cough
    4. 3-year-old is anxious with a high fever, muffled voice, drooling, and progressive respiratory distress

29. Which child is **most** likely to gain therapeutic benefit from blowing bubbles or pinwheels? *(1000)*
    1. 4-year-old diagnosed with cystic fibrosis
    2. 6-year-old with acute epiglottitis
    3. 3-year-old with cough and sore throat
    4. 5-year-old who just had a tonsillectomy

30. The nurse sees that the child takes fluticasone. Which assessment is the nurse **most** likely to perform to evaluate the efficacy of the medication? *(1002)*
    1. Auscultate for bowel sounds.
    2. Auscultate for breath sounds.
    3. Assess for relief of pain.
    4. Assess for relief of itching.

31. A nursing student is participating in the care of a child who is undergoing diagnostic testing for possible Wilms' tumor. When would the supervising nurse intervene? *(1015)*
    1. Student assists the child to obtain a midstream urine specimen.
    2. Student takes the child's weight and compares it to baseline.
    3. Student engages the child in quiet play to conserve energy.
    4. Student palpates the abdominal mass to assess for pain.

32. Which infant is **most** likely to benefit from a pacifier? *(1035)*
    1. Infant who recently had a cleft palate repair
    2. Infant who is being treated for a thrush infection
    3. Infant at risk for sudden infant death syndrome
    4. Infant whose mother abused drugs during pregnancy

33. In teaching a child and family about the dietary management for diabetes, what is the **most** important thing to emphasize? *(1020)*
    1. Avoid candy, desserts, and sodas with sugar.
    2. Maintain a consistent intake and timing of food.
    3. Learn to monitor blood sugar and adjust food accordingly.
    4. Eat the same food at the same time as the rest of the family.

34. The nurse hears in report that the child has nephrotic syndrome. Which assessments is the nurse **most** likely to perform? **Select all that apply.** (1013)
    1. Assess for worsening abdominal pain.
    2. Monitor intake and output.
    3. Check abdominal girth.
    4. Monitor platelet count.
    5. Monitor body weight.

35. The child has a hemoglobin (Hgb) value of 8 g/dL. Which symptom would the nurse expect to see at this Hgb level? (984)
    1. Fatigue
    2. Pallor
    3. Glossitis
    4. "Spoon" fingernails

36. What sign/symptom would be common to both patent ductus arteriosus and septal defects? (979, 981)
    1. Murmurs
    2. Chest pain
    3. Hypotension
    4. Headache

37. What is the **most** likely treatment for the majority of congenital heart defects? (982, 983)
    1. Diet therapy
    2. Exercise
    3. Surgery
    4. Medication

38. The walk-in clinic is conducting screenings on children for blood disorders. Which blood disorder is the **most** likely to be detected during general screenings? (983)
    1. Hemophilia
    2. Sickle cell anemia
    3. Iron deficiency anemia
    4. Idiopathic thrombocytopenic purpura

39. The nurse is instructing the parents of a child with iron deficiency anemia. What enhances iron absorption? (984)
    1. Giving the supplement with milk.
    2. Giving the supplement with citrus juice or fruits.
    3. Offering a chewable form once each day.
    4. Waiting until the child has a full stomach to administer.

40. Which children are **most** likely to need an iron supplement? **Select all that apply.** (984)
    1. A 5-month-old infant who is exclusively breastfed
    2. A healthy toddler with age-appropriate eating habits
    3. A 16-year-old girl who is trying to lose weight
    4. A preterm infant with low birth weight
    5. A 10-month-old infant who eats commercial infant cereal

41. A high school senior with sickle cell disease wants to take a vacation with friends. Which trip would be the **best** choice to avoid the precipitating factors of a sickle cell crisis? (986)
    1. Cross-country ski trip
    2. Hiking in the mountains
    3. Road trip to the beach
    4. Flying to Europe

42. The nurse is talking to the mother of a 10-year-old boy who has hemophilia. Which toy would be the **best** to recommend for this child? (987)
    1. Skateboard
    2. Football
    3. Swim fins
    4. Bicycle

43. Which blood disorder places a child at **greatest** risk for intracranial bleeding if head injury occurs? (987)
    1. Sickle cell anemia
    2. Sickle cell trait
    3. Iron deficiency anemia
    4. Idiopathic thrombocytopenia purpura

44. The child with leukemia has been placed on neutropenic precautions. Which person should **not** enter the room? (989)
    1. A 5-month-old sibling who was born prematurely
    2. A 3-year-old sibling who is coughing and sneezing
    3. A nursing student who is 5 months pregnant
    4. A parent who works at a waste management plant

45. For human immunodeficiency virus testing on a child who is younger than 18 months of age, what is the physiologic explanation for **not** using the standardized testing procedures [Western blot test and enzyme-linked immunosorbent assay (ELISA)]? *(990)*
    1. Infant's immune system is too immature to produce antibodies.
    2. It is unclear whether antibodies are the mother's or the infant's.
    3. The polymerase chain reaction test is safer for infants.
    4. Standardized tests yield too many false negatives for infants.

46. The nurse is talking to a 17-year-old who recently found out that he is human immunodeficiency virus (HIV) positive. He says, "I guess I really messed up. I'm in serious trouble." What is the **most** therapeutic response? *(991)*
    1. "Yes, you made a serious mistake, but you can take the medications."
    2. "You are very young and you shouldn't blame yourself for making a mistake."
    3. "You are thinking about your future and how to live with being HIV positive."
    4. "You sound really scared. Well, don't worry; with treatments, you'll be okay."

47. The child has recently been diagnosed with juvenile idiopathic arthritis. The nurse will prepare an educational brochure for which type of drugs? *(992)*
    1. Tumor necrosis factor blockers
    2. Disease-modifying antirheumatic drugs
    3. Slower-acting antirheumatic drugs
    4. Nonsteroidal antiinflammatory drugs

48. In caring for a neonate who was intubated for respiratory distress syndrome, when does the nurse perform endotracheal tube suctioning? *(994)*
    1. Routinely every 2 hours or according to facility policy
    2. According to the provider's written orders
    3. After auscultation of lungs and noting moisture in the tube
    4. When the neonate begins to secrete and cough up mucus

49. In the acute phase of respiratory distress syndrome, which route of feeding is **most** likely to be used for the neonate? *(994)*
    1. Bottle feeding
    2. Breastfeeding
    3. Parenteral nutrition
    4. Gavage feeding

50. The nurse is reinforcing the instructions to treat the child's viral pharyngitis with lozenges, gargles, and acetaminophen. The mother tells the nurse that she wants a prescription for antibiotics. What is the **best** response? *(996)*
    1. "The provider didn't order any antibiotics."
    2. "Viral pharyngitis is always treated conservatively."
    3. "Let me call the provider so that you can talk to him."
    4. "The throat culture showed no evidence of bacterial infection."

51. Which two conditions can develop if streptococcal infections are inadequately treated? *(996)*
    1. Hydrocephalus and nephrotic syndrome
    2. Rheumatic fever and acute glomerulonephritis
    3. Iron deficiency anemia and gastroenteritis
    4. Bronchopulmonary dysplasia and pneumonia

52. The nurse is caring for a child who had a tonsillectomy. Which report from the unlicensed assistive personnel is the **greatest** concern? *(997)*
    1. "I put the bed flat, because he wanted to go to sleep."
    2. "His pulse is 140 bpm, and earlier in the shift it was 90 bpm."
    3. "I gave him a cup of red soda, because that's what he wanted."
    4. "He got out of bed and has been running up and down the hall."

53. The nurse is assisting an inexperienced provider to examine a child who appears acutely ill with high fever, muffled voice, drooling, and progressive respiratory distress. The nurse would intervene if the provider started to perform which action? *(997)*
    1. Suggested that the mother hold the child on her lap
    2. Called the operating room to alert them about the child
    3. Examined the back of the throat using a tongue blade
    4. Took a history of preceding upper respiratory infection

54. The child presents with a nonproductive, hacking cough that worsens at night. The provider makes the diagnosis of bronchitis. Which instruction will the nurse give to the parent? *(997)*
    1. "Complete all antibiotics as prescribed."
    2. "Cough suppressants will cause drowsiness."
    3. "Use a cool-mist humidifier to relieve cough."
    4. "Withhold fluids at night to decrease secretions."

55. The nurse is working on the pediatric unit and five patients have bronchiolitis caused by respiratory syncytial virus. What infection-control measure should be considered in making care assignments? *(999)*
    1. Health care personnel with minor infections should not be assigned to these patients.
    2. Each patient is placed in a negative pressure room and care is more time-consuming.
    3. All of these patients should be placed in the same room with one nurse to give care.
    4. Nurses who care for these patients should not be assigned to other high-risk patients.

56. For patients with cystic fibrosis, which body system is targeted to prevent the **most** likely complications? *(999)*
    1. Cardiac
    2. Renal
    3. Gastrointestinal
    4. Respiratory

57. Immediately following cleft palate surgery, the infant is to receive nothing by mouth. After the nurse determines that the effects of the anesthesia have disappeared, what is the **first** thing to feed the infant? *(1004)*
    1. Breast milk
    2. Regular formula
    3. Dextrose water
    4. Normal saline

58. For the child experiencing gastroenteritis with diarrhea, which treatment does the nurse anticipate? *(1006)*
    1. Nothing by mouth
    2. Oral rehydration
    3. No solid foods for 48 hours
    4. Traditional BRAT diet

59. There are several different types of hernias that children may experience. What type of hernia usually has spontaneous closure by the time the child is 2 years old? *(1012)*
    1. Hiatal
    2. Inguinal
    3. Umbilical
    4. Diaphragmatic

60. Within hours of delivery, the neonate is diagnosed with the most severe type of hernia that requires immediate surgical repair. What signs/symptoms is the nurse **most** likely to observe with this condition? *(1012)*
    1. Regurgitation after eating
    2. No bowel movements
    3. Outpouching around umbilicus
    4. Difficulty breathing

61. Which pharmacologic treatment does the nurse anticipate for a child who has gastroesophageal reflux? *(1008)*
    1. Prochlorperazine
    2. Calcium chloride
    3. Cimetidine
    4. Fosphenytoin

62. The nurse is caring for an 8-year-old child who has severe diarrhea. IV fluid with potassium is prescribed by the provider and prepared by the pharmacy. Before the nurse hangs the IV solution, which function must be verified? *(1006)*
    1. Auscultate the lungs for the presence of crackles or wheezes.
    2. Check the urine output to ensure that output is at least 30 mL/hour.
    3. Auscultate for bowel sounds to determine presence of peristalsis.
    4. Check blood sugar for evidence of hypoglycemia.

63. A mother brings the 6-year-old child to the clinic for constipation. The mother reports that the child eats what the family eats, takes no medication, has no known health problems, and is very active. What questions will the nurse ask the child? **Select all that apply.** *(1007)*
    1. "What does it feel like when you try to go to the bathroom?"
    2. "When you feel like you have to go, do you go right then or wait?"
    3. "Do you take time to use the bathroom when you are at school?"
    4. "What do you think is making you so constipated?"
    5. "Would you like to eat more fruit, or would you rather take medicine?"

64. The nurse is caring for a child who had hydro-static reduction for intussusception. Which outcome statement indicates that the goal of the therapy was met? *(1010)*
    1. "Barium enema procedure was well-tolerated."
    2. "Parents understand the criteria for surgery if needed."
    3. "Bowel sounds are present; passing stool with barium."
    4. "Nasogastric tube is patent and suction is maintained."

65. Which treatment does the nurse anticipate for the child with nephrotic syndrome? *(1013)*
    1. Frequent ambulation
    2. Increased sodium
    3. Decreased protein
    4. Adrenocortical steroids

66. An infant is diagnosed with hypothyroidism. Which teaching point should be stressed? *(1017)*
    1. Prompt treatment is needed to avoid permanent cognitive impairment.
    2. A delay in treatment could result in damage to the heart and great vessels.
    3. Noncompliance with therapy will result in unusually short stature.
    4. Hypothyroidism will contribute to psychological disorders if untreated.

67. The nurse recognizes that hyperthyroidism is **most** common in which age group? *(1017)*
    1. Neonates
    2. Toddlers
    3. Preschoolers
    4. Adolescents

68. For a child with talipes equinovarus, which care is the nurse **most** likely to provide? *(1023)*
    1. Frequent assessment of breath sounds
    2. Assess for pain and administer medication
    3. Ensure that traction is maintained
    4. Teach parents about cast care

69. The provider asks the nurse for assistance in dealing with the family and examining a 1-year-old child who has a spiral fracture of the right forearm. The x-ray shows an old, healed spiral fracture in the same arm. Based on the nurse's knowledge of musculoskeletal development and fracture pathology, which situation is the nurse prepared to deal with? *(1025)*
    1. Parents will be devastated by possible diagnosis of bone cancer.
    2. Parents must be questioned about possible physical abuse.
    3. Parents must be counseled about possible genetic bone disorder.
    4. Parents need teaching about possible safety issues related to child's age.

70. Which intervention is **most** important for the nurse to implement in the care of a child with varicella? *(1044)*
    1. Initiate airborne and contact precautions.
    2. Use cool-mist humidifier for cough.
    3. Monitor cardiac and respiratory status.
    4. Initiate bleeding precautions.

71. What are the clinical manifestations that the nurse would observe in a school-age child with scoliosis? **Select all that apply.** *(1022)*
    1. Unequal hip and shoulder height
    2. Scapular and rib prominence
    3. Protrusion of the spine in the lumbar region
    4. Posterior rib hump that is visible when bending forward
    5. Taller than expected for age group

72. For a child with strabismus, which condition can develop if the strabismus is not treated? *(1047)*
    1. Myopia
    2. Hyperopia
    3. Presbyopia
    4. Amblyopia

73. After hearing in report that the child has a history of unpredictable sudden-onset status epilepticus, the nurse is **most** likely to check the availability of and obtain a standing as-needed (PRN) order for which medication? *(1030)*
    1. Valproic acid
    2. Phenytoin
    3. Lorazepam
    4. Carbamazepine

74. Which interventions would the nurse use during a child's seizure? **Select all that apply.** *(1031)*
    1. Tell someone to call the provider.
    2. Move the child to the bed when the seizure begins.
    3. Loosen restrictive clothing.
    4. Turn the child's head to the side.
    5. Push a tongue blade between the teeth.
    6. Stay with the child throughout the seizure.

75. What is the **most** important assessment that nurses who work in well-baby clinics should perform to contribute to the early detection of hydrocephalus? *(1027)*
    1. Weigh the infant at every visit and compare to the previous weights.
    2. Routinely measure head circumference and compare for rapid changes.
    3. Check the infant's pupillary response and accommodation.
    4. Ask parents about subtle changes in mental status or behavior.

76. The mother is quite frustrated because the child has attention-deficit/hyperactivity disorder, and it is taking several hours each night to help the child finish his homework. What would the nurse suggest for the mother to try **first**? *(1048, 1049)*
    1. Use a large variety of brightly colored shapes to hold the child's attention.
    2. Create an interactive approach that stimulates all of the senses.
    3. Have the child run and do very active play to tire him out before studying.
    4. Create a calm and quiet space with limited objects and fewer distractions.

77. The nurse anticipates that the child who is depressed could receive which medication? *(1053)*
    1. Fluoxetine
    2. Methylphenidate
    3. Diphenhydramine
    4. Dextroamphetamine

78. Which statement by the parents of a child with an IQ of 40 demonstrates an understanding of the child's capabilities? *(1048)*
    1. "Our child can go to school, but he may have difficulties with abstract concepts."
    2. "Our child can be taught activities of daily living and perform them on his own."
    3. "Our child is likely to have trouble with tasks like swallowing or sitting upright on his own."
    4. "Our child will never be able to perform self-care tasks like bathing on his own."

79. How can the nurse assist and support the parents if the child is experiencing school avoidance? *(1051)*
    1. Reassure parents that the behavior is normal and related to stress.
    2. Tell the parents to allow the child to stay home if he is too stressed.
    3. Tell the child that no one will pressure him if he doesn't want to go.
    4. Suggest getting the homework assignments when he misses school.

80. What are appropriate interventions for a child with autism? **Select all that apply.** *(1051)*
    1. Bring favorite possessions during hospitalization.
    2. Give written material about treatment options for cure.
    3. Vary routine and schedule from day to day.
    4. Provide brief, concrete communication with the child.
    5. Promote increased auditory and visual stimulation.

CRITICAL THINKING ACTIVITIES

81. a. Discuss information that the nurse can share with parents about preventing sudden infant death syndrome (SIDS). *(995)*

    _____

    _____

    _____

    _____

    _____

    _____

    b. Identify risk factors for SIDS. *(995)* _____

    _____

    _____

    _____

    _____

    _____

c.   Describe ways that the nurse could present the information to parents to help prevent SIDS. *(996)*

_____

_____

_____

82. For bronchial asthma, identify the following. *(1001, 1002)*

a.   Signs and symptoms: _____

_____

b.   Diagnostic tests: _____

_____

c.   Medical treatment: _____

_____

d.   Nursing interventions: _____

_____

83. For lead poisoning, identify the following. *(1033)*

a.   Sources of lead: _____

_____

b.   Prevention: _____

_____

c.   Parent guidelines to reduce lead levels: _____

_____

84. The school nurse is talking to a 15-year-old girl. The girl tells the nurse that one of the teachers accused her of using drugs because she thought "I was acting weird." The nurse asks her to describe the "weird behavior" and the girl talks about being withdrawn, with less interest in schoolwork, school activities, or socializing with her friends. Further assessment reveals that the girl often feels sad, down, and empty and has fantasized about committing suicide.

a.   What questions would the nurse ask? *(1054)* _____

_____

_____

b.   How would the nurse determine whether to contact others, such as parents, health-care provider, or school administrators? *(1054)*

_____

_____

_____

Health Promotion and Care of the Older Adult

TABLE ACTIVITY

1. Directions: Fill in the blank boxes to complete the table for comparison of characteristics associated with delirium, dementia, and depression. *(1088)*

	Delirium	Dementia	Depression
Onset	Sudden		
Cognitive impairment		Minimal cognitive impairment initially; progresses to impaired abstract thinking, judgment, memory, thought patterns, calculations, agnosia	
Activity	Increased or decreased; may fluctuate		
Speech and language		Disordered, rambling, or incoherent; struggles to find words	
Reversibility			Can be treated

CLINICAL APPLICATION OF MATH AND CONVERSIONS

Directions: Calculate or make the necessary conversions for math problems encountered in geriatrics.

2. The nurse is performing a physical examination on an 83-year-old resident. On admission to the long-term care unit, the resident weighed 106 lbs. The current weight is 110 lbs. How much weight has the resident gained in kilograms? _____ kg *(1069)*

3. The patient, age 80 years, weighs 130 lbs. To maintain this weight, the patient needs to take in approximately 30 calories per kilogram of body weight per day. How many calories per day should the patient consume? _____ calories *(1069)*

4. An older woman weighed 120 lbs in January. In June, the patient weighs 108 lbs. The patient denies any intentional efforts to lose weight. What percent of the total body weight was lost in 6 months? _____ %

   What should the nurse do? *(1069)* _____

   _____

5. The patient's fluid intake is shown below. What is the total fluid intake in mL? _____ mL

   What should the nurse do? *(1069)* _____

   _____

Time	Amount
700	6 oz of low-fat milk, 6 oz of coffee
1000	8 oz of water
1200	250 mL of water
1400	4 oz of water
1700	250 mL of iced tea
1900	3 oz of juice

6. The nurse is monitoring the patient's urinary output because the patient is on several medications that can be affected by changes in renal excretion. If the patient voids 500 mL over a period of 8 hours, how many mL is the patient producing per hour? _____ mL *(1073)*

MULTIPLE CHOICE

Directions: Select the best answer(s) for each of the following questions.

7. Which assessment finding of the integumentary system is the **most** important to report to the provider or dermatologist? *(1066)*
   1. Tan or brown macule spots
   2. Thick, brittle, yellowed nails
   3. Thin skin with purple patches
   4. Irregular, raised, crusted lesion

8. The nurse determines that a resident is fatigued today, so a partial bath would be acceptable in place of a full bath. Regarding the partial bath, what instructions will the nurse give to the unlicensed assistive personnel(UAP)? *(1067)*
   1. "Assist the patient to wash the perineal area and then the hands."
   2. "Help the resident wash his face, hands, armpits, and perineal area."
   3. "Before breakfast, help the resident wash his hands and face."
   4. "Perform a partial bath on the patient, just for today."

9. The nurse sees that patient is taking a diuretic medication. Which laboratory result is the nurse **most** likely to monitor? *(1092)*
   1. Serum potassium
   2. Urinalysis results
   3. Blood glucose
   4. Serum calcium

10. The nurse is **most** likely to question the prescription for an enteral feeding tube for which patient? *(1071)*
    1. 68-year-old patient who was in an auto accident
    2. 73-year-old patient who has advanced dementia
    3. 65-year-old patient who sustained severe burns
    4. 70-year-old patient who had surgery for lip cancer

11. The UAP tells the nurse that for the past 3 days, a thin brown liquid has been oozing from the resident's rectal area, but there is no formed stool. What should the nurse do **first**? *(1072)*
    1. Tell the UAP to assist the resident to the bathroom every 2 hours.
    2. Instruct the UAP to continue to change the incontinence pants as needed.
    3. Check the resident for a fecal impaction and assess the surrounding skin.
    4. Obtain an order for a stool hemoccult and culture and sensitivity.

12. The patient retired years ago. He was very involved with community, family, and friends, but now appears content to spend more time alone and others support his privacy. Which theory of aging **most** directly explains his behavior? *(1064)*
    1. Disengagement theory
    2. Exchange theory
    3. Continuity theory
    4. Activity theory

13. Which nurse is **most** likely to need an extensive knowledge and understanding of the Patient Self-Determination Act? *(1066)*
    1. Nurse A helps patients and families understand Medicare benefits.
    2. Nurse B cares for patients and families during end-of-life.
    3. Nurse C works at an outpatient surgical and diagnostic center.
    4. Nurse D counsels older people at a community senior citizen center.

14. The patient has a history of peripheral vascular disease. Which symptom is the cause for **greatest** concern? *(1075, 1076)*
    1. Gradual and progressive edema going up both legs
    2. Excessive warmth of the leg on the dominant side
    3. Sudden onset of a cold foot on the non-dominant side
    4. Cramping of the calf muscles after exertion

15. The patient is recovering from a stroke, but some residual symptoms continue. Which statement by a nursing student demonstrates an understanding that precautions need to be taken during meals? *(1071)*
    1. "The aphasia improves as the condition improves."
    2. "Dysphagia creates a risk for developing pneumonia."
    3. "Presbyopia will improve with corrective devices."
    4. "Appropriate exercises will counteract akinesia."

16. The patient reports that nocturia usually occurs once each night, but recently the urge has increased to 4-5 times. What should the nurse suggest as the **first** measure? *(1073)*
    1. Assess the environment for fall hazards.
    2. Take diuretic medication in the morning.
    3. Contact the provider for medical evaluation.
    4. Limit fluids and semisolid foods at bedtime.

17. The UAP is assigned to assist an older adult who is experiencing pruritus with bathing and hygiene. The nurse would intervene if the UAP performs which action? *(1067)*
    1. Uses tepid water for washing and rinsing the body.
    2. Uses an antibacterial soap to reduce potential for infection.
    3. Gives a partial bath of face, hands, axillary, and perineal areas.
    4. Applies a water-based lotion with gentle even strokes.

18. For the older adult patient with dysphagia, which intervention is appropriate to use during mealtimes? *(1071)*
    1. Add thickeners to liquids.
    2. Feed the patient quickly to reduce fatigue.
    3. Place the patient in low Fowler's position.
    4. Provide opportunities for socialization while eating.

19. The patient is taking alendronate. Based on knowledge of this medication, which intervention will the nurse use when caring for the patient? *(1080)*
    1. Handle gently when assisting to move or change position.
    2. Encourage pursed-lip breathing to control breathlessness.
    3. Frequently note the rate, regularity, and strength of the pulse.
    4. Teach the patient how to perform Kegel exercises.

20. The nurse notes that the patient has kyphosis. Which symptom is cause for the **greatest** concern because of the kyphosis? *(1076)*
    1. Heartburn sensation after eating large meal
    2. Weak stream when urinating
    3. Swelling of ankles with prolonged sitting
    4. Difficulty coughing up secretions

21. The nurse is giving a health promotion presentation to a community group of older people. What would be included as primary prevention strategies? **Select all that apply.** *(1061)*
    1. Quit smoking to reduce the risk of heart disease.
    2. Eat a well-balanced diet without excess sugar, fat, or alcohol.
    3. Receive the recommended vaccinations.
    4. Take prescribed medications according to instructions.
    5. Do 20-30 minutes of moderate exercise three to five times a week.

22. Which statement by a senior citizen **best** indicates an understanding of the "donut hole" in her Medicaid prescription plan? *(1065)*
    1. "My dental bills are covered if my dentist prescribes any medication."
    2. "I don't have any money to pay for extra nongeneric medications."
    3. "A percentage of the cost of medications is paid to a certain amount."
    4. "The Affordable Care Act is going to take care of all my medical expenses."

23. The nurse is talking to the daughter of a patient who has dementia. Which comment by the daughter **most** strongly indicates problems related to the caregiver role? *(1091)*
    1. "Would you think I was a horrible person if I asked about respite care?"
    2. "Dealing with Dad is pretty exhausting, but I try to focus on happier times."
    3. "Well, I had to decrease my hours at work, but they do let me telecommute."
    4. "My sister says that I am too impatient with Dad, but she doesn't offer to help."

24. The patient reports feelings of grief related to multiple losses and recent death of her spouse. She appears sad and withdrawn. What is the **best** intervention to help this patient deal with grief and loss? *(1065)*
    1. Role-model cheerful and optimistic behavior.
    2. Encourage alone time and introspection.
    3. Help to set realistic short-term goals.
    4. Suggest temporarily moving in with an adult child.

25. The nurse is caring for a very thin patient who is bedridden. Which intervention is the **best** method to prevent damage to the skin at pressure points? *(1067)*
    1. Gently massage fragile skin with water-based lotion.
    2. Reposition the patient at least every 2 hours.
    3. Use a mechanical lifting device to prevent shearing forces.
    4. Place pressure-reducing pads and aids over bony prominences.

26. The nursing student is caring for a patient with fragile skin. The nurse would intervene if the student performed which actions? **Select all that apply.** *(1067)*
    1. Asks the patient to grab side rail and slide across the bed to change wet linens
    2. Secures the patient's IV with several pieces of tape to prevent dislodgement
    3. Washes dried fecal material from rectal area and rubs to dry moisture
    4. Asks for lifting help when trying to move patient from bed to stretcher
    5. Firmly grasps the patient on the forearm when moving from bed to chair

27. The nurse hears during handover report that the patient has a diminished gag reflex. Which morning assessment would be particularly important? *(1067)*
    1. Checking other reflexes
    2. Auscultating lung fields
    3. Assessing for pain in the neck area
    4. Assessing nutritional status

28. The nurse is encouraging the older adult to reduce calories and consume quality foods. Which breakfast choice is the **best** to supply vitamins, minerals, and fiber? *(1072)*
    1. Biscuits and gravy with coffee and artificial sweetener
    2. Orange juice and a low-fat banana-nut muffin
    3. Bacon with white toast and skim milk
    4. Oatmeal with fresh berries and hot tea

29. The patient reports controlling incontinence by limiting fluid intake. To encourage the patient to meet the minimum daily intake of 1500 mL of fluid, which intervention would be the **most** helpful? *(1073)*
    1. Suggest the use of an adapted cup with a double handle.
    2. Propose voiding every 2 hours during the day and every 4 hours at night.
    3. Divide the 1500 mL of fluid into portions to be taken during waking hours.
    4. Emphasize the importance of adequate fluid for body function.

30. The patient reports sensation of abdominal distention and early satiety. Based on knowledge of how aging affects gastric motility, which intervention would the nurse suggest? *(1095)*
    1. Walking for short distances several times a day
    2. Cooking food with a variety of different seasonings
    3. Preparing homemade frozen dinners with extra portions
    4. Performing oral hygiene to remove offensive tastes and odors

31. Which patient statement is **most** relevant to the medical diagnosis of gastric reflux? *(1070)*
    1. "I have never really liked the taste of milk."
    2. "I have gained a lot of weight within the last year."
    3. "Lately, my stool seems to be a very dark brown color."
    4. "Recently, I noticed a sore in mouth that won't heal."

32. The patient requests a laxative because "I feel constipated." What should the nurse do **first**? *(1071)*
    1. Find out when the last laxative was administered.
    2. Assist the patient to the bathroom and observe afterward.
    3. Ask the patient to describe the typical bowel pattern.
    4. Offer a high-fiber snack of prune juice and bran muffin.

33. The nurse is teaching the patient about self-care measures for modifiable cardiac risk factors. Which teaching points would be included? **Select all that apply.** *(1074)*
    1. Take blood pressure medications as prescribed.
    2. Decrease intake of complex carbohydrates and vegetable proteins.
    3. Perform moderate exercise 30 min/day at least twice a week.
    4. Aim for body mass index of 18.5-24.9 kg/m².
    5. Get adequate sleep and rest.
    6. Avoid exposure to secondhand smoke.

34. The patient with chronic obstructive pulmonary disease states, "I can't cough up this phlegm in the back of my throat." Which intervention is the **best** to address this problem? *(1077)*
    1. Teach purse-lipped breathing.
    2. Promote moderate exercise 3-5 days/week.
    3. Use oxygen therapy as prescribed.
    4. Encourage plenty of fluids to liquefy secretions.

35. A normally cheerful and alert resident in a long-term facility demonstrates lethargy, disorientation, and her skin is very warm. What action should the nurse take **first**? *(1072, 1077)*
    1. Allow the patient to rest for several hours and then reassess mental status.
    2. Increase lighting, give sips of fluid, and control ambient room temperature.
    3. Check vital signs, blood glucose, and pulse oximeter reading.
    4. Use reality orientation and give simple, brief commands.

36. The nurse walks into a room and finds the patient on the floor. The patient reports severe pain in the hip area and the affected leg appears shorter than the other side. What should the nurse do **first**? *(1079)*
    1. Assist the patient back into bed.
    2. Assess for other injuries.
    3. Immobilize the affected side.
    4. Report the findings to the provider.

37. The nurse is interviewing a 56-year-old woman who reports that over the past year she has had frequent minor infections, minor wounds that seem slow to heal, blurred vision, and weight gain. Which laboratory finding is **most** likely to be observed? *(1081)*
    1. Elevated thyroid-stimulating hormone level
    2. Elevated blood glucose level
    3. Elevated estrogen level
    4. Elevated serum cholesterol level

38. The nurse notes that the patient's total cholesterol level is elevated. Which dietary information is the **most** relevant to this laboratory finding? *(1075)*
    1. Elevation of cholesterol is not related to current diet.
    2. Consumption of fluid and fiber should be increased.
    3. Amount of saturated fat in diet should be decreased.
    4. Reduce caloric intake to achieve a body mass index of 18.5-24.9 kg/m².

39. Patient reports "running out of my levothyroxine several weeks ago." What sign/symptom would the nurse expect because the patient has not been taking the medication? *(1082)*
    1. Apathy
    2. Heat intolerance
    3. Diarrhea
    4. Weight loss

40. A newly graduated nurse, age 22, is starting an interview with a 68-year-old patient who presents himself as very proper and conservative. The nurse feels that she will have trouble asking questions related to sexuality. What is the **best** strategy for this situation? *(1082)*
    1. Get another nurse to complete the interview.
    2. Have the patient wait and quickly assess own discomfort.
    3. Ask the patient for permission to initiate the discussion about sex.
    4. Defer the questions until after rapport is established.

41. The nurse is making a home visit and notices that the patient is squinting while reading the newspaper. There is no eye chart available to test the patient's vision. What should the nurse do **first**? *(1084)*
    1. Ask the patient to read the newspaper out loud.
    2. Suggest an appointment with an eye doctor.
    3. Assess the eyes for yellowing of the lens.
    4. Use a small flashlight to check pupil reaction.

42. Which symptom is an **early** sign of primary open-angle glaucoma? *(1084)*
    1. Severe eye pain
    2. Rainbow halo surrounding lights
    3. Pupil dilation
    4. Deteriorating peripheral vision

43. The patient watches the speaker's lips and tilts head towards the person who is speaking. Which position should the nurse assume when interviewing the patient? *(1085)*
    1. Stand near the window, so that there is bright light behind the nurse.
    2. Sit at the patient's eye level and directly face the patient.
    3. Sit beside the patient with mouth at the level of best ear.
    4. Stand over the patient, but lean into eye level when speaking.

44. The nurse works in a long-term care facility and is concerned about the quality of care. Which concern would be supported by the Omnibus Budget Reconciliation Act of 1987? *(1096)*
    1. A resident cannot file a complaint because there is no assigned ombudsman.
    2. A resident's chronic health condition was never assessed or documented.
    3. A resident is treated disrespectfully and there are no consequences for the offender.
    4. A resident dies and the room is immediately assigned to a new resident.

45. A patient has Parkinson's disease. Which long-term outcome is considered the **most** important? *(1089, 1090)*
    1. Adapting to long-term memory loss through reminiscence
    2. Maintaining mobility through exercise and activity
    3. Decreasing confusion by using reality orientation
    4. Managing pain with pharmacologic and nonpharmacologic intervention

46. The patient is slowly recovering from a cerebrovascular accident, but hemianopia has not resolved. Which reminder will the nurse give during mealtimes? *(1090)*
    1. Sit upright before attempting to eat and swallow.
    2. Ask for help if having trouble with utensils or opening wrapped items.
    3. Move head to the right and left when looking at the food tray.
    4. Minimize distractions and focus on chewing and swallowing.

47. Which factors contribute to polypharmacy where the risk for the patient outweighs the benefits? **Select all that apply.** *(1091)*
    1. Takes five or more prescription medications
    2. Sometimes borrows medication
    3. Uses a pill box with pockets for each day of the week
    4. Uses over-the-counter medications including vitamins and herbal preparations
    5. Sees primary care provider on a regular basis
    6. Fills prescriptions at local pharmacies and through the mail

48. The nurse is discharging an older woman to return home to the care of her daughter. Which patient response would prompt the nurse to gather more information about possible elder abuse? *(1093, 1094)*
    1. "My daughter leaves me alone when she goes to work."
    2. "You are nice. Would you come and visit me sometime?"
    3. "Could I have a lunch tray before I go home?"
    4. "When you are old, family can do whatever they want with you."

49. The patient had minor surgery 8 hours ago. He refuses to walk to the bathroom. "I'm old and I just had surgery. You should bring me the urinal. That's what you get paid for." What is the **best** response? *(1095)*
    1. "I'll bring you the urinal, but you have to promise to get up soon."
    2. "Actually, I get paid to make sure that you recover from your surgery."
    3. "Getting up helps prevent constipation, pneumonia, and blood clots."
    4. "Sir, your provider has ordered that you get up and walk around."

50. Which nursing action helps meet goals for older adults according to *Healthy People 2020*? *(1063)*
    1. Checks the patient's blood pressure every 4 hours while in the hospital
    2. Reminds patients that testing stool for occult blood should be done monthly
    3. Teaches fall prevention tips to community-dwelling older adults
    4. Reports onset of new symptoms promptly to the primary care provider

CRITICAL THINKING ACTIVITIES

51. For the following systems, describe changes related to aging.
    a. Integumentary system: *(1067)* _____
    b. Gastrointestinal system: *(1069)* _____
    c. Urinary system: *(1072)* _____
    d. Cardiovascular system: *(1074)* _____
    e. Respiratory system: *(1076)* _____
    f. Musculoskeletal system: *(1078)* _____
    g. Endocrine system: *(1081)* _____
    h. Reproductive system: *(1082)* _____
    i. Neurologic system: *(1086)* _____
    j. Sensory system: *(1083)*
       Vision: _____
       Hearing: _____
       Taste and smell: _____

52. For the following systems, describe the nursing assessment of the older adult.
    a. Integumentary: *(1066)* _____

b. Cardiovascular: *(1074)* _____

_____

c. Respiratory: *(1076)* _____

_____

d. Gastrointestinal: *(1069)* _____

_____

e. Urinary: *(1073)* _____

_____

f. Musculoskeletal: *(1078)* _____

_____

g. Neurologic: *(1087)* _____

_____

h. Vision and hearing: *(1085)* _____

_____

53. The nurse is caring for a 78-year-old woman who comes to the clinic with reports of "problems with my stomach and bowels."

a. What questions would the nurse use to obtain data about the patient's concerns? *(1069)* _____

_____

_____

_____

_____

b. The provider examines the patient and informs the nurse that the patient is likely having gastric reflux and constipation. What nursing interventions may be implemented for the older adult who is experiencing gastric reflux and constipation? *(1070, 1072)*

_____

_____

_____

_____

54. At the beginning of her new job, the nurse is open to any suggestions from others and tries to get along with everyone. As time goes by, she feels comfortable and likes working with a group of younger nurses. There are several older staff members who are nice, but working with them is less stimulating and interesting. In fact, she finds the older staff members to be rigid in their outlook and slow to complete assigned tasks. When the nurse is assigned to precept an older nursing student, she hesitates, because her impression of older people is that they don't make the best nurses.

a. Do you think that this nurse is guilty of ageism? Why or why not? *(1064)* _____

_____

_____

b. How could the nurse create a better situation for herself and others? *(1064)* _____

_____

_____

_____

55. The nurse is making a home visit to a 75-year-old woman who lives with her 80-year-old husband. Both the wife and husband are alert and oriented. Both are taking medication to treat hypertension. The wife has recently returned from a rehabilitation center following a hip fracture that she sustained in a fall. The nurse notes that the home is full of items that reflect a lifetime of living. Many of the rooms in the house tend to be poorly lighted. The house has an upstairs and downstairs bathroom. Identify the factors that are fall risks and make suggestions about how this older couple can prevent future falls. *(1091)*

_____

_____

_____

_____

_____

_____

_____

_____

_____

_____

Concepts of Mental Health

MULTIPLE CHOICE

Directions: Select the best answer(s) for each of the following questions.

1. Which person is acting according to an ascribed role? *(1105)*
   1. Nurse arrives at work 15 minutes before the start of the shift.
   2. Patient with cancer listens as oncologist describes treatment options.
   3. Police officer brings a confused person to the hospital for evaluation.
   4. Child chooses to take dance lessons rather than doing team sports.

2. What are physical signs/symptoms of higher levels of anxiety? **Select all that apply.** *(1105)*
   1. Rapid speech and vocal changes
   2. Increased pulse and respiration
   3. Decreased level of consciousness
   4. Tremors and restlessness
   5. Nausea and occasional vomiting

3. The nursing student expresses a feeling of being overwhelmed by the volume of study, working part-time, and trying to maintain relationships. What is the **best** intervention that the nursing instructor could use to decrease the degree of the student's anxiety? *(1106)*
   1. Allow her to skip a clinical experience.
   2. Ask about her work-study schedule.
   3. Talk about importance of her relationships.
   4. Help her prioritize responsibilities.

4. Which patient is demonstrating the **strongest** motivation to participate in the plan of care? *(1106)*
   1. Patient asks the nurse to show his wife how to change and manage his colostomy bag
   2. Patient does leg exercises because he wants to dance at his 50th wedding anniversary
   3. Patient does a return demonstration of finger exercises for the occupational therapist
   4. Patient tells the nurse he must leave the hospital because his dog is alone at the house

5. Which person is demonstrating the **most** maladaptive behavior? *(1106)*
   1. Nursing student who does poorly on tests places emphasis on skills performance.
   2. Woman is a poor driver and explains that other drivers are too impatient.
   3. Man says his drinking, followed by the occasional sick day, are no big deal.
   4. College student admires her roommate and starts dressing and acting like her.

6. The nurse is assessing a patient's use of defense mechanisms. He reports having a bad day at work and going home and shouting at the children. Which defense mechanism is he displaying? *(1107)*
   1. Projection
   2. Displacement
   3. Identification
   4. Reaction formation

7. Which person is demonstrating regressive behavior? *(1107)*
   1. Victim of sexual abuse laughs while telling about the incident.
   2. Aggressive adolescent participates in a lot of competitive sports.
   3. An 80-year-old acts as if an incident of incontinence did not occur.
   4. An 8-year-old sucks his thumb when hospitalized for the first time.

8. An adolescent female patient tells the nurse that she often feels very "uneasy," but can't identify any specific reasons for this feeling. What is this patient experiencing? *(1105)*
   1. Stress
   2. Anxiety
   3. Crisis
   4. Mental illness

9. Based on factors that possibly affect mental health, which adolescent is **most** likely to have the **best** mental health later in life? *(1100)*
   1. Participates in several school activities and has reasonably good grades
   2. Very competitive in sports and especially eager to be better than older brother
   3. Has a successful father, but mother died shortly after adolescent was born
   4. Has exceptional academic record and parents expect superior performance in all areas

10. A nurse is talking to people who are in a substance abuse support group. Which statement is evidence of the **best** level of mental health? *(1100)*
    1. "I don't have any problems with drinking anymore."
    2. "I just try to avoid drinking, one day at a time."
    3. "As long as my wife doesn't drink, then I won't drink either."
    4. "I have had a really hard time in life and I don't like being judged."

11. What is the **best** rationale for all nurses to study and be familiar with the concepts of basic mental health? *(1100)*
    1. Every nurse must study mental health concepts that are tested for licensure.
    2. Nurses need excellent mental health to help their patients.
    3. Nurses have daily contact with patients who are at risk for mental health problems.
    4. Younger nurses may lack personal experience in dealing with loss or mental illness.

12. Based on Freud's theory of personality development, the superego would cause the nurse to perform which action? *(1104)*
    1. Focus on own duties and ignore extraneous requests to perform additional tasks
    2. Disagree with patient's decision to refuse treatment, but show respect and support
    3. Minimize the importance of a medication error to facilitate patient care
    4. Obtain the continuing education units required to maintain licensure

13. The nurse suffered a terrible traumatic event during childhood, but now appears happy and satisfied with her life and career. According to Freud's theory on preconsciousness, which behavior is the nurse **most** likely to manifest? *(1104)*
    1. Is unable to recall any memory of the traumatic event.
    2. Frequently thinks about the event and experiences growth in reflection.
    3. Remembers the event, but generally represses the unpleasant aspects.
    4. Attempts to experience pleasure and avoids pain at all costs.

14. There is a fire in the facility and the nurse is attempting to instruct patients to go to a safe area. Which patient is **least** likely to be able to understand and appropriately respond to a simple command? *(1105)*
    1. Using a wheelchair to assist bedbound roommate to safe area
    2. Frantically searching through belongings to find her wedding ring
    3. Standing in the corner, crying, and clinging to the bedrail
    4. Walking towards safe area, but arguing about the need to leave

15. Which nursing student is **most** likely to experience stress during the final examination for a course? *(1105)*
    1. Has done well throughout the semester, but didn't get much sleep the night before the exam
    2. Knows that the test is important, but believes that test is just another hurdle to get over
    3. Is smart student, has two children, works full-time, and spouse has chronic illness
    4. Has studied hard for final examination, but graduating is contingent on test results

16. A newly admitted patient appears upset. She says, "I'm going to wear my own clothes. I'm not going to answer any more questions and I'm not giving anyone any blood or pee or anything else!" How should the nurse respond? *(1105)*
    1. "You can wear your own nightgown if you would prefer."
    2. "Let me call your provider so you can talk to her."
    3. "Coming into the hospital is really difficult. What can I do to help?"
    4. "Looks like you are having a bad time. I'll come back later."

17. The home health nurse is visiting an older patient who is socially isolated. The patient is very resistant to talking and rejects all suggestions related to social activities. Based on knowledge of how aging affects mental health, what should the nurse do **first**? *(1108)*
    1. Conclude that the resistance to socialization is an exaggeration of younger behavior.
    2. Assess for physical, financial, or relationship limitations that exist for the patient.
    3. Assist the patient to reminisce about happier times with friends and family.
    4. Locate and contact family members and suggest that they visit the patient.

18. A parent reports that her 8-year-old child has complained of feeling sick on school days, although there is no fever, pain, change in behavior, or any other physical symptoms. Which question should the nurse ask to determine if the child is using the sick role as a coping strategy related to a problem at school? *(1109)*
    1. "Don't you like your school and your teachers anymore?"
    2. "Did something happen at school that made you feel uncomfortable?"
    3. "What will happen if you keep missing school all the time?"
    4. "What do you and your friends like to do during recess and lunch break?"

19. The son of an older woman who lives in a long-term care facility reports that his mother seems to get sick whenever he tries to take vacation time with his wife. He feels frustrated, but also guilty, so he doesn't leave. What should the nurse do **first**? *(1109)*
    1. Validate the son's feelings of frustration and guilt and offer emotional support.
    2. Reassure the mother that she will be well cared for while her son is gone.
    3. Suggest that the son take an overnight trip as a trial run for everyone.
    4. Tell the son that the mother is manifesting a secondary gain by being sick.

20. The provider has just informed a woman that her husband, who is in a coma, is likely to die during the night. The woman is sitting at the husband's bedside and silently weeping. Which action would be the **most** therapeutic? *(1109)*
    1. Silently step outside and call other family members to come and support the wife.
    2. Ask the provider for an order for an anti-anxiety medication for the wife.
    3. Make the patient as comfortable as possible and reassure the wife that he is pain-free.
    4. Quietly stand nearby and watch for the wife's receptiveness to touching or hugging.

CRITICAL THINKING ACTIVITIES

21. Think about times in the past where you have witnessed (or personally experienced) various levels of anxiety. Briefly describe the behaviors that you observed (or feelings that you personally experienced) in each case. *(1105)*

    a. Mild anxiety:_____

    _____

    b. Moderate anxiety: _____

    _____

c. Severe anxiety: _____

_____

d. Panic: _____

_____

e. Refer to the situation of mild anxiety that you just described. What coping responses were used by the individual (or yourself) to deal with stress? *(1106, 1107)*

_____

_____

_____

f. What would you do to strengthen the healthy coping mechanisms and alter or adapt the unhealthy or overused coping mechanism for that person (or yourself)? *(1110)*

_____

_____

_____

22. The nurse is making a home visit with 70-year-old woman who was recently discharged from the hospital. Her husband, who is also in his 70s, confides to the nurse that "Martha just doesn't seem to be herself. The doctor said she is okay to be at home, but she just seems so helpless."

a. How would the nurse go about assessing the wife's emotional state? *(1110)* _____

_____

_____

b. What considerations should be made for the older adult in regard to mental health? *(1108)* _____

_____

_____

23. Based on the characteristics of a mentally healthy individual, select characteristics that currently apply to yourself and give an example of an action, behavior, or event that illustrates your good mental health. *(1110)*

_____

_____

_____

_____

_____

24. Discuss the advantages and disadvantages of the movement to "deinstitutionalize" from the point of view of an individual with a chronic mental illness. *(1102)*

_____

_____

_____

_____

_____

_____

Care of the Patient With a Psychiatric Disorder

MATCHING

Directions: Match the therapy to the correct description. Indicate your answers in the spaces provided.

Therapy	Description of Therapy

_____ 1. electroconvulsive therapy *(1132)*

_____ 2. behavior therapy *(1131)*

_____ 3. cognitive therapy *(1131)*

_____ 4. group therapy *(1132)*

_____ 5. play therapy *(1132)*

_____ 6. hypnosis *(1132)*

_____ 7. psychoanalysis *(1132)*

_____ 8. adjunctive therapies *(1132)*

a. Breaking negative thought patterns and developing positive feelings about memories

b. Using toys, such as a puppet, to be a "spokesperson" for feelings

c. Helps recover deeply repressed emotions

d. A very small amount of electrical current used to trigger a tonic-clonic seizure

e. Group of patients with similar problems gain insight through discussion

f. Includes occupational, recreational, music, magnetic, and art therapies, and hydrotherapy

g. Intense therapy that brings unconscious thoughts to the surface

h. Conditioning and retraining of behavioral responses by repetition

MULTIPLE CHOICE

Directions: Select the best answer(s) for each of the following questions.

9. The nursing students are preparing to enter a clinical rotation on an acute care psychiatric unit. What types of disorders are the students **most** likely to observe during this clinical experience? **Select all that apply.** *(1115, 1116)*
   1. Major depressive disorder
   2. Psychotic disorder
   3. Neurotic disorder
   4. Neurocognitive disorder
   5. Bipolar disorder
   6. Panic attack disorder

10. A nurse is working at a walk-in clinic when a Good Samaritan brings an unidentified, confused older woman found wandering in the street. The woman is dressed in clean clothes, but is disoriented to self, place, and time. She can't give appropriate answers to simple questions. What assessments can the nurse perform to help differentiate dementia from delirium? **Select all that apply.** *(1114)*
    1. Use pulse oximeter and count respirations.
    2. Give simple directions and assess for response.
    3. Check blood pressure and assess peripheral pulses.
    4. Use glucometer to check blood glucose.
    5. Check temperature and assess for dehydration.

11. In a care plan for a patient with paranoid schizophrenia, a nursing student correctly includes "observe for signs of agitation and ensure safety." During the clinical day, when would the nursing instructor intervene? *(1115)*
    1. Student reports that patient tilts his head adopts a listening pose when there is no one around.
    2. Student observes that patient is pacing and muttering and helps other patients to move away.
    3. Student suggests to the patient that they go to his room and spend quiet time talking together.
    4. Student assists the medication nurse to administer medication and watches for pouching.

12. The nurse has a family member who is diagnosed with cyclothymic disorder. What is the **primary** reason that the nurse would encourage follow-up visits with the psychiatrist? *(1122)*
    1. Many patients with cyclothymic disorder progress to bipolar disorder.
    2. Cheerfulness will progress to poor judgment and provocative behavior.
    3. If untreated, delirium may lead to death from exhaustion.
    4. Cyclothymic disorder is prodromal to major depressive disorder.

13. Which educational brochure is the nurse **most** likely to prepare for a patient who has seasonal affective disorder? *(1122)*
    1. "SSRIs: A New Class of Antidepressant Medications"
    2. "How Phototherapy Helps to Relieve Your Symptoms"
    3. "The Benefits and Risks of Hydrotherapy"
    4. "How to Make Selections for Your Music Therapy"

14. Which psychiatric disorder is **most** likely to manifest signs/symptoms that are similar to a myocardial infarction? *(1123)*
    1. Somatoform disorder
    2. Anorexia nervosa
    3. Schizophrenia
    4. Panic attack

15. Which intervention is recommended to prevent posttraumatic stress disorder? *(1126)*
    1. Initiating group therapy for survivors of trauma
    2. Reviewing pre-event instructions with participants
    3. Debriefing immediately after a traumatic event
    4. Identifying people at risk for anxiety disorders

16. The nurse is assessing a patient and notices tooth erosion and calloused knuckles. Which behavior would the nurse watch for around mealtimes? *(1129)*
    1. Hiding the food or throwing it away
    2. Pushing the food around the plate
    3. Eating an extraordinarily large amount
    4. Self-induced vomiting

17. Which patient has a sexual disorder that could be treated with surgery? *(1127)*
    1. Patient A has premature ejaculation.
    2. Patient B has transvestic fetishism.
    3. Patient C has transsexualism.
    4. Patient D has hypoactive sexual desire.

18. The nurse is reviewing the patient's medication list and sees that the he has been taking olanzapine for several years. Which patient response indicates that the medication therapy is successful? *(1134)*
    1. Says that nightmares and flashbacks have decreased
    2. Reports that his compulsive behavior is under control
    3. Says he still misses his dead wife, but doesn't ruminate
    4. Smiles as he tells the nurse about his new job

19. The nurse has just finished taking shift report. Which patient should the nurse check on **first**? *(1134)*
    1. Patient has a serum lithium level of 1.5 mEq/L with slurred speech.
    2. Patient has bizarre movements of the face with torticollis and oculogyric crisis.
    3. Patient has hyperthermia, muscle rigidity, and labile blood pressure.
    4. Patient has rigidity, resting tremors. and a shuffling gait.

20. The nurse is caring for an older resident in a long-term care facility who develops confusion, delirium, agitation, and mutism. The nurse sees that the patient takes sertraline. Which additional assessment findings would accompany serotonin syndrome? *(1133)*
    1. Blood pressure fluctuation and ataxia
    2. Headaches and anxiety
    3. Vomiting and muscle pain
    4. Crying spells and irritability

21. The patient is in the manic phase of bipolar affective disorder. What is the **primary** aim of the nurse's therapeutic communication? *(1116, 1121)*
    1. To reinforce assertive behaviors
    2. To provide focus and consistency
    3. To orient to surroundings and time
    4. To encourage expression of feelings

22. Which medication is **most** likely to be prescribed for a patient with an obsessive-compulsive disorder? *(1118)*
    1. Lithium carbonate
    2. Haloperidol
    3. Chlorpromazine
    4. Clomipramine

23. For a patient who is receiving lithium therapy, which electrolyte level is **most** important to monitor? *(1122)*
    1. Calcium
    2. Sodium
    3. Magnesium
    4. Potassium

24. A patient tells you that he is hearing voices right now that are telling him not to eat. What is the **best** response? *(1115)*
    1. "What specifically did the voices tell you not to eat?"
    2. "Did the voices say why they didn't want you to eat?"
    3. "Just ignore the voices. Lunch is served at 1:00 PM."
    4. "I don't hear any voices. What you are experiencing now?"

25. Based on the information provided in the change-of-shift report, which patient will the nurse see **first**? *(1121, 1122)*
    1. Patient had electroconvulsive therapy 30 minutes ago.
    2. Patient has refused to take the morning medication.
    3. Patient has said, "I am going to meet my [dead] wife."
    4. Patient identified "voices" with a message from God.

26. The patient was admitted to the acute care facility for drug-induced psychosis. He tells the nurse that he has smelled his own flesh rotting for the past 2 days. Which positive symptoms is the patient is experiencing? *(1120)*
    1. Delusion
    2. Avolition
    3. Akathisia
    4. Hallucination

27. What are typical signs and symptoms of schizophrenia? **Select all that apply.** *(1115)*
    1. Phobias
    2. Delusions
    3. Mania
    4. Paranoia
    5. Redoing

28. Which patient statement would indicate a compulsion? *(1125)*
    1. "I can't stop thinking about my hand towels being out of place on the towel rack."
    2. "I had to drive back home eight times this morning to be sure I locked my front door."
    3. "Those voices in my head are driving me crazy. Can you make them stop?"
    4. "It terrifies me to think about going fishing; I know there may be spiders in the boat."

29. A woman has bipolar disorder and is currently displaying an outgoing personality, productivity in her work, and great optimism. What phase of bipolar disorder is she experiencing? *(1121)*
    1. Manic
    2. Depressive
    3. Cyclothymic
    4. Hypomanic

30. A wife complains that her husband must be neurotic. What signs and symptoms would the nurse expect the husband to display? **Select all that apply.** *(1113)*
    1. Nervousness
    2. Low self-esteem
    3. Out of touch with reality
    4. Phobias
    5. Impaired judgment

31. The patient asks the nurse not to tell anyone that he wants to end his life. What should the nurse tell the patient? *(1132)*
    1. "Information must be shared with the rest of the health care team."
    2. "All disclosures from patient to nurse are always confidential."
    3. "Consider talking to a spiritual advisor before acting impulsively."
    4. "Information is documented in writing, but not verbally discussed."

32. The unlicensed assistive personnel (UAP) reports that an older patient said, "You have been kind and I want you to remember me," and then she gave the UAP her grandmother's necklace. What should the nurse do **first**? *(1122)*
    1. Investigate the relationship between the patient and the UAP.
    2. Instruct the UAP to return the necklace to the patient.
    3. Talk to the patient about the gesture of gift-giving to employees.
    4. Praise the UAP for having trust and rapport with the patient.

33. Which patient is **most** likely to be experiencing a panic attack? *(1123)*
    1. Patient A reports fear of being followed and demonstrates hypervigilance.
    2. Patient B reports an excruciating headache with blurred vision and nausea.
    3. Patient C reports an aura that is followed by tonic-clonic seizure activity.
    4. Patient D reports chest pain, fear of going crazy, sweating, and trembling.

34. It's lunchtime and a staff member walks into the dayroom of an acute psychiatric unit and announces, "It's chow time folks! Hop on down." Which patient is **most** likely to start physically hopping? *(1120)*
    1. Major depression with apathy and flat affect
    2. Disorganized schizophrenia with concreteness
    3. Panic disorder with agoraphobia and anxiety
    4. Dysthymic disorder with suicidal ideations

35. The nurse's neighbor has a teenage son who displays poor hygiene and odd excessive religious beliefs. Before referral to the provider, what could the nurse do to try to differentiate between prodromal phase schizophrenia and normal adolescent behavior? *(1130, 1131)*
    1. Help the neighbor compare current behavior to childhood behaviors.
    2. Talk directly to the teenager and ask about his beliefs and interests.
    3. Assess and compare the parent's religious beliefs to the teen's.
    4. Ask the neighbor if there is a family history of mental illness.

36. The patient reports nausea, vomiting, and stomach pain. She has a new job with a lot of responsibilities, many people to supervise, and two projects that are due within the month. If physical causes are ruled out, these symptoms are consistent with which mental health disorder? *(1127)*
    1. Somatoform disorder
    2. Posttraumatic stress disorder
    3. Generalized anxiety disorder
    4. Bulimia nervosa

37. The nurse is trying to assess a patient who is newly diagnosed with schizophrenia. The patient refuses to speak, but whispers, "They are listening to my conversations through the intercom." What should the nurse do? *(1130, 1131)*
    1. Conduct the interview in whispers or by writing.
    2. Walk over to the intercom and turn it off.
    3. Suggest that they move to the garden area.
    4. Acknowledge his feelings of fear and anxiety.

38. The patient says, "The man on the television is telling me to buy that motorcycle." What is the **most** therapeutic response? *(1130, 1131)*
    1. "It's just a television program; he wasn't really talking to you."
    2. "You can't buy a motorcycle right now; you are in the hospital."
    3. "Have you been thinking about buying a motorcycle?"
    4. "Television advertisements try to persuade us to buy products."

39. The nurse is caring for a patient who is scheduled to have surgery in the morning, but she also happens to have an anxiety disorder. What should the nurse do **first** to decrease stimuli for this anxious patient? *(1130, 1131)*
    1. Close the door and give the patient some privacy.
    2. Ask if sounds, light, or movement are disturbing.
    3. Turn off the lights so that the patient can sleep.
    4. Limit the number of visitors to decrease noise.

40. Which information is appropriate when preparing a patient for electroconvulsive therapy? **Select all that apply.** *(1123)*
    1. "Pain will be experienced, but it only lasts a few seconds."
    2. "Confusion may last for a few hours."
    3. "A grand mal seizure occurs, but it is very brief."
    4. "Temporary memory loss is experienced after treatment."
    5. "Most patients are kept in the hospital for 2-3 days afterward."

CRITICAL THINKING ACTIVITIES

41. The nurse is working in a long-term care facility. There are two residents who have been living there for several years. Both are showing signs of new-onset mental health change. A resident with quadriplegia was recently admitted to the hospital for treatment of pressure injuries. He returned to the long-term care facility several weeks ago, but now he seems sullen and withdrawn and frequently talks about death. The other resident is an older man with no family. He has a history of chronic depression. He is ambulatory and able to independently perform most activities of daily living. He has been talking about the loss of friends and family and his desire to join them. He mentions feeling "lonely, old, and useless." He asked the nurse if she would "give him a few extra pills."

    a. What warning signs of suicide are these two residents currently showing? What are other signs to watch for? *(1122)*

    _____

    _____

    _____

    _____

    b. Compare and contrast precautions that should be taken for these two residents who are suicidal. *(1122)*

    _____

    _____

    _____

    _____

    _____

    _____

    _____

42. The nurse is caring for a patient with chronic pain who displays sadness, loss of interest in activities, and pessimistic thoughts. The nurse reports these findings. A consulting psychiatrist makes the medical diagnosis of depression.

    a. Identify possible patient outcomes for this patient who is experiencing depression. *(1124)* _____

    _____

    _____

    _____

    _____

    _____

    b. What specific treatments for depression should the nurse anticipate? *(1132, 1133)* _____

    _____

    _____

    _____

    _____

    _____

    _____

    _____

c. Give examples of medications that are typically used to treat depression. *(1133)*_____

_____

_____

_____

d. For antidepressant medications, what side effects could the patient experience, and what are the nursing actions to address these effects? *(1135)*

_____

_____

_____

_____

_____

_____

_____

Care of the Patient With an Addictive Personality

chapter **36**

TABLE ACTIVITY

1. Directions: On the table below, indicate at least one or two disorders that are associated with chronic alcohol use for each body system. *(1144)*

Disorders Associated with Alcoholism

System	Disorders
Gastrointestinal	
Hepatic	
Cardiovascular and blood disorders	
Respiratory	
Uroreproductive	
Musculoskeletal	
Neurologic	

SHORT ANSWER
Directions: Using your own words, answer each question in the space provided.

2. CAGE is an assessment tool that is used to identify problems with alcohol abuse. Two or more affirmations to the four questions indicate probable alcoholism. What are the four questions? *(1144)*

   a. _____
   b. _____
   c. _____
   d. _____

3. Identify the four elements that are included in the definition of *addiction*. *(1140)*

   a. _____
   b. _____
   c. _____
   d. _____

MULTIPLE CHOICE

Directions: Select the best answer(s) for each of the following questions.

4. A patient comes into the walk-in clinic for a prescription refill. She admits to recently taking a hit of "Molly." What assessment findings would the nurse expect? *(1151)*
   1. Pinpoint pupils and memory loss
   2. Increased pulse and blood pressure
   3. Slurred speech and listlessness
   4. Confabulation and lack of coordination

5. Which person is displaying the five personality traits that are associated with an addictive personality? *(1142)*
   1. Stay-at-home mom feels dependent, insecure, and easily upset. She is frequently depressed and sees herself as having no marketable skills.
   2. Manager feels overwhelmed by work. She overcompensates, is aggressive and competitive, and frequently displays false bravado around others.
   3. College student is quiet, shy, and unsure of herself around others. She studies and stays at home to avoid social situations.
   4. Woman feels angry about her husband's infidelity. She becomes flirtatious and has a series of one-night stands to express her hostility towards men.

6. Which person is **most** likely to develop alcohol dependency? *(1141)*
   1. A 50-year-old French female who drinks after death of a spouse
   2. A 30-year-old Irish female who does recreational drinking and cocaine
   3. A 14-year-old Native American male who drinks and father is an alcoholic
   4. A 42-year-old Jewish male with depression related to liver cancer

7. In the United States, there has been a decrease in alcohol use over the years. According to experts, there are factors that account for this decrease. Which nursing action is consistent with these identified factors? *(1141)*
   1. Nursing assessment includes standardized tools to identify alcohol abuse.
   2. Nursing programs include substance and alcohol abuse in the curriculum.
   3. There are increased roles for nurses at residential treatment centers.
   4. Patient teaching includes short- and long-term health effects of alcohol abuse.

8. What behaviors are seen in the **early** stage of substance dependency? **Select all that apply.** *(1142)*
   1. Stops using to prove control over substance use
   2. Makes light of concerns expressed by family or friends
   3. Socializes more with other users and less with family
   4. Takes the substance to just feel "normal"
   5. Demonstrates mood swings, guilt, and resentment

9. Infective endocarditis is **more** likely to occur with which route of substance abuse? *(1142)*
   1. Smoking a bong
   2. Snorting opioids
   3. Huffing inhalants
   4. Injecting drugs

10. When a person is drinking an alcoholic beverage, which function of the central nervous system will be affected **first**? *(1143)*
    1. Frontal cortex is affected and person experiences memory loss and loss of judgment.
    2. The limbic system is affected and disrupts regulation of hunger, thirst, and sexual desire.
    3. Higher centers of the brain are affected, and person starts to lose self-control.
    4. Basal ganglia of the brain are affected, and this leads to obsessive-compulsive behavior.

11. The nurse is talking to a group of people who are likely to be in denial about alcohol abuse, but each is describing a typical drinking pattern for a Saturday night. Which person has the **highest** amount of reported alcohol intake for a single day? *(1143)*
    1. Drinks a six-pack of beers (12 ounces per can)
    2. Drinks three glasses of red wine (4 ounces per glass)
    3. Drinks one beer (12-ounces) and two glasses of wine (4 ounces per glass)
    4. Drinks three mixed drinks (1 1/2 ounces hard liquor per drink)

12. The nurse hears in report that the patient is receiving thiamine for Wernicke encephalopathy. Which assessment finding indicates the thiamine is effective? *(1143)*
    1. Hallucinations cease and delirium are resolved.
    2. Memory and muscle coordination show improvement.
    3. Tremors are decreased and there is no seizure activity.
    4. Vomiting, cramps, and diarrhea have resolved.

13. A patient has a blood alcohol level of >500 mg/dL (>0.50%). Which action is the nurse likely to use **first**? *(1154)*
    1. Assess for changes in mental status.
    2. Assist with ambulation because of clumsiness.
    3. Set limits for loosening of inhibitions.
    4. Assist provider with intubation.

14. A coworker states that he consumes too much caffeine and wants to eliminate it from his diet. Which question would the nurse ask **first**? *(1150)*
    1. "Are you aware that you will have withdrawal symptoms?"
    2. "Do you take any supplements or over-the-counter medications?"
    3. "Have you ever tried to give up or cut down on your consumption?"
    4. "What would you typically eat and drink during a 24-hour period?"

15. The patient is initiating smoking cessation. Which symptom is associated with withdrawal from nicotine? *(1150)*
    1. Lethargy
    2. Improved concentration
    3. Decreased heart rate
    4. Decreased appetite

16. The nurse is working at a facility that assists workers who have substance abuse problems. Which worker is **least** likely to need help or assistance to get through withdrawal? *(1154)*
    1. Person A has been smoking cannabis for several years.
    2. Person B admits to a steady increase in amphetamine use.
    3. Person C reports using heroin whenever it is available.
    4. Person D frequently uses hallucinogens on the weekends.

17. A college student who has used marijuana since early high school is diagnosed with amotivational cannabis syndrome. Which behavioral characteristics is he **most** likely to display? **Select all that apply.** *(1152)*
    1. Unusual irritability
    2. Frequent mood swings
    3. Physical aggression
    4. Psychosis
    5. Depression

18. A patient was prescribed an opiate analgesic for a fractured femur. He states that he has noticed that he doesn't seem to get the relief that he used to, despite the fact that his leg is healing. What should the nurse tell the patient? *(1149)*
    1. "Tolerance to opioids develops rapidly, but abstinence reverses tolerance."
    2. "You should switch to nonsteroidal antiinflammatory medications."
    3. "Addiction to opioid medications is common for those who have chronic pain."
    4. "This is an expected effect; I will contact the provider to increase your dosage."

19. The nurse's friend tells her that she thinks her boyfriend may have an alcohol problem. Which question will elicit indicators of the **early** stage of alcoholism? *(1142)*
    1. "What form of alcohol does he drink?"
    2. "Is the drinking controlling him?"
    3. "What makes you think there's a problem?"
    4. "Have you talked to him about this?"

20. The nurse is caring for a teenager who crashed his parents' car while he was intoxicated. The mother, wracked with guilt, confides that she knew he had a drinking problem, but didn't do anything about it. What is the **most** therapeutic response? *(1145)*
    1. "You can't watch your kids all of the time, especially when they are teenagers."
    2. "The accident may be a blessing; now you can get help for his drinking."
    3. "You feel like you are to blame, but it was his choice to drink and drive."
    4. "It's hard for parents to really believe that their child has a drinking problem."

21. The nurse is a assessing a patient who has been in the middle stage of substance abuse for years. Which factor is likely to hasten the progression from the middle stage to the late stage? *(1142)*
    1. Poor family relationships
    2. Multiple substance abuse
    3. Gastrointestinal problems
    4. Substance abuse on the job

22. From a cultural standpoint, which patient is the **least** likely to develop alcoholism? *(1142)*
    1. Asian
    2. Irishman
    3. Mormon
    4. Inuit

23. Which patient represents the leading national health problems in the United States? *(1142)*
    1. An infant who has birth defects and fetal alcohol syndrome
    2. An adolescent with cancer who smokes medicinal cannabis
    3. An executive who uses cocaine to counter-act his depression
    4. An older patient who is an alcoholic with heart disease

24. What is the physiologic reason for the vitamin B_1, folic acid, and vitamin B_{12} deficiencies that occur in alcoholism? *(1143)*
    1. Alcohol affects the intestinal mucosa and results in decreased absorption.
    2. One ounce of alcohol provides 200 kcal but has no other nutritional value.
    3. Alcohol has a diuretic effect, so most nutrients are excreted in the urine.
    4. The liver metabolizes most of the alcohol; thus the liver is damaged.

25. The nurse is caring for a postoperative patient who has a history of alcoholism. The patient demonstrates restlessness, tachycardia, and mild diaphoresis. How could the nurse differentiate between suspected alcohol withdrawal and postoperative complications, such as bleeding or infection? *(1144)*
    1. Call the provider and obtain an order for blood alcohol level.
    2. Monitor vital signs and assess for pain related to the surgery.
    3. Explain concerns and then ask the patient about alcohol use.
    4. This differentiation is beyond the nurse's scope of practice.

26. Which substance has the **most** potential for danger during withdrawal? *(1143)*
    1. Alcohol
    2. Heroin
    3. Amphetamine
    4. Nicotine

27. The nurse is interviewing a patient who has an alcohol problem and his wife has decided to file for divorce. Which patient statement typifies the **most** common defense mechanism used by substance abusers? *(1156)*
    1. "My wife is the one who has a drinking problem. I am glad she is gone."
    2. "I don't have a drinking problem. My wife just used that as an excuse."
    3. "Have you ever been married? I wouldn't recommend it to anyone."
    4. "My wife got on my nerves, so sometimes I would have a few drinks."

28. Which laboratory findings are likely to be seen for a patient who has chronic alcoholism? **Select all that apply.** *(1144)*
    1. Elevated liver enzymes
    2. Decreased hemoglobin
    3. Electrolyte imbalances
    4. Abnormal blood proteins
    5. Hyperglycemia
    6. Abnormal clotting times

29. A person is brought to the hospital for an acute opioid overdose, which is probably a suicide attempt. The patient is difficult to arouse, and the family is hysterical. What is the **priority** action? *(1148)*
    1. Assess for time of ingestion.
    2. Check airway and respirations.
    3. Calm the family to obtain a history.
    4. Administer IV naloxone.

CRITICAL THINKING ACTIVITIES

30. A daughter of a home health patient very hesitantly approaches the nurse and asks for information about alcohol abuse. At first, the daughter is very vague and claims to be asking out of general interest. As rapport develops, the daughter discloses that her mother (home health patient) and her stepfather seem to be drinking more alcohol. The daughter is not sure if they are true "alcoholics," but is worried about how their drinking is affecting the rest of the family.

    a. The nurse decides to collect data to determine if the family members have risk factors that could contribute to alcoholism. What are some contributing factors? *(1142)*

    _____

    _____

    _____

b. What can the nurse tell the daughter about the effects that alcoholism can have on relationships between family members who abuse alcohol and family members who do not? *(1142)*

_____

_____

_____

_____

31. The nurse suspects that something unusual is happening during the night shift. The patients frequently complain that the pain medication that they receive at night seems ineffective. These complaints seem to occur when the same two nurses are working together; however, the nurse hesitates to report these complaints because he recognizes that subjective reports of pain could be influenced by a number of factors.

a. What should the nurse do? *(1153)* _____

_____

_____

_____

_____

b. What are the specific role-related signs or behaviors that may be seen if nurses are chemically impaired? *(1155)*

_____

_____

c. The nurse recognizes that reporting a chemically impaired nurse may be a way for that nurse to get assistance in overcoming the problem and prevent possible dangers to patients. What assistance is available? *(1155)*

_____

_____

_____

_____

_____

d. What is the Healthcare Integrity and Protection Data Bank (HIPDB) and how does it impact the chemically impaired nurse? *(1155)*

_____

_____

_____

_____

_____

32. How would you feel about reporting a friend/coworker for stealing opioid medication? *(1155)* _____

_____

_____

_____

_____

_____

Home Health Nursing

MULTIPLE CHOICE

Directions: Select the best answer(s) for each of the following questions.

1. Which patient is **most** likely eligible for Medicare coverage for home health services? *(1160)*
   1. 71-year-old who needs help with bathing, grooming, and toileting
   2. 67-year-old who is discharged from the hospital after hip surgery
   3. 83-year-old who has dementia and needs around-the-clock supervision
   4. 45-year-old who needs prefilling of insulin syringes and diabetes education

2. Which nursing action indicates that the nurse understands how diagnosis-related groups impact nursing practice? *(1160)*
   1. Collaborates with RN to ensure that the nursing diagnoses align with the medical diagnosis
   2. Reviews the pathophysiology and chronic effects of medical diagnosis for all assigned patients
   3. Does focused assessments related to medical diagnosis and reports findings to prevent complications
   4. Reinforces information about the medical diagnosis and teaches self-care measures to prevent relapse

3. Which patient situation is an example of the major impact that diagnosis-related groups has on hospitalized patients? *(1160)*
   1. Patient A has to select a different provider for insurance purposes.
   2. Patient B has a medical diagnosis that is not covered by Medicare.
   3. Patient C has more out-of-pocket costs because of medical diagnosis.
   4. Patient D is discharged, but still needs ongoing home care.

4. For families and patients who receive Medicare home services, what is the significance of the 60-day period? *(1164)*
   1. The family or patient must pay for the first 60 days of home services, then Medicare coverage starts.
   2. The patient must need skilled nursing or therapy for at least 60 days to be eligible for home care coverage.
   3. Recertification by physician and primary disciplines must be completed for each subsequent 60-day period.
   4. Persons who are eligible for Medicare get a maximum coverage of 60 days of home care each year.

5. The nurse is making a home visit with an older woman who has an indwelling urinary catheter because of urinary retention. The nurse notes that the urine has a strong, foul odor and the woman seems lethargic and listless. What should the nurse do **first**? *(1165)*
   1. Call the supervising RN and ask for a second opinion about possible urosepsis.
   2. Take vital signs, and do a head-to-toe assessment to identify sources of infection.
   3. Clamp the catheter and then obtain a fresh urine specimen using sterile technique.
   4. Remove the indwelling catheter and save the tip of the catheter for culture.

6. Which evaluative statement indicates that the "improvement" goal of service is being met for a patient who has type 2 diabetes mellitus and was recently discharged after a toe amputation related to a diabetic foot ulcer? *(1164)*
   1. Patient loses 5 lbs after adherence to exercise routine and healthy eating.
   2. Wound edges are well approximated; tissue is pink with no evidence of infection.
   3. Patient gives return demonstration of inspection, cleaning, and care of feet.
   4. Patient resumes routine blood glucose testing and self-administration of insulin.

7. The nurse is visiting a patient who uses a mask for delivery of home oxygen therapy. What assessments will the nurse perform? **Select all that apply.** *(1165)*
   1. Check the patient's skin underneath the straps.
   2. Observe the tops of ears for skin breakdown.
   3. Assess oral and mucous membranes.
   4. Observe the amount and quality of secretions.
   5. Check and replace the oxygen equipment as needed.

8. Following a stroke, a patient exhibits difficult swallowing and is at high risk for aspiration. Which member of the health care team should be consulted to give expert assistance to this patient? *(1166)*
   1. Speech-language therapist
   2. Ear, nose, and throat specialist
   3. Occupational therapist
   4. Physical therapist

9. The LPN/LVN is reviewing documentation and sees that it has been a month since the RN made a visit to the patient's home or interacted directly with the home health aide. What should the LPN/LVN do? *(1167)*
   1. Contact the director of the agency to review the documentation.
   2. Assess the patient, supervise the aide, and update the documentation.
   3. Remind the RN that the onsite visit and supervision of the aide are overdue.
   4. Continue to provide care and documentation under the existing plan.

10. Which nurse is demonstrating the **best** collaboration with the patient, family, and Spanish interpreter to improve communication? *(1170)*
    1. Nurse A speaks a little Spanish but defers to the interpreter.
    2. Nurse B asks the interpreter to use very simple language.
    3. Nurse C gives all information directly to the interpreter.
    4. Nurse D speaks directly to the patient and family.

11. The nurse observes that the home health patient has trouble with tasks that require fine motor skills such as writing or manipulating eating utensils. Which member of the health care team is **best** able to assist the patient with these problems? *(1166)*
    1. Physician
    2. Physical therapist
    3. Home health aide
    4. Occupational therapist

12. The home health nurse is reviewing use of home oxygen with the patient and family. Which information should be included? *(1165)*
    1. Use petrolatum-based lubricant on the lips.
    2. Place "No Smoking" signs where they are clearly visible.
    3. Change disposable equipment once a month.
    4. Use wool blankets to provide warmth and static control.

13. Which home health patient would be the **best** candidate for a telehealth program? *(1168)*
    1. Lacks fine motor control to perform ostomy care
    2. Needs infusion of total parenteral nutrition every morning
    3. Recently prescribed insulin and blood glucose monitoring
    4. Requires assessment of home environment for safety

14. What do Medicare and Medicaid require for the patient to be entered into the formalized system? *(1164)*
    1. An evidence-based clinical pathway that relates to the primary medical diagnosis
    2. A standardized nursing care plan that is linked to the hospital discharge diagnosis
    3. An individualized nursing care plan that is developed by the RN and LPN/LVN
    4. An interdisciplinary treatment plan that is reviewed and signed by the physician

15. Which evaluative statement indicates that the "restorative" goal of service is being met? *(1164)*
    1. Patient who had a stroke 4 weeks ago is now able to feed self without signs of choking
    2. Patient who had smoking cessation classes reports no smoking for past 2 months
    3. Patient who had bariatric surgery reports exercising routinely with no weight gain
    4. Patient who has hypertension reports compliance with low-cholesterol, low-sodium diet

16. The LPN/LVN who is working under the supervision of the RN has been assigned to do home care for an older patient with diabetes and hypertension. Which nursing actions are within the scope of practice of the LPN/LVN? **Select all that apply.** *(1165)*
    1. Conduct the admission assessment in the home environment.
    2. Prefill insulin syringes.
    3. Perform fingersticks for blood glucose readings.
    4. Monitor blood pressure and weight.
    5. Reinforce therapeutic diabetic diet information.
    6. Evaluate the patient at the end of the 60-day period.

17. An older patient who has emphysema requires respiratory and physical therapy. His daughter is trying to determine if her father can continue to live independently in his own home and if he qualifies for any Medicare home health coverage. Which set of activities is **most** likely to require out-of-pocket payment? *(1166)*
    1. Bathing and oral hygiene
    2. Walking and transfers
    3. Shopping and cooking
    4. Eating and toileting

18. A home health aide has been assigned to assist a patient with a bath several times a week. Which instruction is appropriate for the nurse to give to the aide? *(1167)*
    1. "Try to do everything for the patient, so he feels nurtured."
    2. "Ask the patient if he prefers a shower, tub bath, or a partial bath."
    3. "If you or the patient has any problems, just let me know."
    4. "Watch for redness of the skin, particularly on the buttocks and back."

19. A nurse is spending 3 or more hours with each patient for home visits. The supervisor sees this as a problem. What should the supervisor do **first**? *(1167, 1168)*
    1. Explain that clinical efficiency is critical within the industry.
    2. Describe how the current Medicare prospective payment system works.
    3. Ask the nurse to describe what happens on a typical home visit.
    4. Review the nurse's documentation for evidence of how the time is spent.

20. For home health care, what are the purposes of documentation? **Select all that apply.** *(1168)*
    1. Provides an accurate picture of the type and quality of care
    2. Replaces verbal nursing reports that are used in facilities
    3. Allows the health care team to make internal evaluations as needed
    4. Provides evidence required for reimbursement and payments
    5. Serves as a legal document that is subject to close scrutiny
    6. Allows family to have access to all patient information

CRITICAL THINKING ACTIVITIES

21. A 63-year-old woman had several toes amputated because of complications of diabetes. The patient also takes medication for high blood pressure. She was recently discharged from the hospital and needs home health care. The home health care team includes an RN, LPN/LVN, physical therapist, and a home health aide. The patient is having trouble with balance and ambulation and currently needs some assistance with hygiene.

    a. What is the role of the LPN/LVN in home health care of this patient? *(1165)* _____
    _____
    _____

    b. What activities may be delegated to a home health aide? *(1166, 1167)* _____
    _____
    _____

    c. What are the Medicare requirements for the following services? *(1166)*

        i. Physical therapy: _____

          _____

        ii. Home health aide: _____

          _____

22. Compare the admission process to home health service to the admission process of an acute care facility. *(1167)*

    _____

    _____

    _____

    _____

    _____

    _____

23. Today, the home health patient with heart failure seems short of breath, has 4+ pitting edema in the lower extremities, and a weight gain of 5 lbs within a week. The pulse oximeter reading is 89% on oxygen at 4 L/min per nasal cannula. The nurse calls the provider and receives an order to have the patient transported by ambulance to the hospital for an exacerbation of heart failure. The nurse informs the patient about the provider's plan. The patient says, "I don't want to go to the hospital. Can you stay with me and give me an IV diuretic? That's all they will do at the hospital."

    a. What should the nurse do first? *(1170)* _____

        _____

        _____

    b. If the patient continues to refuse to go to the hospital despite the nurse's best efforts to convince him, do **you** think that the nurse should stay? If so, for how long and under what conditions should the nurse continue to stay with the patient? *(1170)*

        _____

        _____

        _____

        _____

    c. What additional resources could the nurse call upon? *(1160)* _____

        _____

        _____

        _____

        _____

24. Identify qualities/attributes in yourself that would indicate that a career in home health would either be suitable (or not) for you. *(1164)*

    _____

    _____

    _____

    _____

    _____

Long-Term Care

SHORT ANSWER
Directions: Using your own words, answer each question in the space provided.

1. List four or five services that are available to support older community-dwelling adults who live alone or with family members. *(1177)*

   _____

   _____

   _____

   _____

   _____

2. Identify at least four ethical/legal issues related to long-term care services. *(1183)* _____

   _____

   _____

   _____

   _____

   _____

MULTIPLE CHOICE
Directions: Select the best answer(s) for each of the following questions.

3. Which person is **most** likely to qualify for Program of All Inclusive Care for the Elderly (PACE)? *(1178)*
   1. 73-year-old woman with moderate Alzheimer's disease who lives with 77-year-old spouse
   2. 60-year-old woman with mild dementia who needs adult daycare when her daughter is at work
   3. 80-year-old man who needs tube feedings and respiratory treatments every 6 hours
   4. 55-year-old man who lives in a rural area and needs transportation to the veteran's hospital

4. The LPN/LVN staffing coordinator receives an incomplete report about an older person (Mr. X) who is requesting home care. Which question is the **most** important to ensure appropriate scheduling and assignment? *(1178)*
   1. "Has Mr. X ever had home health before? If so, would he like the same caregiver?"
   2. "What is Mr. X's medical diagnosis and what is the name of his primary care provider?
   3. "Does Mr. X need assistance with activities of daily living or skilled nursing care?"
   4. "How many days of the week and hours per day does Mr. X need care and assistance?"

5. Which outcome statement indicates that the **primary** goal of hospice care has been met? *(1178)*
   1. Family is notified to attend patient because death is near.
   2. Family is aware of and agrees with plan of care.
   3. Patient signals readiness to let go and then dies.
   4. Patient is clean, dry, comfortable, and pain-free.

6. Which patient is **most** likely to benefit from palliative care? *(1178)*
   1. Patient who sustained a hip fracture needs additional time for rehabilitation.
   2. Patient with a feeding tube and oxygen therapy shows slow but steady deterioration.
   3. Patient with dementia frequently cries, but no organic cause of pain is identified.
   4. Patient with rheumatoid arthritis has chronic pain and long-term disabilities.

7. The nurse is giving anticipatory guidance to a woman who provides around-the-clock care for an older grandmother with early stage Alzheimer's disease. Which action would the nurse suggest to avoid a "precipitating event" that would lead to sudden long-term care placement for the grandmother? *(1181)*
   1. Check home for safety hazards.
   2. Ask family/friends to visit frequently.
   3. Reminisce and decorate with nostalgic items.
   4. Establish a simple daily routine.

8. The LPN/LVN is caring for 60 residents at a long-term care facility with a team of four certified nursing assistants (CNAs) and two certified medication aides (CMAs). What role/responsibilities related to medication administration is the LPN/LVN **most** likely to assume? *(1182)*
   1. CMAs will administer all medications and LPN/LVN will supervise all CNA and CMA actions.
   2. LPN/LVN will administer opioids, non-opioids, enteral tube, and as-needed (PRN) medications.
   3. LPN/LVN and CMAs can give medications, so each caregiver administers to 20 residents.
   4. LPN/LVN can delegate medication administration to CMAs or CNAs if they have experience.

9. What is an example of a person who requires assistance with instrumental activities of daily living? *(1179)*
   1. Able to stand, but can't independently ambulate to the bathroom
   2. Can brush own teeth if someone applies the toothpaste
   3. Can pay bills by check, but doesn't understand online payments
   4. Owns a car, but vision and psychomotor coordination are poor

10. Before a clinical rotation at a long-term care center, the nursing instructor advises a group of first-year nursing students to do some reading about health problems that are likely to be found among the older adult residents. Which list represents the **most** common disorders that the students will see? *(1181)*
    1. Cardiovascular disease, hypertension, depression, dementia, and type 2 diabetes
    2. Chronic obstructive pulmonary disease, paraplegia, and hip or long bone fractures
    3. Amyotrophic lateral sclerosis, stroke, urinary incontinence, and end-stage renal failure
    4. Hypothyroidism, schizophrenia, traumatic injury, and peripheral vascular disease

11. The nurse is training a new CNA at a long-term care facility. Which topics would the nurse include in the CNA's training regarding activities of daily living? **Select all that apply.** *(1177, 1179)*
    1. Equipment needed for bathing or showering
    2. Ways to maintain independence in brushing teeth
    3. Communication techniques to encourage socialization
    4. Safety measures to use during ambulation
    5. Money management during shopping
    6. Ways to maintain privacy during toileting

12. A patient requires extensive wound care and intravenous antibiotics due to an infection of a surgical wound. Which type of care will **best** meet his needs? *(1180)*
    1. Long-term care facility
    2. Subacute unit
    3. Residential care facility
    4. Hospice unit

13. Which nursing action reflects the positive influence of the Omnibus Budget Reconciliation Act (OBRA) on long-term care? *(1182)*
    1. Instructs CNA to safely apply safety reminder devices
    2. Reviews and updates the residents' advance directives
    3. Reviews the qualifications of a CNA who applied for a job
    4. Ensures that each resident qualifies for Medicaid or Medicare

14. An older couple needs assistance with bathing, dressing, and taking their medication. Both are always alert and oriented. They are mobile but suffer from arthritis. Which setting would be the **most** beneficial for this couple? *(1179)*
    1. Skilled nursing facility
    2. Subacute unit
    3. Adult daycare facility
    4. Assisted-living community

15. The interdisciplinary team at a long-term care facility is meeting to discuss the care plan of one of the residents. Who should attend this meeting? **Select all that apply.** *(1181)*
    1. Physical therapist
    2. Activities director
    3. CNA
    4. Nursing unit manager
    5. Other interested residents
    6. Resident

16. The nurse is talking to a nursing student who is doing a clinical rotation in a nursing home facility. What is the **priority** concept that the nurse will emphasize during the student's orientation to the facility? *(1184)*
    1. Respectful communication
    2. Complete documentation
    3. Residents' safety and security
    4. Assistance with activities of daily living

17. What is the purpose of a resident assessment instrument? *(1184)*
    1. Facilitates assessment of functional, medical, mental, and psychosocial status
    2. Allows residents to self-assess and report on what they can do for themselves
    3. Identifies the problems that residents will have in communicating needs
    4. Used by surveyors during unannounced visits to assess residents' quality of life

18. How does documentation in a long-term care facility differ from that in a hospital setting? *(1184)*
    1. Documentation occurs at the beginning and end of each 24-hour period.
    2. The assistants do most of the physical care, so they do most of the documentation.
    3. Summaries of resident status over a longer time, usually monthly, are recorded.
    4. Documentation occurs only if there is a sudden change in a resident's status.

19. An older patient is alert, ambulatory, and can independently perform activities of daily living. Recently, he has started wandering and today the police had to bring him back home. Which question would the nurse use **first** to help the family determine if long-term care is needed? *(1184)*
    1. "Who has the power of attorney for health care?"
    2. "What are the current living arrangements for family members?"
    3. "What kinds of options have you considered for your dad?"
    4. "Is there any way to plan 24-hour care among the family?"

20. An interdisciplinary team meeting is planned to discuss the needs and goals of a resident who is very hostile about being in the long-term care facility. The CNA who has the best relationship with the resident is not invited to attend. What should the nurse do? *(1182)*
    1. Ask the resident to invite the CNA.
    2. Advocate for the CNA to attend.
    3. Ask the CNA to do a written statement.
    4. Inform the CNA of the outcomes.

CRITICAL THINKING ACTIVITIES

21. You are considering applying for a job in a long-term care facility. Your clinical experiences in nursing school included acute care and long-term care facilities. You recognize that part of selecting a job is to match your interests and experiences with the setting, patients, other caregivers, and philosophy of the institution.

   a. What is the profile of the patient/resident who requires long-term care in an institutional setting? Envision yourself working with this type of patient/resident. Is it a good fit for you? *(1175)*

   _____

   _____

   _____

   _____

   _____

   b. The administration of medications in long-term care facilities is different than in acute care. Describe the differences and state ways to increase your comfort level with this process. *(1182)*

   _____

   _____

   _____

   _____

   _____

22. Your grandmother has reached a stage where your family has decided that she requires more care than the family is able to give her at home.

   a. Discuss points about choosing a nursing home. *(1181)* _____

   _____

   _____

   _____

   _____

   _____

   b. How will your family finance the nursing home care for your grandmother? *(1182, 1183)*_____

   _____

   _____

   _____

23. Why would a nurse who works in long-term care actually need a better understanding of legal aspects, such as advance directives and power of attorney or guardianship, compared to a nurse who works in an acute care facility? *(1183)*

   _____

   _____

   _____

   _____

   _____

   _____

Rehabilitation Nursing

SHORT ANSWER
Directions: Using your own words, answer each question in the space provided.

1. Identify and briefly define five circumstances where rehabilitation is needed. *(1189)*

   a. _____

   b. _____

   c. _____

   d. _____

   e. _____

2. What are the six goals of rehabilitation? *(1190)*

   a. _____

   b. _____

   c. _____

   d. _____

   e. _____

   f. _____

MULTIPLE CHOICE
Directions: Select the best answer(s) for each of the following questions.

3. An older patient who had a stroke has multiple residual symptoms. The spouse wants more therapy for her husband so he can "be like himself." What should nurse do **first**? *(1190)*
   1. Advocate for the provider to recertify physical therapy and increase frequency of speech therapy.
   2. Point out that some patients with stroke never fully recover to preexisting health state.
   3. Assess what spouse means by "be like himself" and her expectations of additional therapy.
   4. Ask the medical director to clarify goals and then compare those to the spouse's goals.

4. Which patient action is the **best** demonstration of a functional outcome? *(1190)*
   1. Patient states that his quality of life has improved after therapy.
   2. Patient agrees to biweekly physical therapy appointments.
   3. Patient knows signs/symptoms for when to call the provider.
   4. Patient independently ambulates around the house.

5. Which outcome statement **best** indicates that the goal of rehabilitation has been successfully met? *(1190)*
   1. Patient telecommutes for work, regularly attends church, and joins a chess club.
   2. Patient regularly performs exercises as instructed by the occupational therapist.
   3. Patient demonstrates ability to maintain colostomy care and diet therapy.
   4. Patient completes activities of daily living with partial assistance.

6. The physiatrist tells the nurse that the patient with a spinal cord injury may be developing heterotopic ossification in the right knee. How would the nurse use this information in planning care for this patient? *(1199)*
   1. Instruct the certified nursing assistant to handle the patient very gently.
   2. Ask the physical therapist about type and frequency of range-of-motion exercises.
   3. Frequently check the right leg for perfusion, pulse, temperature, pallor, and edema.
   4. Elevate the leg on a pillow and apply ice packs to reduce swelling and discomfort.

7. Which patient needs interventions that are based on the habilitative approach? *(1200)*
   1. Man who had a myocardial infarction
   2. Woman who had carpal tunnel surgery
   3. Older man who had knee replacement surgery
   4. Child who was born with spina bifida

8. The nurse is assisting a patient with a spinal cord injury to move into a wheelchair. What should the nurse do **first** to prevent postural hypotension? *(1197, 1198)*
   1. Take the blood pressure and pulse to establish a baseline.
   2. Ask the patient if he feels dizzy or lightheaded.
   3. Make sure the patient is well hydrated and well nourished.
   4. Raise the head of the bed 15-20 minutes before moving him.

9. The nurse works at a rehabilitation unit and is assigned four patients with the following medical conditions: arthritis, spinal cord injury, stroke, and multiple sclerosis. What basic nursing measure is common to the care of these four patients? *(1192)*
   1. Maintaining body alignment and position changes
   2. Assessing for pain and administering pain medication
   3. Assessing for orthostatic hypotension and dizziness
   4. Initiating bladder training and monitoring incontinence

10. Which patient is **most** likely to need cues and reminders to accomplish activities of daily living? *(1199)*
    1. Has chronic obstructive pulmonary disease
    2. Has traumatic brain injury (TBI)
    3. Has spinal cord injury
    4. Has posttraumatic stress disorder

11. The patient experienced a spinal cord injury at the T1–T5 level. What should the patient be able to do? *(1196)*
    1. Assist with activities of daily living.
    2. Ambulate with the use of assistive devices.
    3. Resume normal sexual activities.
    4. Control bowel and bladder function.

12. A construction worker sustained an injury to C3 after a fall at a work site. What does the nurse anticipate that this patient will demonstrate? *(1196)*
    1. Use of the arms, but not the legs
    2. Control of bladder, but not bowels
    3. Potential for respiratory failure and infections
    4. Problems understanding and following instructions

13. The spouse reports that her husband tripped and bumped his head. He never lost consciousness but seemed confused for a few minutes after the accident. Which assessment finding does the nurse expect? *(1199)*
    1. Headache and vertigo
    2. Difficulty with judgment and reasoning
    3. Posttraumatic amnesia and aggressiveness
    4. Appears awake, but does not respond

14. The patient has a spinal cord injury above the level of T5. While assisting with hygienic care, the nurse notices that the patient is diaphoretic and shivering, and he states that he has a headache. Upon assessment, it is found that his blood pressure is elevated. What should the nurse do **first**? *(1199)*
    1. Reposition to a position of comfort.
    2. Inform the provider.
    3. Check for bladder distention.
    4. Give an antihypertensive medication.

15. The nurse anticipates that the patient with a spinal cord injury is at risk for venous thrombosis. Which interventions will be used for prevention? **Select all that apply.** *(1199)*
    1. Fluid restriction
    2. Passive and active range-of-motion exercises
    3. Application of heat
    4. Administration of anticoagulants
    5. Application of elastic stockings
    6. Assessment for swelling, redness, and heat in extremities

16. The nurse is assessing a patient who had a stroke and was recently admitted to the rehabilitation unit. What is the **best** method to determine how much assistance is required for hygienic care? *(1193)*
    1. Ask the unlicensed assistive personnel (UAP) to assist as needed.
    2. Ask the patient how much he feels like he can do for himself.
    3. Read the documentation from the transferring facility.
    4. Observe the patient as he performs tasks such as eating.

17. The older patient with a hip fracture has a self-care deficit related to bathing due to problems with ambulation and balance. Which action would the nurse use to foster independence, while ensuring safety? *(1198)*
    1. Help the patient sit in the bathtub and bathe self, rather than attempt to stand and balance in the shower.
    2. Have the UAP stay with the patient during shower, but tell the UAP to let the patient wash herself.
    3. Have the patient remain in bed and bring her a basin of water and towels and allow her to wash her own hands and face.
    4. Assist the patient to sit in a stable chair in the shower stall and adjust the water temperature of the handheld shower spray.

18. Which patient is **most** likely to need minimization of distractions that would prevent participation in therapy? *(1199, 1200)*
    1. Patient who has been depressed for several months
    2. Patient who had a myocardial infarction
    3. Patient who had a traumatic brain injury
    4. Patient who has chronic obstructive pulmonary disease

19. A patient had cardiac surgery. His condition is much improved, but it seems unlikely that he will be able to return to his job. The spouse expresses fears that her husband will die if she doesn't quit her job and stay home to take care of him. In this case, what would be considered the **best** outcome? *(1190)*
    1. Patient continuously works toward resuming his old job.
    2. Spouse acknowledges patient's ability to independently stay at home.
    3. Spouse quits her job, and fears about husband's death are alleviated.
    4. Patient acknowledges spouse's fears, and encourages her to stop worrying.

20. A patient was involved in an explosion at a chemical factory and sustained polytrauma/blast-related injury. What types of injuries would the health care team expect to find? **Select all that apply.** *(1195)*
    1. Burns
    2. Fractures of extremities
    3. Chemical pneumonitis
    4. Brain injury
    5. Myocardial infarction
    6. Hearing loss

CRITICAL THINKING ACTIVITIES

21. The patient who sustained a TBI was admitted to an acute care facility then transferred to a rehabilitation facility. Now the patient is alert, stable, and ambulatory but he suffers residual effects from the TBI.

   a. In the rehabilitative assessment of this patient, what may the nurse expect to find? *(1199)* _____

   _____

   _____

   _____

   _____

   _____

   _____

   b. What type of interventions does the nurse anticipate for the patient with a TBI? *(1201)*_____

   _____

   _____

   _____

   _____

22. The nurse is caring for a patient who needs post-stroke care and rehabilitation. The patient has residual right-sided weakness in the arm and leg. The physical therapist and the occupational therapist are optimistic that the patient can recover some function, but probably not return to pre-stroke status. The patient is currently discouraged and is focused on loss and disability. He shows little interest in performing the exercises or in learning how to do self-care.

   a. What should the nurse do first? *(1193)* _____

   _____

   _____

   _____

   _____

   b. Identify several ways that the nurse can encourage independence. *(1190, 1192)* _____

   _____

   _____

   _____

   _____

Hospice Care

MULTIPLE CHOICE

Directions: Select the best answer(s) for each of the following questions.

1. An older adult resident under hospice care resides in a long-term care facility and end of life is imminent. The primary care provider has ordered an IV fluid bolus to correct hypotension and dehydration. The hospice nurse questions the order and the facility nursing staff are not sure what to do. Who should be contacted to mediate this situation? *(1208)*
   1. Director of nursing services for the facility
   2. Family member who has power of attorney
   3. Medical director of the core interdisciplinary team
   4. Supervisor of the hospice nurse

2. The family of an older adult is struggling with the financial issues related to long-term care versus losing household income if someone quits work to provide full-time end-of-life care. Which member of the core interdisciplinary team would be **most** helpful in advising the family? *(1208)*
   1. Social worker
   2. Nurse coordinator
   3. Medical director
   4. Admissions nurse

3. Which outcome statement **best** indicates that the goal of bereavement counseling has been met? *(1210)*
   1. Widow reports that family missed her dead husband during the holidays, but he was fondly remembered.
   2. Older widow appreciates bereavement counselor and a deep personal relationship develops.
   3. Widow calls bereavement counselor several times a month for several years after the death of spouse.
   4. Bereavement counselor sends cards and messages, but never hears from the widow of the deceased.

4. The nurse hears in report that the patient received hypodermoclysis. Which assessment is the nurse **most** likely to perform to evaluate efficacy of this therapy? *(1214)*
   1. Assess for bowel sounds and abdominal distention.
   2. Assess mucous membranes and skin turgor.
   3. Assess for relief of local pain and general discomfort.
   4. Assess for nausea and frequency of vomiting.

5. Which factors contribute to constipation in terminally ill patients? **Select all that apply.** *(1214)*
   1. Poor dietary intake
   2. Poor fluid intake
   3. Hyperglycemia
   4. Hyponatremia
   5. Opioids for pain control
   6. Decreased activity

6. The nurse is looking at the patient's chart and a Physician Orders for Life-Sustaining Treatment (POLST) form and a Do Not Resuscitate (DNR) order are both included. Under what circumstance would the nurse need to compare the POLST to the DNR to clarify nursing interventions? *(1217)*
   1. Patient has terminal illness and refuses to eat.
   2. Patient is having chest pain with trouble breathing.
   3. Patient has no pulse and is not breathing.
   4. Patient is difficult to arouse with faint pulse.

7. Which patient **best** meets the criteria for admission to hospice? *(1206)*
   1. The patient is in very poor health, homeless, and prognosis is uncertain; no family caregivers are available for support.
   2. The patient is undergoing cancer treatments, but pain and symptoms are currently difficult for the family to manage.
   3. The patient has less than 6 months to live and patient and caregiver are willing to participate in the planning of care.
   4. The family wants the patient to receive around-the-clock skilled nursing care and emergency life support as needed.

8. The family of a dying patient is feeling physically and emotionally exhausted while taking around-the-clock shifts to care for their loved one. Which hospice service would be the **best** benefit for the family? *(1209)*
   1. Respite care service
   2. Palliative care consultation
   3. Bereavement counseling
   4. Hospice ethics committee

9. The provider orders oral opioid medication for the terminally ill patient for pain control. What other medications would the nurse expect the provider to order? **Select all that apply.** *(1212, 1215)*
   1. Anticholinergics
   2. Anticonvulsants
   3. Anticoagulants
   4. Antiemetics
   5. Antihypertensives
   6. Anxiolytics

10. The hospice nurse performs a pain assessment and gives different amounts of pain medication to the patient rather than the same dose each time. What is the **best** rationale for this practice? *(1212)*
    1. Determining the right dose of medication is difficult, so different amounts are tried to determine a safe dose.
    2. As a person is dying, the organs begin to shut down and absorption and metabolism of medication decreases.
    3. Every patient is different in how he or she responds to the medication, so it is administered by trial and error.
    4. The dosage is titrated to manage pain while keeping the patient alert enough to interact with the family.

11. Which nursing intervention would help the patient/family to meet the hospice goals? *(1218)*
    1. Encourage the family to consider putting the patient into long-term care.
    2. Remind the cancer patient that hoping for remission is therapeutic and beneficial.
    3. Reassure the primary caregiver that going out to a movie is not being selfish.
    4. Reinforce that eating and drinking as much as possible facilitates healing and recovery.

12. The hospice nurse is working with a patient and family who are from a different culture than the nurse's own. The family insists on performing some rituals that seem to be making the patient physically uncomfortable and emotionally distraught. What should the nurse do **first**? *(1209)*
    1. Graciously respect the patient's and family's cultural beliefs and allow them to continue.
    2. Politely ask the patient if he wants to continue or if he would like the family to stop.
    3. Humbly attempt to understand the benefit of the rituals from a cultural point of view.
    4. Respectfully inquire if there is a way to modify the rituals to make them less traumatic.

13. The hospice volunteer tells the nurse that he is thinking about quitting. "I like the patient, but the wife has me doing the shopping, the yardwork, and walking the dog. Now she wants me to paint the house." What should the nurse do? *(1209)*
    1. Talk to the wife and explain the role and responsibilities of the volunteer.
    2. Call the volunteer coordinator and ask for additional help to paint the house.
    3. Ask the patient how he has been getting along with the volunteer.
    4. Instruct the volunteer to explain the situation to the volunteer coordinator.

14. The hospice nurse notices that the patient and hospice aide joke and talk and seem to have a close relationship. The nurse suspects that the patient is disclosing more feelings and concerns to the aide than he is to the rest of the staff. What is the **most** important thing that the nurse should do? *(1210, 1211)*
    1. Praise the hospice aide for having a supportive rapport with the patient.
    2. Have frequent contact with the aide to get updates on the patient's concerns.
    3. Remind the aide about scope of practice and staff-patient boundaries.
    4. Try to spend more time with the patient to develop a better rapport and trust.

15. The patient is a large man who needs assistance to move and transfer to a wheelchair. His wife, the caregiver, is a relatively small woman. Which team member can **best** assist the wife with this issue? *(1211)*
    1. Physiatrist
    2. Hospice aide
    3. Physical therapist
    4. Nurse coordinator

16. The nurse reads in the documentation that the Edmonton Symptom Assessment System (ESAS) was used when the patient was first admitted into hospice. Which current assessment findings could be compared to the baseline established by ESAS? *(1211)*
    1. Patient's satisfaction with plan of care and recommendations for improvement
    2. Patient's subjective feeling of pain, tiredness, and overall feeling of well-being
    3. Patient's cognitive, intellectual, and perceptual status and ability to make judgments
    4. Patient's ability to perform activities of daily living and home maintenance

17. The patient is having significant pain, but refuses to take oral morphine. "Because it makes me feel confused and I hallucinate." What should the nurse do **first**? *(1212)*
    1. Encourage taking the medication for now, but promise to call the provider.
    2. Offer a prescribed nonopioid drug and try several nonpharmacologic options.
    3. Call the pharmacist to see if alternative routes of administration cause fewer side effects.
    4. Give the patient a lower dose and observe for confusion or other side effects.

18. Patient has nausea that is likely to be related to a mechanical obstruction caused by the progressive growth of a tumor and the nausea is exacerbated by the patient's anxiety. Which medication, if prescribed, would the nurse question? *(1210)*
    1. Promethazine: suppository 30 minutes before meals
    2. Prochlorperazine: oral dose as needed for nausea
    3. Lorazepam: oral dose as needed every 6-8 hours for anxiety
    4. Senna: oral dose two times per day

19. The patient is having nausea and vomiting, so the nurse gives the patient an antiemetic and the vomiting subsides. What should the nurse offer the patient **first**? *(1214)*
    1. Diluted bouillon
    2. Plain white rice
    3. Vanilla pudding
    4. Favorite food

20. The patient has not had a bowel movement. What is the **initial** nursing action? *(1214)*
    1. Explain to the patient that a decreased oral intake decreases the amount of stool.
    2. Assess the amount and frequency of opioid usage.
    3. Advise the patient to increase fiber and fluids in the diet.
    4. Assess discomfort, bowel sounds, and firmness of the abdomen.

21. The nurse notes that the patient is weak and emaciated and determines that stomatitis is contributing to the problem. Which intervention would be the **most** helpful? *(1215)*
    1. Administer an antiemetic medication 30 minutes before meals.
    2. Weigh the patient after meals and point out small improvements.
    3. Assist with oral hygiene and use water-soaked swabs before and after meals.
    4. Have family bring in meals, rather than cook at home.

22. The provider has informed the hospice patient, family, and nurse that there is an invasive untreatable tumor that is contributing to the patient's anorexia. Which intervention is the **best** for the patient? *(1215)*
    1. Emotional support
    2. Artificial hydration
    3. Total parental nutrition
    4. Tube feedings

23. The nurse gets a phone call from the caregiver who reports hearing the "death rattle." What instructions should the nurse give to the caregiver? *(1215)*
    1. "I will get an order for a bronchodilator medication and bring it to the house."
    2. "Apply oxygen and stay with him. I will come to the house right now."
    3. "Sit the patient upright in bed, apply oxygen, and call 911."
    4. "This is expected: mucus and fluids will pool in the back of his throat."

24. The caregiver reports that the patient is having a hard time managing excessive secretions especially at night, which causes a lot of coughing and choking. He is unable to sit up by himself. What is the **best** intervention to suggest for this problem? *(1215)*
    1. Teach the patient to cough and deep-breathe.
    2. Obtain an order for droperidol.
    3. Teach the caregiver to perform oral-tracheal suctioning.
    4. Obtain an order for transdermal scopolamine.

25. The hospice aide was devastated when the patient died and the nurse discovers that the aide has been visiting the caregiver on daily basis for the past 12 months. What should the nurse do? *(1216)*
    1. Assess the caregiver's feelings about the frequent visits from the aide.
    2. Report the hospice aide's behavior to the nurse coordinator.
    3. Assess the hospice aide's feelings and motivations for behavior.
    4. Suggest that the hospice aide contact the bereavement counselor.

26. The nurse makes a home visit and the caregiver, who is normally calm and eager to participate in the plan of care, is very angry and insists that the plan needs to be changed because "Nothing is working and I can't go on like this!" What should the nurse do **first**? *(1217)*
    1. Contact the interdisciplinary team so that the plan can be reevaluated.
    2. Call the nurse coordinator to come and assess the situation.
    3. Check the patient for changes in physical, emotional, or behavioral status.
    4. Use therapeutic communication and encourage the caregiver to express concerns.

CRITICAL THINKING ACTIVITIES

27. The family of a patient with terminal cancer has requested information about hospice care. The patient has severe pain and potential curative treatments have been exhausted.

    a. How would the nurse assess the patient's pain? *(1211)* _____

    _____

    _____

    _____

    b. In addition to assessment, what are the other nursing responsibilities for management of a hospice patient's pain? *(1212)*

    _____

    _____

    _____

    _____

    c. For pain relief or reduction, identify the types of medications that may be used for the following. *(1212)*

       i. Mild to moderate pain: _____

    _____

    ii. Severe pain: _____

_____

    iii. Long-lasting results:_____

_____

  d. What nonpharmacologic measures may also be implemented to relieve or reduce pain? *(1212)*

_____

_____

_____

_____

_____

28. The patient is an 86-year-old man who has Alzheimer's disease. His 80-year-old wife has been taking care of him at home for the past 10 years. He was recently diagnosed with an aggressive and inoperable cancer. His family agrees that he should be in hospice, but they are unable to agree on who should be the primary caregiver. The wife insists that she has been taking care of her husband for 10 years and is capable. The eldest son has been responsible for paying the bills and overseeing his parents' finances; he thinks that his sister, who is a nurse but lives in a different state, should move back and be the caregiver. The sister thinks that the grandson who is living with his grandparents and attends the university should be the caregiver. The grandson agrees that he is at the house most often, but is reluctant to take the responsibility. Discuss how the hospice team can assist this family in the decision-making process. *(1209)*

_____

_____

_____

_____

_____

_____

_____

_____

_____

Introduction to Anatomy and Physiology

CROSSWORD PUZZLE

1. Directions: Use the clues to complete the crossword puzzle.

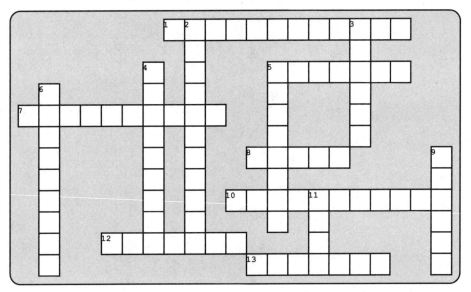

Across

1. Engulf and digest foreign material *(1227)*
5. Cell division *(1226)*
7. Movement of water and particles through a membrane by force from either pressure or gravity *(1228)*
8. Several kinds of tissues united to perform a more complex function *(1231)*
10. Extracellular fluid taken into the cell and digested *(1227)*
12. Diffusion of water through a selectively permeable membrane in the presence of at least one impermeant solute *(1228)*
13. Largest organelle within the cell *(1225)*

Down

2. Body's internal environment is relatively constant *(1224)*
3. Perform more complex functions than any one organ can perform alone *(1224)*
4. Internal living material of cells *(1225)*
5. Thin sheets of tissue that serve many functions in the body *(1229)*
6. Solid particles in a fluid move from an area of higher concentration to an area of lower concentration *(1228)*
9. Groups of similar cells that work together to perform a specific function *(1228)*
11. Smallest living unit of structure and function in the body *(1232)*

FIGURE LABELING

Planes of the Body

2.   Directions: Label the figure below with the correct names of the body planes and anatomical directionality of the body: sagittal, coronal, ventral, dorsal, transverse, caudal, and cranial. *(1222)*

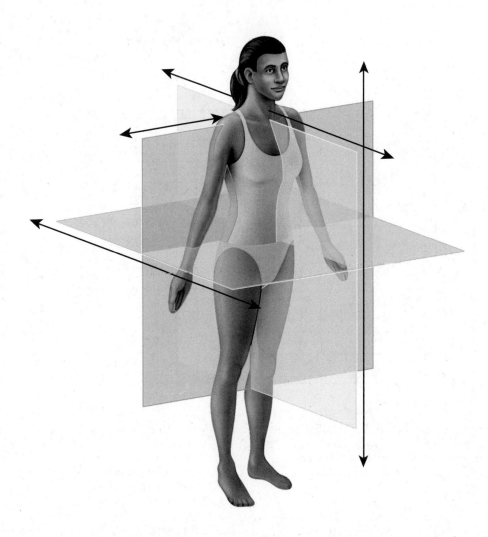

TABLE ACTIVITY

3. The table below lists one part of each of the major systems of the body. Identify the major system and then identify at least one function. *(1231)*

One Body Part of Major System	Major System	Function
Lungs		
Blood vessels		
Brain		
Stomach		
Kidneys		
Bones		
Voluntary muscles		
Skin		
Thyroid gland		
Lymph nodes		
Gonads		

MULTIPLE CHOICE

Directions: Select the best answer(s) for each of the following questions.

4. The patient reports, "I ran into the coffee table and bruised my shin." Which sample of documentation **best** reflects the nurse's knowledge of anatomy and medical terminology? *(1221)*
   1. Skin damage noted on the right lower leg in the shin area
   2. Patient reports running into coffee table and bruising shin
   3. Moderate bruising noted on the patient's right leg just below knee
   4. 4-cm ecchymosis on mid-anterior of right tibia-fibula

5. The patient needs assistance to turn and move in bed and is at risk for the complications of immobility. The nurse documents with date and signature: 10:00 Assisted into a right lateral side-lying position; 12:00 Assisted into supine position; 14:00 Assisted into left lateral side-lying position. What is the **best** rationale for this type of documentation? *(1221)*
   1. Documentation shows that needs were met and the goal was achieved.
   2. Documentation reflects actions taken to prevent complications of immobility.
   3. Nurse is following standard documentation guidelines.
   4. Nurse is demonstrating a professional knowledge of terminology.

6. The nurse reads in the chart that the neglected infant sustained a superficial sunburn on the dorsal body surface. What instructions would the nurse give to the unlicensed assistive personnel? *(1221)*
   1. "You will see a thin film of cream on the baby's perineal area."
   2. "If you see peeling or blistering on the front of the chest, let me know."
   3. "Use tepid water and gently wash the baby's back and pat dry."
   4. "The baby's face and the top of his head may appear red and flaky."

7. The nurse is checking peripheral pulses on a patient who has peripheral vascular disease. Which pulse is the **most** distal in the lower extremities? *(1222)*
   1. Dorsalis pedis
   2. Popliteal
   3. Posterior tibial
   4. Femoral

8. Which anatomical structure is in the medial portion of the chest? *(1221)*
   1. Lungs
   2. Heart
   3. Sternum
   4. Clavicles

9. Which part of the cell has distinct surface proteins that play an important role in tissue typing to determine compatibility for organ transplant? *(1225)*
   1. Protoplasm
   2. Nucleus
   3. Cytoplasm
   4. Plasma membrane

10. One type of cell in the body relies on the action of the ion pump to move nearly all calcium ions to special compartments or out of the cell. What bodily function is **most** affected by this process? *(1228)*
    1. Muscle contraction
    2. Digestion of food
    3. Protection against infection
    4. Secretion of hormones

11. The health care provider tells the nurse that the patient has a hematopoietic disorder. Which laboratory result would the nurse expect to see? *(1230)*
    1. Decreased potassium
    2. Decreased red blood cell count
    3. Increased glucose
    4. Increased blood urea nitrogen

12. For a patient with a history of splenectomy, which topic is the nurse **most** likely to review to ensure that the patient has a good understanding of the self-care related to loss of the spleen? *(1231)*
    1. Blood glucose monitoring
    2. Dietary sources of fiber
    3. Infection control measures
    4. Fall prevention

13. The patient reports pain in the right upper abdomen just inferior to the ribs. Based on the nurse's knowledge of anatomy, which organ is **most** likely to be contributing to the patient's discomfort? *(1223)*
    1. Small intestine
    2. Spleen
    3. Gallbladder
    4. Cecum

14. The nurse suspects that the patient has urinary retention and must assess for bladder distention. Which region of the patient's abdomen will the nurse palpate? *(1223)*
    1. Umbilical region
    2. Hypogastric region
    3. Right hypochondriac region
    4. Left iliac region

15. The patient has a stomach ulcer. Based on knowledge of anatomy, the nurse recognizes that the patient is likely to report pain or discomfort in which region of the abdomen? *(1223)*
    1. Epigastric region
    2. Right iliac region
    3. Left lumbar region
    4. Hypogastric region

16. The patient is diagnosed with appendicitis. The health care provider orders ice to the abdomen pending emergency surgery. Where will the nurse place the prepared ice bag? *(1224)*
    1. Left lower quadrant
    2. Right lower quadrant
    3. Left upper quadrant
    4. Right upper quadrant

17. In the case of bowel obstruction, which condition is **most** likely to cause the first episodes of vomiting if the patient is consuming solid foods? *(1224)*
    1. Distal large intestine obstruction
    2. Proximal large intestine obstruction
    3. Distal small intestine obstruction
    4. Proximal small intestine obstruction

18. The patient sustains injury to the epidermis. Which problem will the nurse anticipate and try to prevent? *(1230, 1231)*
    1. Risk for infection
    2. Loss of strength
    3. Decreased secretion of mucus
    4. Loss of insulation

19. The patient is in a coma and has continuous open-mouthed breathing, which causes dry mucous membranes of the mouth. What is the **most** important rationale for the nurse to perform good oral hygiene for this patient? *(1231)*
    1. Preserve patient's dignity
    2. Lubricate food for digestion
    3. Prevent respiratory infection
    4. Maintain condition of teeth

20. The patient tells the nurse that he has a history of bursitis. Which focused assessment is the nurse **most** likely to perform that relates to this information? *(1231)*
    1. Auscultate the bowel sounds and palpate the abdomen.
    2. Auscultate the lung sounds and watch respiratory effort.
    3. Put joints through range of motion and ask about discomfort.
    4. Ask patient to balance on right leg and then on left leg.

CRITICAL THINKING ACTIVITIES

Activity 1

21. Why is it important for the nurse to have knowledge of anatomy and physiology? *(1221)* _____

_____

_____

_____

_____

Activity 2

22. The patient says, "I have a bruise on the tip of my right big toe." Document the patient's report using anatomical terminology. *(1221)*

_____

_____

_____

_____

_____

Activity 3

23. Discuss how the accurate usage and correct spelling of anatomical terminology enhances the credibility of your nursing documentation. *(1221)*

_____

_____

_____

_____

_____

Care of the Surgical Patient

TABLE ACTIVITY

1. Directions: The patient has just returned from gastric surgery. Next to each assessment, list normal findings and the frequency of data collection. *(1263, 1264, 1265, 1268, 1269, 1270)*

Assessment	Normal Findings	Frequency
a. Vital signs		
b. Incision		
c. Respiratory effort		
d. Pain		
e. Urinary function		
f. Neurovascular		
g. Activity		
h. Gastrointestinal function		

MATCHING

Directions: Match the term or suffix on the left with the meaning on the right. (1236)

	Term		**Meaning**
_____	2. anastomosis	a.	Surgical removal of
_____	3. -ectomy	b.	Direct visualization by a scope
_____	4. -lysis	c.	Opening into
_____	5. -orrhaphy	d.	Surgical joining of two ducts or blood vessels to allow flow from one to another; to bypass an area
_____	6. -oscopy	e.	Surgical repair of
_____	7. -ostomy	f.	Destruction or dissolution of
_____	8. -otomy	g.	Opening made to allow the passage of drainage
_____	9. -pexy	h.	Plastic surgery
_____	10. -plasty	i.	Fixation of

MULTIPLE CHOICE

Directions: Select the best answer(s) for each of the following questions.

11. After surgery, which foods would the nurse suggest to the patient that are specific for building and repairing body tissue? *(1238)*
    1. Variety of foods but avoid processed sugar
    2. Lean meat and low-fat dairy products
    3. Whole grain breads and cereals
    4. Seasonal fruits and leafy green vegetables

12. The newly hired nurse is told that generally morning medications are withheld on the day of surgery. The nurse is **most** likely to clarify withholding which medication? *(1240)*
    1. Phenytoin
    2. Warfarin sodium
    3. Ranitidine
    4. Acetaminophen

13. Which preoperative patient teaching topics are a nursing responsibility? **Select all that apply.** *(1239)*
    1. Gastrointestinal cleansing preparation
    2. Need for assistive devices postoperatively (e.g., crutches)
    3. Date and time of the surgery
    4. Risks and benefits of the procedure
    5. Written pre- and postoperative instructions

14. The nurse is reviewing the presurgical laboratory results for a patient who has a history of cardiac problems. Which abnormal result is of **greatest** concern? *(1243)*
    1. Sodium: 146 mEq/L
    2. Blood glucose: 130 mg/dL
    3. Blood urea nitrogen: 25 mg/dL
    4. Potassium: 5.8 mEq/L

15. The nurse is interviewing the patient to obtain a medical history prior to a surgical procedure. Which patient report warrants further investigation because of a possible latex allergy? *(1245)*
    1. Had sore throat after having a nasogastric tube inserted for stomach decompression
    2. Developed a large hematoma in the antecubital fossa after donating blood
    3. Experienced severe swelling of the labia after urinary catheterization
    4. Had skin irritation after dermabrasion to remove a small precancerous growth

16. Which data set is **most** important to note prior to starting the skin preparation before surgery? *(1245)*
    1. Temperature, turgor, and dryness of skin; history of dehydration and electrolyte imbalance
    2. Presence of infection, irritation, bruises, or lesions on skin; history of skin allergies
    3. Underlying structures such as veins, arteries, or nerves; history of peripheral vascular disease
    4. Color of skin, sensation to touch, and hair distribution; history of peripheral neuropathy

17. The patient is in the postanesthesia care unit and is having difficulty maintaining a patent airway after extubation. Which intervention would be used to maintain a patent airway until the patient is fully conscious? *(1257)*
    1. Ventilate using a bag-valve-mask
    2. Use an oral suction catheter
    3. Give oxygen per nasal cannula
    4. Insert an oral airway

18. What is the significance of the nurse's signature on the preoperative checklist? *(1259)*
    1. Specifies that the preoperative medication was given
    2. Delegates care on the list to the appropriate staff members
    3. Indicates the nurse assumes responsibility for care on the list
    4. Confirms that the patient understands the preoperative care

19. What postoperative assessments would the nurse make to comply with the facility policy based on the "times 4" factor? *(1264)*
    1. Takes vital signs, checks IV, incisional sites, and any tubes 4 times every hour for 4 hours, then every hour times 4 hours, then every 4 hours times 4 days
    2. Does vital signs and general assessments every 15 minutes times 4 (for 4 times), every 30 minutes times 4, every hour times 4, then every 4 hours
    3. Takes pulse, blood pressure, respiratory rate, and pulse oximeter readings every 15 minutes times 4 (for 4 times), then every hour until assessments approximate baseline
    4. Does vital signs, checks IV, incisional sites, tubes, and postoperative orders every 15 minutes times 4 (for 4 times), then delegates vital signs every hour times 4 hours

20. The postsurgical patient manifests hypotension; tachycardia; restlessness; apprehension; and cold, moist, pale skin. How does the nurse interpret these findings and what action would the nurse take **first**? *(1265)*
    1. Suspects hypoglycemia and administers IV 10% dextrose per standard protocol
    2. Suspects a panic attack and administers a PRN (as needed) dose of lorazepam
    3. Suspects airway obstruction and inserts an oral airway using nursing judgment
    4. Suspects hypovolemic shock and administers oxygen per standard protocol

21. The patient is in the induction stage of anesthesia. Which activity will **most** likely be taking place? *(1257)*
    1. Positioning the patient to perform the surgical procedure
    2. Decreasing the dosage of anesthetic agents
    3. Cleaning, shaving, and preparing the skin
    4. Establishing and verifying placement of the endotracheal tube

22. During the preoperative teaching session, a patient voices concerns about waking up during surgery. Which response should the nurse give to the patient? *(1257)*
    1. "The anesthesia given during surgery will not wear off and allow you to wake up."
    2. "The anesthesiologist is able to monitor for this and will provide medications as needed."
    3. "There is a very small chance of waking towards the end of the surgical procedure."
    4. "Don't be concerned; emergence from anesthesia is very rare."

23. The patient is scheduled to undergo a urologic procedure in the surgical suite. The patient will be conscious during the procedure. What type of anesthesia will **most** likely be used? *(1257)*
    1. Nerve block
    2. Epidural anesthesia
    3. Spinal anesthesia
    4. Local anesthesia

24. The patient is scheduled to undergo the removal of a benign cyst from his hand in the health care provider's office. The nurse is aware that the provider will **most** likely use which type of anesthesia? *(1258)*
    1. Regional anesthesia
    2. Local anesthesia
    3. Moderate sedation
    4. Intrathecal anesthesia

25. The nurse is preparing to assist the surgeon who is performing a procedure using moderate sedation. Which nursing action is the **most** important during the procedure? *(1258)*
    1. Monitoring intake and output
    2. Administering the medication
    3. Reassuring the patient
    4. Assessing vital signs

26. The nurse is preparing an in-service for nursing staff about moderate sedation. What should be emphasized in the presentation? *(1259)*
    1. There will be temporary paralysis and loss of sensation in the legs.
    2. There is a risk of aspiration and laryngeal spasm after extubation.
    3. Resuscitation equipment should be readily available.
    4. Patients have a risk for thrombus because of prolonged positioning.

27. When developing the plan of care for an Arab American undergoing surgery, what is a cultural consideration? *(1240)*
    1. Stoicism during pain and discomfort
    2. Expected submissive role of women
    3. Need for a written consent for surgery
    4. Avoidance of sustained eye contact

28. When is the **best** time to perform preoperative teaching? *(1240, 1242)*
    1. 1 to 2 days before surgery
    2. Morning of surgery
    3. At least 2 weeks preoperatively
    4. When the nurse has extra time

29. Before surgery on the bowel, what is the purpose of administering neomycin, sulfonamides, or erythromycin? *(1243)*
    1. Decreases likelihood of bowel perforation
    2. Prevents urinary tract infections
    3. Detoxifies the gastrointestinal tract
    4. Reduces the risk of pneumonia

30. The nurse is providing care for a patient in the postanesthesia care unit after emergency surgery. The patient has been on antihypertensive medications for a long time. What side effects related to use of these medications should the nurse monitor for? *(1256)*
    1. Bradypnea
    2. Hypotension
    3. Tachycardia
    4. Diaphoresis

31. The patient is instructed to discontinue taking nonsteroidal antiinflammatory drugs (NSAIDs) for several days before surgery. What is the **best** explanation for the need to hold this medication? *(1256)*
    1. "NSAIDs increase susceptibility to postoperative bleeding."
    2. "NSAIDs impair healing during the postoperative period."
    3. "NSAIDs interact with the medications used for anesthesia."
    4. "NSAIDs are associated with an increase in postoperative infections."

32. A mastectomy is scheduled for an 81-year-old patient. What is the **highest** priority during the immediate postoperative recovery period? *(1264)*
    1. Assessing for confusion
    2. Airway management
    3. Pain management
    4. Monitoring bleeding

33. The patient is being prepared to go to the operating room. With proper instructions, which tasks can be delegated to the unlicensed assistive personnel (UAP)? **Select all that apply.** *(1237)*
    1. Compare current vital signs to baseline measurements.
    2. Assist the patient to remove personal clothing and don a hospital gown.
    3. Check the IV pump rate and the IV insertion site.
    4. Assist the patient to move from the bed to the stretcher.
    5. Ensure that the preoperative checklist is complete.
    6. Apply antiembolic stockings.

34. The nurse is performing preoperative teaching for a patient who must undergo a breast biopsy. The patient begins to cry softly and says, "I can't believe this is happening to me." What response should the nurse use **first**? *(1238)*
    1. "Do you need more information about the procedure?"
    2. "The biopsy is a minor procedure, there are very few risks."
    3. "Don't worry, everything will be okay; we'll take care of you."
    4. "You seem scared; tell me what you are thinking about."

35. Which patient is **most** likely to have problems related to medications that are given in the perioperative setting? *(1238)*
    1. A 23-year-old woman who believes in alternative and complementary therapies
    2. A 73-year-old woman who takes multiple medications for several chronic conditions
    3. A 56-year-old man who has recently started an oral antidiabetic medication
    4. A 7-year-old child who occasionally uses a rescue inhaler for asthma

36. The patient tells the nurse that he has been smoking for years and is likely to continue to smoke before and after his surgery. Which piece of equipment will the nurse emphasize during the preoperative teaching? *(1240)*
    1. Normal range for pulse oximeter
    2. Use of incentive spirometer
    3. Use of patient-controlled analgesia pump
    4. Operation of the call bell

37. The nurse is evaluating the patient's understanding of the preoperative teaching. Which question should the nurse ask? *(1241)*
    1. "Do you have any questions about the postoperative care?"
    2. "Would you like written information about the care plan?"
    3. "Did you understand everything I told you about the care?"
    4. "What questions do you have about the postoperative care?"

38. The surgeon is preparing to explain a procedure to the patient and obtain informed consent. Which information is the **most** vital to relate to the surgeon before he/she enters the patient's room? *(1243)*
    1. Patient has been talking about refusing the surgery.
    2. Patient had a hypoglycemic episode 3 hours ago.
    3. Patient's laboratory reports are not available yet.
    4. Patient received morphine and a sedative 1 hour ago.

39. The patient is to have nothing by mouth (NPO) starting at midnight the night before surgery. Which task can be delegated to the UAP? *(1243)*
    1. Give the patient small sips of water if he reports thirst.
    2. Assist with oral care, but instruct the patient not to swallow fluids.
    3. Obtain small hard candy for the patient to suck on.
    4. Check the patient's intravenous fluids every 2 hours.

40. Which patient should not be instructed to cough after surgery? *(1248)*
    1. The patient who had abdominal surgery
    2. The patient who had pneumonia before surgery
    3. The patient who had intracranial surgery
    4. The patient who had thoracic surgery

41. The patient had surgery at 10:00 AM. At 6:00 PM, the nurse notes that the patient has not voided since returning from surgery. What should the nurse do **first**? *(1268)*
    1. Help the patient to the toilet and open the faucet so that water runs.
    2. Palpate the symphysis pubis to determine if the bladder is distended.
    3. Call the surgeon and obtain an order for catheterization.
    4. Help the patient get up and ambulate to stimulate urination.

42. The patient is undergoing spinal anesthesia and the patient's position has to be slightly adjusted during the procedure. Which occurrence is cause for **greatest** concern? *(1257)*
    1. Slight decrease in blood pressure
    2. Loss of sensation in both feet
    3. Slowing of respiratory rate
    4. Inability to freely move the legs

43. A patient who had surgery on the left hip tells the nurse, "You might think I am crazy, but my right arm kind of hurts since I had my surgery." What should the nurse do **first**? *(1259)*
    1. Check the operating records for patient's position during the operation.
    2. Call the surgeon and inform him/her of the new-onset arm pain.
    3. Assess the arm for pulse, sensation, movement, pain, and temperature of skin.
    4. Give the patient a mild pain medication and elevate the arm on a pillow.

44. Which instruction is the nurse **most** likely to give to the patient before administering the preoperative medication? *(1259)*
    1. "Please go to the bathroom and void."
    2. "Let me mark the operative site."
    3. "I am going to draw a blood sample."
    4. "Please sign the consent form."

45. The patient will soon be transferred from the postanesthesia care unit to the nursing unit. Which tasks can be delegated to the UAP? **Select all that apply.** *(1237)*
    1. Place the bed in a high position with side rails in appropriate position.
    2. Obtain a clean gown and extra pillows for positioning.
    3. Set up suction equipment and test function.
    4. Get stethoscope, thermometer, and sphygmomanometer.
    5. Check the function of the IV pump.
    6. Place bed pads to protect linens from drainage.

46. The anesthesiologist has written the order to transfer the patient from the postanesthesia care unit to the nursing unit. Which assessment finding would delay the transfer? *(1263)*
    1. Patient is awake, but nausea and some vomiting continue.
    2. Patient is breathing normally, but reports a sore throat and cough.
    3. Patient is crying and reports pain related to the surgical incision.
    4. Patient has a decreased blood pressure and pulse is increasing.

47. The patient had surgery 10 hours ago. The UAP tells the nurse that the blood pressure (BP) is 96/60 mm Hg and the patient says, "My blood pressure is usually 120/78." What should the nurse do **first**? *(1265)*
    1. Check the patient for signs and symptoms of hypovolemic shock.
    2. Tell the UAP to go back and repeat the BP and report back.
    3. Tell the UAP to take and report BP and pulse every 5 minutes for 15 minutes.
    4. Call the surgeon and report the low reading of 96/60.

48. Which task is the responsibility of the scrub nurse? *(1263)*
    1. Sends for the patient at the proper time
    2. Checks medical record for completeness
    3. Performs and confirms patient assessment
    4. Assists with surgical draping of patient

49. The nurse is preparing to discharge a patient from an ambulatory surgery setting. How does the nurse determine when the patient is ready to be discharged? *(1273)*
    1. Patient states he is ready to drive himself home.
    2. Patient is groggy, but readily arouses to normal stimuli.
    3. Patient reports that pain is controlled and nausea has ceased.
    4. Family is available and willing to take responsibility.

50. The nurse is caring for a postoperative patient who has preexisting type 2 diabetes. Which assessment is **most** relevant to a complication associated with diabetes? *(1238)*
    1. Impaired communication
    2. Bloody emesis
    3. Poor wound healing
    4. Hypoventilation

CRITICAL THINKING ACTIVITIES

Activity 1

51. Discuss latex allergies. Include types, influencing factors, risk factors, and methods of preventing problems for patients who have latex allergies. *(1245)*

_____

_____

_____

_____

_____

_____

_____

Activity 2

52. Describe how the nurse can use the ABCDEF mnemonic device to ascertain serious illness or trauma in the preoperative patient. *(1238)*

_____

_____

_____

_____

_____

_____

_____

Activity 3

53. Discuss four or five considerations for older adults who require surgery. *(1238)* _____

_____

_____

_____

_____

_____

Care of the Patient With an Integumentary Disorder

SHORT ANSWER

Directions: Using your own words, answer each question in the space provided.

1. What are the functions of the skin? *(1276, 1277)* _____

   _____

   _____

   _____

   _____

2. When performing an assessment of an integumentary problem, what should be included using "PQRST"? *(1284)*

   _____

   _____

   _____

   _____

   _____

3. When performing an assessment of a mole, what characteristics should be included using "ABCDE" for assessment of skin lesions? *(1284)*

   _____

   _____

   _____

   _____

4. The nurse is assessing the skin of several patients. What are the physiologic factors that influence skin color? *(1279)*

   _____

   _____

5. The patient is a very dark-skinned individual who has low hemoglobin and hematocrit. How would the nurse assess this patient for pallor? *(1284)*

   _____

6. The darker-skinned patient reports an itching sensation, but the nurse cannot detect a rash with visual inspection. What technique can the nurse use? *(1284)*

_____

FIGURE LABELING

Rule of Nines

7. Directions: Label the body according to the rule of nines. *(1315)*

8. Calculate the percentage of burns for each of the situations listed below using the rule of nines. *(94, 95)*

   a. A 19-year-old was burned while playing with fireworks. He has burns on both of his arms (anterior and posterior) and his anterior chest and abdomen. _____%

   b. A 70-year-old man was burned when he backed up into an open-flame heater. He has burns on the posterior of his body from his ankles to his neck. He also has burns on the anterior portion of his legs. _____%

   c. The patient, who has diabetes mellitus, stepped into a hot shower and has burns on his back and buttocks. _____%

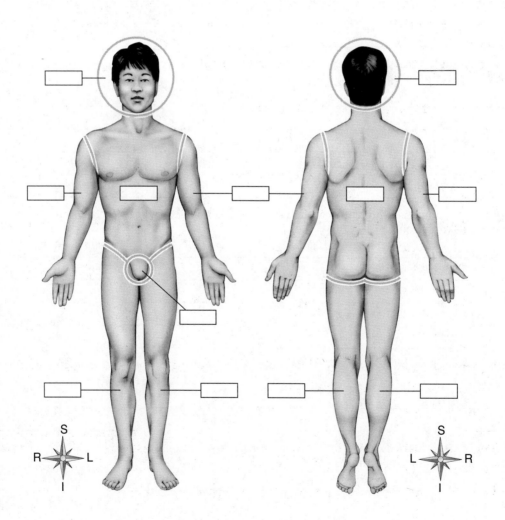

MULTIPLE CHOICE

Directions: Select the best answer(s) for each of the following questions

9. The nurse hears in report that the patient has anemia. Based on this information, what would the nurse expect to observe when assessing the patient's integumentary system? *(1279)*
   1. Cyanosis in the periphery
   2. Yellow tinge of conjunctivae
   3. Pallor of mucous membranes
   4. Brown concentration of melanin

10. What would be considered **early** signs/symptoms of a pressure injury (Stage 1)? *(1285)*
   1. Shallow, open, shiny, dry injury; pink-red wound bed without sloughing or bruising
   2. Full-thickness tissue loss, subcutaneous fat visible; possible undermining and tunneling
   3. Full-thickness tissue loss, slough and black eschar in wound bed with undermining and tunneling
   4. Intact skin with nonblanchable redness, painful, warm, soft localized area over a bony prominence

11. Which neonate has the **greatest** risk of being infected by herpes virus during childbirth? *(1286)*
   1. Mother has chronic genital herpes, but was never treated.
   2. Mother contracted genital herpes during first half of pregnancy.
   3. Mother previously had severe genital herpes outbreaks.
   4. Mother acquired genital herpes near the time of delivery.

12. A patient is prescribed oral acyclovir for type 1 herpes simplex virus. What is the expected outcome if the patient is compliant with the medication regimen? *(1288)*
   1. Prevents complications, such as meningitis or pneumonitis
   2. Shortens the outbreak and lessens the severity of symptoms
   3. Eliminates the likelihood of spreading the infection to others
   4. Decreases the probability of recurrent outbreaks

13. Which people have the **greatest** risk for serious complications secondary to herpes zoster infection? **Select all that apply.** *(1293)*
   1. Healthy middle-aged adult who never had chickenpox
   2. Older adult who takes large doses of prednisone for a chronic condition
   3. Middle-aged adult who just started taking chemotherapy
   4. Nurse who recently received the first dose of varicella vaccine
   5. Young adult who is positive for the human immunodeficiency virus

14. The nurse must assess several patients who have skin disorders. Which disorder can manifest signs/symptoms that could be mistaken for venous thrombosis? *(1294)*
   1. Cellulitis
   2. Pityriasis rosea
   3. Spider angioma
   4. Tinea corporis

15. What is the common factor for etiology and pathophysiology of folliculitis, furuncles, and carbuncles? *(1295, 1296)*
   1. Superficial infections are caused by fungus.
   2. Parasites get underneath the skin.
   3. Hair follicles are infected or inflamed.
   4. There is an allergic response to an allergen.

16. Which question would the nurse ask to assist the health care provider to determine the cause of contact dermatitis? *(1298)*
   1. "Have you used any new soaps or detergents?"
   2. "Are you currently sexually active?"
   3. "Is anyone in the household having similar symptoms?"
   4. "Have you had a recent febrile illness?"

17. The patient comes to the walk-in clinic and reports noticing itching shortly after eating shrimp. The nurse observes that the patient has wheals over the anterior neck and chest. Which assessment would the nurse perform **first**? *(1300)*
   1. Check orientation and observe for change in mental status.
   2. Auscultate heart sounds for pericardial friction rub.
   3. Take vital signs and observe for hypovolemic shock.
   4. Count respiratory rate and auscultate breath sounds.

18. The nurse instructs the patient on use of lindane. What additional instructions will the nurse give? *(1308)*
    1. If skin lesion starts to bleed or ooze or feels different (swollen, hard, lumpy, itchy, or tender to the touch), report symptoms to the health care provider.
    2. Apply broad-spectrum sunscreens with a sun protection factor of 15 or greater approximately 15 minutes before sun exposure and after swimming.
    3. Furniture, carpeting, and car interiors must be cleaned. Wash bed linens in hot water; then use dryer. Put stuffed toys in hot dryer for a full cycle.
    4. Use neutral soaps and avoid hot water and vigorous rubbing. Skin and hair should be washed to remove excess oil and excretions and to prevent odor.

19. Which data set represents the signs/symptoms of an exacerbation of systemic lupus erythematosus? *(1306)*
    1. Vesicles preceded by pain, generally in the thoracic region
    2. Fever, rash, cough, or increasing muscle and joint pain
    3. Erythema, pain, and tenderness over an area of skin
    4. Vesicles appear, ulcerate, rupture, and encrust

20. The nurse hears in report that a young female patient is very upset because of alopecia; she cannot focus on the overall cancer treatment plan. In addition to therapeutic communication, which intervention could the nurse use? *(1312)*
    1. Suggest therapeutic baths using colloid solution.
    2. Teach the patient about use of scarves or wigs.
    3. Suggest shaving, tweezing, or rubbing with pumice.
    4. Advise the patient to use lotion immediately after bathing.

21. The health care provider has diagnosed a patient with paronychia. Which assessment is the nurse **most** likely to perform before administering the ordered therapy? *(1313)*
    1. History of allergies to antibiotics
    2. Rating of pain on a pain scale
    3. Baseline range of motion
    4. Feelings about body image

22. A patient reports hair loss (hypotrichosis). Which assessment is the nurse **most** likely to conduct to assist the health care provider to determine the etiology of hypotrichosis? *(1313)*
    1. Type of hair-care products
    2. Use of herbal supplements
    3. Smoking history
    4. Dietary assessment

23. A patient is admitted for pain and tenderness in his lower right leg. The nurse's assessment reveals that the extremity is warm, swollen, and has a slightly pitted appearance. Which measure would the nurse use to relieve the discomfort? *(1294)*
    1. Assist the patient to ambulate as much as possible.
    2. Administer cool compresses or a covered ice bag.
    3. Elevate the leg with pillows to reduce edema.
    4. Assist with a therapeutic bath and gently pat skin to dry.

24. The nurse is assisting a mother to plan meals for a child who was recently diagnosed with eczema. Which foods should the nurse mention as common allergens associated with eczema? *(1300)*
    1. Strawberries and cured meats
    2. Eggs, rye, and preservatives
    3. Orange juice, wheat, and eggs
    4. Wheat, sugar, and bananas

25. The nurse knows that the health care provider frequently prescribes isotretinoin for patients with acne. Which question is the **most** important to routinely ask? *(1289)*
    1. "Are you pregnant or contemplating a pregnancy in the near future?"
    2. "Do you have a history of kidney problems or frequent urinary tract infections?"
    3. "How often do you sunbathe? Are you willing to abstain during treatment?"
    4. "Do you have any problems with your liver or a history of hepatitis?"

26. The nurse is interviewing an older adult. Which statement is cause for the **greatest** concern? *(1310)*
    1. "My toenails are tough and thick."
    2. "This black mole on my neck is itching."
    3. "My hair is thinning and I have a bald spot."
    4. "I have a lot of 'age spots' on my hands."

27. The nurse notes that the patient has clubbing of the fingertips. Based on this finding, which question would the nurse ask? *(1284)*
    1. "Have you been diagnosed with a respiratory disorder?"
    2. "Do you take medication for high blood pressure?"
    3. "Do you have a family history of diabetes mellitus?"
    4. "Are you taking medication for osteoporosis?"

28. To assess the temperature and texture of the patient's skin, which technique would the nurse use? *(1284)*
    1. Use the fingertips and gently palpate the affected area.
    2. Use the palms of the hands and compare opposite body areas.
    3. Use a cotton-tipped applicator and apply gentle pressure.
    4. Use a gloved finger to touch skin and ask about sensations.

29. The school nurse is assessing a 15-year-old girl and notices multiple linear superficial cuts over the girl's anterior forearms. What should the nurse do **first**? *(1284)*
    1. Call child protective services to report possible abuse.
    2. Notify the girl's parents about the finding.
    3. Ask the girl directly what happened to her arms.
    4. Initiate protective measures to prevent self-harm.

30. The nurse is assessing a patient who was recently transferred from home to a skilled nursing facility. The nurse sees a pressure injury with full-thickness tissue loss, which is covered by a thick, black layer of eschar. What should the nurse do **first**? *(1285, 1286)*
    1. Gently remove the eschar and check for tunneling and depth.
    2. Document the size and location of this stage IV injury.
    3. Contact the wound care specialist for wound management.
    4. Leave eschar intact; collaborate with RN to develop care plan.

31. The home health aide phones the nurse and says, "Yesterday, I helped the patient bathe. I wore gloves during the bath, but then afterwards he said that he was just diagnosed with herpes zoster." Which question would the nurse ask **first**? *(1291, 1292)*
    1. "Are you having a painful burning rash with itching?"
    2. "Did the patient have fluid-filled vesicles on the back or trunk?"
    3. "Have you received two doses of varicella vaccine?"
    4. "How long were you in contact with the patient?"

32. The nurse hears during shift report that the patient was admitted for penicillin-induced dermatitis medicamentosa. Which question is the **most** important to ask? *(1299)*
    1. Was the affected area immediately washed and rinsed?
    2. Has the patient been medicated for pain and itching?
    3. Has the patient had any respiratory distress?
    4. Does the patient have any fever or other signs of infection?

33. The nurse would be prepared to administer epinephrine as needed for which patient? *(1300)*
    1. Has burning sensation and a dry crusty lesion on the lip
    2. Has a single pink, scaly patch that resembles a large ringworm
    3. Has skin maceration, fissures, and vesicles around the toes
    4. Has raised red wheals and hives and an expiratory wheeze

CRITICAL THINKING ACTIVITIES

Activity 1

34. Discuss the nursing care of a patient who has sustained a major burn through the emergent phase, acute phase, and rehabilitation phase. *(1316-1320)*

    a.   Emergent phase:_____

        _____

        _____

    b.   Acute phase: _____

        _____

        _____

    c.   Rehabilitation phase:_____

        _____

        _____

Activity 2

35. Discuss teaching points for self-examination of skin, scalp, moles, blemishes, and birthmarks. *(1311)*

36. Discuss teaching points for skin cancer prevention. *(1311)*

Care of the Patient With a Musculoskeletal Disorder

FIGURE LABELING

1. Directions: Label the figure of the anterior view of skeleton below with the correct names of the bones of the body. *(1329)*

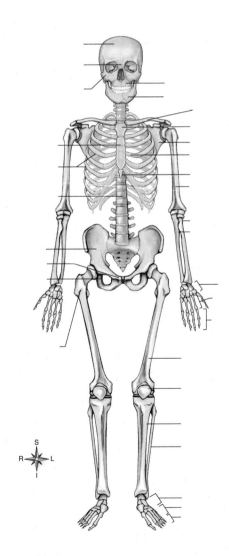

SHORT ANSWER

Directions: Using your own words, answer each question in the space provided.

2. List five functions of the skeletal system. *(1328)*

   a. _____

   b. _____

   c. _____

   d. _____

   e. _____

3. List three functions that muscles perform when they contract. *(1332)*

   a. _____

   b. _____

   c. _____

4. Discuss neurovascular assessment and include the seven Ps of orthopedic assessment. *(1363)* _____

   _____

   _____

   _____

   _____

5. What does "RICE" mean in relation to the treatment for sprains? *(1377)* _____

   _____

MULTIPLE CHOICE

Directions: Select the best answer(s) for each of the following questions.

6. The nurse is planning care for several patients on the orthopedic unit. Which patients will need frequent neurovascular checks during the shift? **Select all that apply.** *(1357)*
   1. Patient has a long leg cast for fracture sustained in an automobile accident.
   2. Older patient had elective hip replacement surgery secondary to arthritis.
   3. Construction worker sustained a crush injury to the lower leg.
   4. Patient has Volkmann's contracture of the right upper extremity.
   5. Young athlete sustained a dislocated shoulder during a football game.

7. The nurse sees that the patient has a new prescription for alendronate. In addition to medication teaching, which self-care measure is the nurse **most** likely to review with the patient? *(1348)*
   1. Fluid intake of at least 2000 mL daily
   2. Postural and breathing exercises
   3. Weight-bearing exercise, such as walking
   4. Application of heat and cold packs for pain

8. The home health nurse is reviewing the medication reconciliation list for a patient who has osteoarthritis. The list includes tramadol, acetaminophen, lisinopril, cortisone, and ibuprofen. Which drug-drug combination is cause for **greatest** concern? *(1345)*
   1. Lisinopril and tramadol
   2. Lisinopril and acetaminophen
   3. Lisinopril and cortisone
   4. Lisinopril and ibuprofen

9. What information would the nurse teach about sleep hygiene for a patient who has fibromyalgia? **Select all that apply.** *(1351)*
   1. Take a long, hot bath just before bedtime.
   2. Keep the sleeping environment dark, quiet, and comfortable.
   3. Keep a diary of sleep patterns.
   4. Exercise regularly every day.
   5. Have a protein snack just before going to bed.

10. Which patient needs to be monitored for shock? *(1365)*
    1. Patient reports pain in the muscles, bones, and joints; headaches, altered thought processes, and stiffness.
    2. Patient reports chest pain, especially on inspiration; nurse observes irritability, restlessness, and stupor.
    3. Patient experiences deep, unrelenting, progressive, and poorly localized pain unrelieved by analgesics.
    4. Patient appears anxious, weak, and lethargic; nurse observes hypotension, tachycardia, and diaphoresis.

11. A patient is prescribed colchicine to treat gout. The nurse would assess for which potential medication side effects? *(1346)*
    1. Diarrhea, nausea, and vomiting
    2. Seizures and dysrhythmias
    3. Fluid retention and sodium retention
    4. Hypercalcemia and orthostatic hypotension

12. Which foods should the nurse recommend as good sources of calcium for a 59-year-old woman who is concerned about her risk for osteoporosis? **Select all that apply.** *(1348)*
    1. Milk
    2. Spinach
    3. Potatoes
    4. Sardines
    5. Organ meats

13. The nurse is interviewing a young woman who injured her ankle while playing soccer. Considering the diagnostic testing most likely to be ordered, which question is **most** important to ask? *(1331)*
    1. "Do you have allergies to seafood or iodine?"
    2. "Is there any chance you could be pregnant?"
    3. "Are you currently taking any medications?"
    4. "Do you have a history of radiation exposure?"

14. The nurse is assessing a patient who had a myelogram 3 hours ago. Which patient comment causes the **greatest** concern? *(1332)*
    1. "My head hurts. Could I get an aspirin or a Tylenol tablet?"
    2. "I am thirsty. Would it be okay if I drank a soda or some juice?"
    3. "My foot feels numb and I can't move my toes very well."
    4. "I am not used to lying in bed all day long; I'd like to walk around."

15. The nurse hears in report that the patient has a medical diagnosis of ankylosing spondylitis. What will the nurse include in the focused assessment for this patient? *(1342)*
    1. Perform the 7 Ps of orthopedic assessment.
    2. Assess for back pain and vision changes.
    3. Frequently check for change in mental status.
    4. Check for urinary retention and overflow incontinence.

16. The patient says to the nurse, "I have excruciating pain in my big toe at night." Which assessment question is the nurse **most** likely to ask? *(1346)*
    1. "Have you noticed a change in your bowel movements?"
    2. "How much exercise would you normally get in a week?"
    3. "Do you eat organ meats, yeast, herring, or mackerel?"
    4. "Do you notice jaw tension, excessive fatigue, or anxiety?"

17. The patient is admitted for acute osteomyelitis of the left lower extremity. Which instruction should the nurse give to the unlicensed assistive personnel (UAP)? *(1350)*
    1. Use drainage and secretion precautions when caring for the patient.
    2. Assist the patient to ambulate in the hall every 2-3 hours.
    3. Anticipate that movement is more difficult in the morning.
    4. Refresh the patient's ice pack every 2 hours or as needed.

18. The nurse is caring for a patient who had unicompartmental knee surgery. Which interventions will the nurse use in the postoperative period? **Select all that apply.** *(1352)*
    1. Encourage deep-breathing and coughing every 2 hours.
    2. Begin with a clear liquid diet and advance to regular as tolerated.
    3. Inspect the skin at the edge of the cast for erythema.
    4. Assess the patient's ability to use an assistive device such as a walker.
    5. Monitor IV fluids and effectiveness of antibiotics.
    6. Administer intraarticular injections of corticosteroids.

19. The patient had a hip arthroplasty and returned from the postanesthesia care unit several hours ago. The patient is now restless and anxious. What is the nurse's **first** action? *(1367)*
    1. Decrease anxiety by reassuring the patient that everything is going as expected.
    2. Initiate vital signs every 15 minutes, compare to baseline, and monitor trends.
    3. Look at the urinary output and compare the total to baseline.
    4. Call the patient's family and invite them to spend time at the bedside.

20. A fiberglass cast has been applied to the forearm of a 6-year-old child to treat and stabilize a greenstick fracture. Which teaching point is the **most** important to emphasize with the child? *(1366)*
    1. Instructing the child to keep the cast dry
    2. Teaching the child to report pain to the parents
    3. Showing the child how to test capillary refill
    4. Reminding the child to wiggle the fingers

21. The nurse is supervising a nursing student in caring for a patient who had internal fixation for a hip fracture. The nurse would intervene if the student performed which action? *(1358)*
    1. Assessed the amount of drainage in the Jackson-Pratt drain
    2. Encouraged coughing and the use of the incentive spirometer
    3. Removed the antiembolism stocking to assess the skin
    4. Placed the patient in high Fowler's position prior to eating

22. The nurse is providing care for a patient who has just had a hip replacement. Which comment from the patient indicates the need for further education? *(1354)*
    1. "I need to be on bedrest for the first 72 hours."
    2. "I need to obtain a seat riser for my toilet at home."
    3. "I should never sit with my legs crossed."
    4. "I'll have limitations in hip position for 2-3 months."

23. A nurse is checking on an older neighbor who just fell down. The man cheerfully tells the nurse, "I just tripped on the carpet and took a spill. No harm done!" Based on mechanism of injury, which assessment is the nurse **most** likely to perform if the neighbor will allow it? *(1362)*
    1. Head-to-toe to detect occult injury
    2. Palpation and range of motion for wrist injury
    3. Mental status examination for head injury
    4. Environmental assessment for other hazards

24. The patient was in a car accident and reports pain over the pelvic region with difficulty raising legs in a supine position. The nurse notes ecchymosis over the pelvic region. Which laboratory test is the **primary** concern in the immediate phase of care? *(1365)*
    1. Hemoglobin and hematocrit
    2. Blood type and Rh
    3. Urinalysis
    4. Stool for occult blood

25. The patient with a cast on the lower extremity reports pain at 7/10. What should the nurse do **first**? *(1357)*
    1. Reposition the leg so that elevation is maintained.
    2. Administer pain medication as prescribed.
    3. Report potential compartment syndrome to RN.
    4. Perform the 7 Ps of orthopedic assessment.

26. The nurse hears in report that the patient has Volkmann's contracture of the dominant upper extremity. Which intervention would the nurse plan to use? *(1367)*
    1. Frequently assess using the 7 Ps of orthopedic assessment.
    2. Assess the patient's abilities to perform activities of daily living.
    3. Teach the patient to report pain, loss of sensation, or swelling.
    4. Instruct the UAP on proper position and alignment.

27. The nurse is caring for a patient with a long bone fracture. The laboratory reports the following arterial blood gas results. What should the nurse do **first**? (1368)

pH	7.4
Paco$_2$	40 mm Hg
Pao$_2$	95 mm Hg
HCO$_3$	26 mEq/L
Sao$_2$	98%

1. Assess the patient for signs of fat embolism and respiratory distress.
2. Report these normal results to the health care provider.
3. Place the patient in high Fowler's position to ease respirations.
4. Check the vital signs and continue to monitor the patient.

28. A computer data entry clerk reports paresthesia in the thumb, index finger, and middle finger and pain that increases during the night. The clerk has an appointment with a health care provider next week. In the meantime, what self-care measure would the nurse advise? (1381)
1. Use warm packs and sleep with hands on a pillow.
2. Frequently change position and stretch hands while working.
3. Use a mild analgesic such as ibuprofen or aspirin.
4. Wrap the wrist snugly with an elastic bandage.

29. The patient who had a laminectomy reports abdominal discomfort with a gaseous, bloated feeling and mild nausea. What should the nurse do **first**? (1383)
1. Offer clear liquids.
2. Encourage ambulation.
3. Listen for bowel sounds.
4. Administer an antiemetic.

30. The patient reports long bone pain that increases with weight bearing. The health care provider tells the nurse that the patient has an elevated serum alkaline phosphatase. The nurse prepares to give emotional support because the provider must tell the patient that additional diagnostic testing is needed to rule out which condition? (1303)
1. Phantom limb pain
2. Compartment syndrome
3. Fibromyalgia
4. Osteogenic sarcoma

CRITICAL THINKING ACTIVITIES

Activity 1

31. Discuss factors that contribute to osteoporosis and the nurse's role in helping patients prevent bone loss and fractures. (1347-1349)

_____

_____

_____

_____

_____

Activity 2

32. A 32-year-old woman has been told that she might have fibromyalgia syndrome; however, the health care provider tells her that this is just a possibility and that additional diagnostic testing would be needed. The patient is angry at first and then she begins to cry and confides in the nurse, "I am just so frustrated with these doctors and I just want to be able to live a normal life." Discuss fibromyalgia syndrome from the patient's point of view. *(1350, 1351)*

Activity 3

33. The home health nurse is visiting a thin, older woman who lives alone. The three-story house is a little cluttered with old belongings. Her bedroom and bathroom are on the second floor. The rugs are worn and the hallways are poorly lit. The woman cheerfully reports that she has a cane, a walker, and eyeglasses, but frequently misplaces "all of the 'old person' stuff." The woman has a small friendly dog; he jumps at her legs and she frequently bends down to pet him. Discuss the potential for hip fracture for this woman. *(1356)*

Student Name_____ Date_____

Care of the Patient With a Gastrointestinal Disorder

45

FIGURE LABELING

1. Directions: Label the digestive organs. (1392)

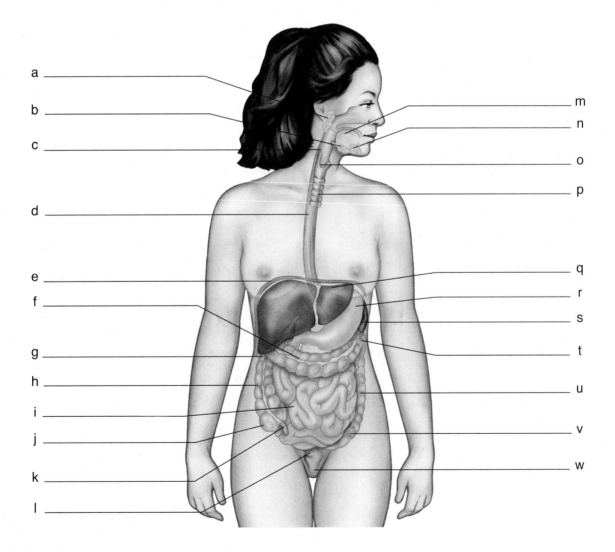

a _____
b _____
c _____
d _____
e _____
f _____
g _____
h _____
i _____
j _____
k _____
l _____

m _____
n _____
o _____
p _____
q _____
r _____
s _____
t _____
u _____
v _____
w _____

SHORT ANSWER

Directions: Using your own words, answer each question in the space provided.

2. List three functions of saliva. *(1393)*

   a. _____

   b. _____

   c. _____

3. List four major functions of the large intestine. *(1394)*

   a. _____

   b. _____

   c. _____

   d. _____

4. The liver is a complex organ that has many functions; name four or five of these functions. *(1395)*

   _____

   _____

   _____

   _____

MULTIPLE CHOICE

Directions: Select the best answer(s) for each of the following questions.

5. According to research, removal or disease of the appendix could theoretically affect which function? *(1394)*
   1. Immunologic response
   2. Red blood cell production
   3. Fluid and electrolyte balance
   4. Vitamin B$_{12}$ production

6. The large intestine is the site of bacterial action that produces vitamin K. Potentially, loss of the large colon or disruption of this bacterial action could disrupt which body function? *(1395)*
   1. Color vision
   2. Bone formation
   3. Intestinal absorption
   4. Blood clotting

7. What is the **most** important postprocedure instruction to give to a patient who has had an upper gastrointestinal study with barium? *(1398)*
   1. Watch for and report bleeding.
   2. Monitor temperature.
   3. Increase fluid intake.
   4. Eat a low-residue diet.

8. The nurse is planning care for several patients who will be undergoing diagnostic testing for disorders of the gastrointestinal system. Which patient is going to require the **most** time for postprocedural care? *(1397)*
   1. Patient must undergo capsule endoscopy to confirm diagnosis of celiac disease.
   2. Patient needs an esophagogastroduodenoscopy for evaluation of an ulcer.
   3. Patient is scheduled for a barium swallow to evaluate extent of hiatal hernia.
   4. Patient is tested for *H. pylori*: breath, serum antibody test, and fecal assay antigen.

9. The patient reports a substernal burning sensation that radiates into the neck and jaw. He says, "I think it's heartburn." The nurse decides to check vital signs and conduct further assessments of the pain. What is the **best** rationale for the nurse's decision? *(1403)*
   1. Pain assessment is performed before and after offering medication or nonpharmacologic interventions.
   2. Report to the health care provider should include vital signs and a description of the signs/symptoms.
   3. Heartburn can lead to more serious conditions, such as hemorrhage, sepsis, or cancer.
   4. The subjective sensations mimic angina and a potential cardiac condition should not be overlooked.

10. Which patient situation **most** strongly indicates the need for further investigation as a potential public health problem? *(1417)*
    1. Patient develops symptoms of acute gastritis after excessive drinking at a local bar.
    2. Patient has bloody diarrhea after eating a grilled hamburger that was served at a fundraiser.
    3. Patient has a burning sensation and regurgitation after eating spicy food at an ethnic restaurant.
    4. Patient has abdominal bloating and muscle aches after eating pastry at a local bakery.

11. What are the common causes of fecal incontinence? **Select all that apply.** *(1441)*
    1. Normal changes of aging
    2. Injury during anal intercourse
    3. Surgical trauma to anal sphincter
    4. Injury during childbirth
    5. Spinal cord lesions
    6. Voluntary inhibition of defecation

12. When planning care for a patient with a motor paralysis, which intervention is the **most** important as a long-term solution for the patient's defecation? *(1441)*
    1. Teach the family and patient the logroll to clean fecal incontinence.
    2. Include the patient and family in planning a bowel training program.
    3. Contact social services to find funds for incontinence pads and briefs.
    4. Arrange for home health services for assistance with hygiene and toileting.

13. Which patient is the **best** candidate for a bowel training program that will incorporate biofeedback? *(1441)*
    1. Patient has structural damage to the rectum secondary to a fistula.
    2. Patient has a motility disorder but is alert and motivated.
    3. Patient is ambulatory but has mild dementia and forgetfulness.
    4. Patient is passing liquid stool secondary to a fecal impaction.

14. The patient is practicing a bowel training program. Which food will the nurse encourage the patient to eat? *(1441)*
    1. Lean chicken meat
    2. Low-fat milk
    3. Whole-grain cereal
    4. Red meat

15. A patient is being treated with sucralfate for gastroesophageal reflux disease. Which teaching point would the nurse emphasize? *(1411)*
    1. Oral anticoagulants, theophylline, and propranolol may require dosage reductions.
    2. Coating action may interfere with the absorption of other drugs—separate by 2 hours.
    3. Contraindicated during pregnancy; women of childbearing age must use reliable contraception.
    4. Avoid driving or other hazardous activities until accustomed to sedating effects.

16. A patient had a partial gastrectomy. Because this surgery creates an increased risk for pernicious anemia, which teaching point is important to emphasize? *(1416)*
    1. Blood serum vitamin B_{12} level should be measured every 1 to 2 years.
    2. Hemoglobin and hematocrit should be measured every 1 to 2 months.
    3. Injections of iron dextran are given because of intestinal ulceration.
    4. Increase fresh fruits and vegetables and decrease intake of fat and red meat.

17. The risk of cancer of the stomach is associated with which factors? **Select all that apply.** *(1414)*
    1. Hyperkalemia
    2. Hypochlorhydria
    3. Chronic atrophic gastritis
    4. Diet high in smoked and preserved foods
    5. Gastric ulcers
    6. Diet low in fresh fruits and whole grains

18. When caring for a patient diagnosed with Crohn's disease, what signs and symptoms does the nurse expect to observe? **Select all that apply.** *(1426)*
    1. Nausea and vomiting
    2. Diarrhea and abdominal pain
    3. Weight gain and lactose intolerance
    4. Weight loss and malnutrition
    5. Fatigue and fever

19. The nurse is providing care to a patient suspected of having acute appendicitis. Which interventions may be included in the care? **Select all that apply.** *(1428)*
    1. Apply heating pad to the abdomen.
    2. Maintain bedrest and nothing by mouth (NPO).
    3. Administer antacids as needed to decrease gastric acidity.
    4. Monitor vital signs including temperature.
    5. Administer antibiotics as prescribed.
    6. Administer enemas until clear.

20. The patient had an esophagogastroduodenoscopy several hours ago and now reports abdominal pain and tenderness. What should the nurse do **first**? *(1397)*
    1. Auscultate for bowel sounds.
    2. Administer pain medication.
    3. Assess the abdominal pain.
    4. Check for melena.

21. The patient had capsule endoscopy. Which discharge instruction should the nurse give to the patient? *(1397)*
    1. The capsule will pass with bowel movement in 2-3 days; no need to retrieve.
    2. Use gloves and examine stool for several days to retrieve pill camera device.
    3. Use a mild laxative and increase liquids to facilitate expulsion of pill camera.
    4. Small amounts of light red blood and thick mucus in the stool are expected.

22. The nurse inserts a nasogastric tube so a patient can undergo the Bernstein test to determine the cause of esophageal pain. Which outcome is considered a positive test result? *(1397)*
    1. Administering nitrates relieves pain.
    2. Taking an antacid has no effect on pain.
    3. Decompressing the stomach relieves pain.
    4. Instilling hydrochloric acid causes pain.

23. The patient needs to have a series of tests of the gastrointestinal system. Which test must be scheduled last? *(1399)*
    1. Barium studies
    2. Stool sample for ova and parasites
    3. Colonoscopy
    4. Flat plate of the abdomen

24. The nursing student reports seeing a pearly, bluish-white "milk-curd" on the mucous membranes of the older patient's mouth. The nurse would intervene if the student performs which action? *(1400)*
    1. Checks for angular cheilitis at the corner of the mouth
    2. Removes the plaques with a soft toothbrush
    3. Observes the quantity and type of food consumed
    4. Offers the patient unsweetened yogurt

25. The nurse is talking to a neighbor who says that she has had a sore on her lip for about 3 weeks. What advice should the nurse give? *(1401)*
    1. Use lipstick or lip balm that has a sunscreen.
    2. Advise rinsing the mouth with diluted hydrogen peroxide.
    3. Consult the health care provider because of the duration of the sore.
    4. Increase intake of fresh fruits and vegetables for vitamin content.

26. The health care provider has recommended a conservative approach to manage the patient's gastroesophageal reflux disease. What would be included in the nurse's instructions to support the provider's recommendation? *(1403)*
    1. Give the patient a brochure about Nissen fundoplication.
    2. Suggest methods for elevating the head of the bed at home.
    3. Teach the signs and symptoms of Barrett's esophagus.
    4. Give the patient a reminder card for endoscopy and biopsy.

27. The nurse is caring for a patient who was admitted for peptic ulcer disease. Which abnormal finding is the **greatest** concern? *(1408)*
    1. Fecal assay antigen test is positive for *H. pylori*.
    2. Stool for occult blood is positive.
    3. White blood cell count is elevated.
    4. Pain is present during the hydrochloric acid test.

28. The patient who had surgery for a peptic ulcer several weeks ago reports experiencing an episode of diaphoresis, nausea, vomiting, epigastric pain, explosive diarrhea, and dyspepsia. Which question is **most** relevant to the symptoms and the surgical history? *(1416)*
    1. "Can you describe the pain? Where was it and how long did it last?"
    2. "Did you eat before the symptoms? And if so, what did you eat?"
    3. "Have you been taking your medications according to instructions?"
    4. "Did you ever experience these symptoms before the surgery?"

29. The patient is admitted for hemorrhagic colitis caused by the *E. coli* pathogen. Which order would the nurse question? *(1417)*
    1. Encourage oral fluids as tolerated
    2. Dextrose 5% in normal saline at 150 mL/hour
    3. Loperamide 2 mg after unformed stool
    4. Initiate contact isolation

30. The older adult patient has been put into contact isolation because of watery diarrhea. Laboratory results are pending, but the *C. difficile* pathogen is suspected. What instruction should the nurse give to the unlicensed assistive personnel? *(1417)*
    1. Cluster care and limit the amount of time spent in the room.
    2. Use diluted bleach solution to clean the toilet bowl after each use.
    3. Wear a mask during patient care and discard upon exiting the room.
    4. Use soap and water to wash hands, rather than the antiseptic hand rub.

31. The nurse is assisting a patient who is newly diagnosed with celiac disease. Which lunch tray would be the **best** choice? *(1419)*
    1. Whole grain pasta with marinara and a green salad
    2. Chicken breast sandwich on rye bread and an apple
    3. Chicken noodle soup and crackers with fruit salad
    4. Stir-fry vegetables with rice and orange slices

32. The patient confides in the nurse that she feels angry because the health care provider has hinted that irritable bowel syndrome (IBS) might be the problem but offers no definitive medical diagnosis. What is the **most** therapeutic response? *(1420)*
    1. "IBS is hard to diagnose. It is more a process of excluding other disorders."
    2. "I'll ask the health care provider to talk to you about your concerns."
    3. "You seem really frustrated. What has the provider told you so far?"
    4. "I can get some literature about IBS; maybe additional information will help."

33. The patient is admitted for an exacerbation of ulcerative colitis and the nurse hears in report that the patient had 20 liquid stools within the past 24 hours. Which laboratory result is the **most** important to follow up on? *(1422)*
    1. Electrolyte levels
    2. Liver function studies
    3. Hemoglobin and hematocrit
    4. Fecal occult blood

34. The nurse enters the room of a young woman and sees that she is crying. The patient states, "The doctor told me I need surgery and an ileostomy. I'll be pooping into a bag! I'm leaving the hospital right now!" What should the nurse do **first**? *(1438)*
    1. Obtain a leaving Against Medical Advice form and contact the provider.
    2. Sit with the patient and help her verbalize her fears and concerns.
    3. Arrange for the patient to meet another person who has an ostomy.
    4. Contact the enterostomal therapist to talk with the patient.

35. Which medical diagnosis requires that the nurse be extra vigilant for concurrent urinary tract infections? *(1426)*
    1. Crohn's disease
    2. Appendicitis
    3. Ulcerative colitis
    4. Peptic ulcer disease

36. A parent says, "I think my son has an appendicitis. He won't eat and he says he has pain just to the right of his belly button." If the nurse places the child on an examination table, which position is the child **most** likely to assume if the mother is correct about appendicitis? *(1428)*
    1. Prone with head supported by forearm
    2. Supine with arms and legs extended
    3. Sits upright, with chest extended
    4. Side-lying with knees flexed

37. The patient is admitted for acute diverticulitis. The nurse would intervene if a nursing student performed which action? *(1429)*
    1. Advises to avoid heavy lifting
    2. Assists with a meal tray
    3. Assesses bowel sounds
    4. Checks the white blood cell count

38. A patient sustained blunt trauma to the abdomen. Several hours after being admitted for observation, the patient reports severe abdominal pain with exquisite tenderness to light palpation. What should the nurse do **first**? *(1431)*
    1. Take vital signs and perform additional assessment of the abdomen.
    2. Place the patient in a semi-Fowler's position to localize purulent drainage.
    3. Call the health care provider and report possible peritonitis.
    4. Administer an as-needed pain medication and reevaluate pain in 30 minutes.

39. The nurse is caring for a patient who had a right hemicolectomy for colorectal cancer. Which postoperative interventions will the nurse use in the care of this patient? **Select all that apply.** (1438)
    1. Monitor vital signs, pain level, and return of bowel sounds.
    2. Check dressings for drainage and bleeding and change as ordered.
    3. Discontinue the urinary catheter when the patient is discharged.
    4. Encourage the patient to cough, deep-breathe, and turn.
    5. Maintain bedrest while the nasogastric tube is on suction.
    6. Keep accurate intake and output records to monitor fluid balance.

40. An obese male truck driver comes to the clinic and reports intense rectal itching. The health care provider determines that the patient has hemorrhoids. What nonsurgical approach can the nurse teach the patient to help manage the condition? (1439)
    1. Suggest a low-fiber diet.
    2. Advise the use of a hydrocortisone cream.
    3. Increase fluid intake.
    4. Recommend rubber-band ligation.

41. What is considered an **early** sign of mechanical obstruction of the intestines? (1434)
    1. Loud, frequent, high-pitched bowel sounds
    2. Intermittent periods of decreased or absent bowel sounds
    3. Decreased blood pressure with tachycardia
    4. Abdominal distention and vomiting

42. Which sign/symptom should be investigated as an **early** warning of colorectal cancer? (1436)
    1. Abdominal distention
    2. Rectal bleeding
    3. Nausea
    4. Weight loss

CRITICAL THINKING ACTIVITIES

Activity 1

43. The patient reports a burning sensation in the mid-epigastric area after eating, and occasionally experiences a feeling of warm fluid moving up the throat with a sour taste in the mouth. The health care provider makes the medical diagnosis of gastroesophageal reflux disease and suggests trying lifestyle modifications. Discuss the dietary interventions and lifestyle modifications that the nurse will reinforce. (1404)

_____

_____

_____

_____

_____

_____

Activity 2

44. A 24-year-old male patient presents with weakness, loss of appetite, abdominal pain and cramps, inter-mittent low-grade fever, sleeplessness caused by diarrhea, and stress. The health care provider recom-mends diagnostic colonoscopy and laboratory testing and identifies the medical diagnosis of Crohn's disease and sulfasalazine is prescribed. The dietitian is consulted and provides extensive teaching about dietary strategies to manage the disease process. Discuss Crohn's disease from the patient's point of view. *(1426, 1427)*

_____

_____

_____

_____

_____

_____

Activity 3

45. The nurse has taken a new job at a long-term care center. With regards to the gastrointestinal system, what are some of the lifespan considerations that the nurse is likely to observe while caring for this group of older adults? *(1433)*

_____

_____

_____

_____

_____

Activity 4

46. The nurse is providing care to a patient suspected of having an intestinal obstruction. *(1433-1435)*

    a. When performing an assessment on the patient, what objective data should be included?

    _____

    _____

    b. What diagnostic tests may be performed to confirm the presence of an intestinal obstruction?

    _____

    _____

    c. What are the goals of treatment for an intestinal obstruction?_____

    _____

    _____

    d. Compare mechanical and nonmechanical intestinal obstruction. _____

    _____

    _____

Care of the Patient With a Gallbladder, Liver, Biliary Tract, or Exocrine Pancreatic Disorder

chapter

46

SHORT ANSWER

Directions: Using your own words, answer each question in the space provided.

1. Identify at least five modifiable risk factors for pancreatic cancer. *(1470)*

   _____

   _____

   _____

   _____

MULTIPLE CHOICE

Directions: Select the best answer(s) for each of the following questions.

2. The nurse hears in report that the patient has a total bilirubin of 2.8 mg/dL. What would the nurse expect to observe during the morning assessment? *(1445)*
    1. Jaundice of the sclera and mucous membranes
    2. Pallor of the palms of hands and soles of feet
    3. Cyanosis of the lips with minor exertion
    4. Cherry red discoloration of the face and chest

3. The home health nurse sees that the patient's albumin level is 3.4 g/dL. Based on this information, which assessment is the nurse **most** likely to perform? *(1446)*
    1. Frequency and type of exercise and physical activity
    2. Dietary preferences and typical intake for 24-hour period
    3. Frequency of using tobacco or illicit substances
    4. Occupational or other environmental exposure to toxins.

4. The nurse is responsible for the postprocedural care of several patients who had diagnostic testing. The unlicensed assistive personnel (UAP) reports that one of the patients is having shortness of breath; rapid, shallow breathing; and a rapid pulse. Which patient is **most** likely to develop these signs/symptoms as a postprocedural complication? *(1448)*
    1. Patient had a radioisotope scan of the liver.
    2. Patient had ultrasonography of the pancreas.
    3. Patient had computed tomography of the abdomen.
    4. Patient had a needle biopsy of the liver.

5. The nurse is caring for an older patient who becomes confused and combative under stressful situations or during changes in routine. The health care provider has ordered several diagnostic tests. The nurse is **most** likely to contact the provider before scheduling which test? *(1450)*
   1. 2-hour spot urine for urine amylase
   2. Serum ammonia test
   3. Endoscopic retrograde cholangiopancreatography
   4. Total protein and serum albumin

6. The patient has a damaged liver and is therefore unable to correctly metabolize protein. Loss of this function results in portal hypertension, hypoalbuminemia, and hyperaldosteronism. Based on the nurse's knowledge of pathophysiology, what would the nurse expect to observe when assessing the patient? *(1452)*
   1. Flatulence
   2. Ascites
   3. Asterixis
   4. Cachexia

7. What are **early** signs/symptoms of cirrhosis of the liver? *(1452)*
   1. Esophageal varices
   2. Spider angiomas
   3. Ascites
   4. Flulike symptoms

8. The home health nurse is visiting a patient who has cirrhosis of the liver. Which patient behavior is cause for **greatest** concern? *(1456)*
   1. Patient nicked his face several times while using a razor blade for shaving.
   2. Patient bumped his head on the doorway and now seems mildly confused.
   3. Patient noticed bleeding from the gums after brushing teeth and flossing.
   4. Patient has ecchymotic spots on his forearms and back of the hands.

9. The health care provider may prescribe a protein-restricted diet for which patient? *(1448)*
   1. Patient is recovering from acute hepatic encephalopathy.
   2. Patient is in the early stage of cirrhosis of the liver.
   3. Patient is being treated conservatively for cholecystitis.
   4. Patient is recovering from hepatitis A, contracted 3 months ago.

10. Which people should be advised to get the hepatitis B vaccine (HBV)? **Select all that apply.** *(1460)*
    1. Nurse who works in the emergency department
    2. Person who injects illicit substances
    3. Groundskeeper who works at an inner city park
    4. Newborn who is having a 2-month well-baby examination
    5. Older resident who lives in a long-term care facility
    6. Military person who is stationed in a developing country

11. The nurse hears in report that the patient has hepatic encephalopathy and is receiving lactulose. What will the nurse observe if the medication therapy is successful? *(1455)*
    1. Improved mental status
    2. Decreased ascites
    3. Improved appetite
    4. Decreased jaundice

12. What instructions should be given to the UAP about the care of a patient with viral hepatitis? **Select all that apply.** *(1459)*
    1. Perform scrupulous hand hygiene.
    2. Wear gown and gloves when handling excreta.
    3. Exercise caution when putting needles in the sharps box.
    4. Wear a mask if bedside care is extensive or prolonged.
    5. Organize care to reduce time and exposure to the patient.

13. The patient had a laparoscopic cholecystectomy yesterday and is schedule to be discharged today. Which assessment finding would delay the discharge? *(1466)*
    1. Patient reports mild shoulder pain.
    2. Patient reports pain when T-tube is clamped.
    3. Patient notices bile leakage from the puncture site.
    4. Patient eats but his appetite is not at baseline.

14. The nurse is providing teaching to a patient scheduled to undergo a needle biopsy of the liver. During the examination, what will the patient be told to do? *(1457)*
    1. Deeply inhale and hold breath until instructed to exhale.
    2. Cough forcefully as the needle is withdrawn.
    3. Inhale and exhale slowly and evenly as the needle is inserted.
    4. Exhale and hold breath as the needle is inserted.

15. A T-tube was inserted during a cholecystectomy. What does the nurse expect to observe when assessing the patient? *(1467)*
    1. Greenish-yellow drainage from the tube
    2. Localized inflammation around the tube site
    3. Significant postoperative pain until the tube is removed
    4. Moderate amount of light-red bleeding from the tube

16. After a laparoscopic cholecystectomy, the patient reports shoulder pain. What should the nurse do? *(1466)*
    1. Perform gentle range-of-motion exercises to reduce shoulder discomfort.
    2. Assist the patient to ambulate to clear the residual carbon dioxide.
    3. Explain that the pain is an expected side effect of anesthesia.
    4. Reassure that the pain is expected and give an analgesic as prescribed.

17. When caring for a patient with acute pancreatitis, which laboratory finding is the **best** indicator of the disorder? *(1468)*
    1. Low albumin
    2. Elevated lipase
    3. Increased blood glucose
    4. Elevated amylase

18. Which behavior places a person at **greatest** risk to contract hepatitis E? *(1459)*
    1. Eating raw shellfish or drinking water in Mexico
    2. Engaging in unprotected anal and vaginal sex
    3. Sharing and reusing needles for illicit drug injection
    4. Getting tattooed with nonsterile equipment

19. The nurse hears in report that the patient had lithotripsy for gallstones. Which postprocedural assessment is the nurse most likely to perform? *(1464-1465)*
    1. Assess for drainage at the incision site
    2. Assess level of pain and discomfort
    3. Assess for nausea and amount of emesis
    4. Assess ability to do activities of daily living

20. A young woman who is pregnant is having symptoms of cholecystitis and the health care provider has informed her that diagnostic testing is required. Which educational brochure will the nurse prepare for this patient? *(1447)*
    1. "What You Need to Know About Ultrasonography of the Gallbladder"
    2. "Frequently Asked Questions About Oral Cholecystography"
    3. "Intravenous Cholangiography: A Patient's Guide for Decision-making"
    4. "Computed Tomography of the Abdomen as a Diagnostic Tool"

21. The patient had a hepatobiliary iminodiacetic acid (HIDA) scan. What instructions should the nurse give to the UAP who is assisting the patient with hygiene? *(1447)*
    1. Immediately flush all urine and stool.
    2. Wear your personal dosimeter at all times.
    3. Give care as usual; there are no special considerations.
    4. Watch for and report any bleeding at the puncture site.

22. The nurse hears in report that several patients are scheduled for diagnostic testing. The nurse must plan to frequently take vital signs (every 15 minutes x 2, then every 30 minutes x 4 , and then every hour x 4) after which test? *(1448)*
    1. Serum ammonia test
    2. Needle liver biopsy
    3. Oral cholecystography
    4. Radioisotope liver scan

23. The nurse is instructing the UAP about assisting several patients with morning hygiene. Which patient needs to use a soft toothbrush with very gentle brushing action? *(1456)*
    1. Recently diagnosed with hepatitis A
    2. Surgery pending for cholelithiasis
    3. In later stage of cirrhosis of the liver
    4. Nothing by mouth for acute pancreatitis

24. A first-semester nursing student tells the nurse that she would like to teach and coach coughing and deep-breathing to several patients. Which patients would be **best** for the nurse to recommend to the student? **Select all that apply.** *(1454)*
    1. Scheduled to have a cholecystectomy in 2 days
    2. Looks forward to having a liver transplant from a living donor
    3. Has cirrhosis of the liver and esophageal varices
    4. Prescribed several weeks of bedrest for chronic hepatitis
    5. Is on bedrest for acute pancreatitis with severe pain

25. The patient has symptoms of hepatic encephalopathy and the health care provider wants to be called about laboratory results. Which laboratory result should the nurse seek out to validate the suspected condition? *(1448)*
    1. Serum bilirubin
    2. Serum albumin
    3. Ammonia level
    4. Blood glucose

26. The health care provider orders an intramuscular immune serum globulin for a hospital employee who was exposed to hepatitis A. A dosage of 0.2 mL/kg of body weight is ordered. The employee weighs 155 lbs. How many mL should the nurse draw up? _____ mL *(1460)*

27. A patient with acute pancreatitis is refusing to have a nasogastric tube inserted and wants to leave the hospital. What can the nurse say to help the patient to accept the therapy? *(1469)*
    1. "I can give you pain medication before or after the procedure."
    2. "Let me call the health care provider so he can explain the therapy."
    3. "The tube will be inserted by our most experienced nurse, so don't worry."
    4. "The tube will decrease the nausea, vomiting, pain, and abdominal distention."

CRITICAL THINKING ACTIVITIES

Activity 1

28. A 34-year-old patient with a history of end-stage liver disease related to chronic hepatitis has been added to the waiting list to receive a liver transplant. During his preoperative education classes, he voices many questions and concerns. *(1461)*

    a. What are the primary risks associated with the planned transplant? _____

    _____

    b. For which postoperative complications will the patient be at risk? _____

    _____

    _____

    c. How will the risk of organ rejection be handled? _____

    _____

    _____

    _____

    d. Discuss the appropriate postoperative nursing care. _____

    _____

    _____

    _____

Activity 2

29. A 49-year-old patient comes to the emergency department for right upper-quadrant pain. She reports that the pain began a few hours after eating French fries, a hamburger, and an ice cream sundae at a local fast-food restaurant. Upon assessment, the abdomen is distended. The patient also has nausea and vomiting. *(1463, 1464)*

    a. What does the nurse expect the patient to be diagnosed with? _____

    b. What are some other signs and symptoms that may develop? _____

    _____

c.   What diagnostic examinations may be used to help diagnose this patient? _____

_____

_____

_____

Activity 3

30. a.   Based on knowledge of the etiology and clinical course of pancreatic cancer, discuss some of the psychological challenges that a patient could face. *(1470, 1471)*

_____

_____

_____

_____

b.   What can the nurse do to assist the patient with these psychological challenges? *(1470, 1471)* _____

_____

_____

_____

_____

Care of the Patient With a
Blood or Lymphatic Disorder

chapter
47

SHORT ANSWER

Directions: Using your own words, answer each question in the space provided.

1. What are the three main functions of blood? *(1476)* _____
   _____
   _____
   _____

2. What are three functions of the lymphatic system? *(1480)* _____
   _____
   _____

3. What are two main functions of the lymph glands? *(1481)* _____
   _____

4. What are five functions of the spleen? *(1481)* _____
   _____
   _____
   _____
   _____

TABLE ACTIVITY

5. Directions: Complete the table below with the normal values for selected blood tests. *(1476)*

Blood Test	Normal Values	
Red blood cells (RBCs)	Males:	Females:
Hemoglobin	Males:	Females:
Hematocrit	Males:	Females:
Platelet count		
White blood cells (WBC) actual cell count		
Prothrombin time (PT)		
International Normalized Ratio (INR)		
Partial thromboplastin time (PTT)		

MULTIPLE CHOICE

Directions: Select the best answer(s) for each of the following questions.

6. There was a major catastrophe in the city and health care facilities are being overwhelmed with trauma victims. Based on the concept of universal recipient, which patient theoretically has the **best** chance of getting a unit of blood if there is a shortage in the blood banks? *(1479)*
    1. Has blood type O and is Rh negative
    2. Has blood type A and is Rh positive
    3. Has blood type B and is Rh negative
    4. Has blood type AB and is Rh positive

7. During physical assessment, the nurse detects swelling in the cervical lymph nodes and the patient's skin feels hot to the touch. Which question is the nurse **most** likely to ask to follow up on the assessment findings? *(1481)*
    1. "Do you have a personal or family history of cancer?"
    2. "Have you ever been told that you were anemic?"
    3. "Have you been exposed to any infectious disorders?"
    4. "Do you take any anticoagulant medications?"

8. Which patient has the **greatest** risk for developing a complication related to the penetration of underlying structures during a bone marrow biopsy or aspiration? *(1482)*
    1. An older patient had a bone marrow biopsy from the posterior iliac crest.
    2. A very thin patient had a bone marrow aspiration from the sternum.
    3. A child had a bone marrow aspiration from the posterior iliac crest.
    4. An obese patient had a bone marrow aspiration from the tibia.

9. Which objective finding indicates that the healthy adult's body is compensating for a blood loss of less than 750 mL? *(1483)*
    1. Urine output is scant.
    2. Blood pressure is low.
    3. Has slight increase in pulse.
    4. Is stuporous and confused.

10. The patient is admitted for an exacerbation of polycythemia vera. Which patient report is cause for **greatest** concern? *(1493)*
    1. Reports pain in lower leg with redness and swelling
    2. Has generalized pruritus after taking a hot shower
    3. Reports fullness and satiety after eating a small salad
    4. Has burning sensation of the hands and feet

11. Which lunch tray is the **best** choice for providing nutrients needed for erythropoiesis? *(1490)*
    1. Fried egg, potato and cheese burrito, low-fat milk, and an apple
    2. Chicken breast sandwich with fries, low-fat milk with vanilla yogurt
    3. Fresh fruit salad with whole-grain roll and strawberry smoothie
    4. Spinach salad with nuts and strawberries and tuna on whole-grain bread

12. The nurse is caring for a young patient who is usually very healthy, but has vomiting and diarrhea secondary to food poisoning. What would be an expected laboratory result for this patient? *(1476)*
    1. Elevated hemoglobin and hematocrit
    2. Normal hemoglobin and hematocrit
    3. Low platelet count
    4. Increased prothrombin time

13. The health care provider tells the nurse that the laboratory results show that the patient has bandemia. The nurse will plan to be extra vigilant for which condition? *(1478)*
    1. Venous thrombosis
    2. Thrombocytopenia
    3. Sepsis or septic shock
    4. Allergic response

14. Which patient is **most** likely to require testing for anti-D antibodies and/or an injection of Rh immunoglobulin? *(1480)*
    1. An Rh-positive mother who is at 28 weeks gestation
    2. Any woman who has an ectopic pregnancy
    3. An Rh-negative mother who had a miscarriage
    4. An Rh-positive mother impregnated by an Rh-negative father

15. When caring for patients who are Jehovah's Witnesses, which information applies for use of blood products? *(1484)*
    1. Some Jehovah's Witnesses may permit the use of certain blood volume expanders.
    2. It is not legal for this patient to refuse transfusions if the bleeding is truly life-threatening.
    3. Some Jehovah's Witnesses may consent to homologous blood transfusions.
    4. Jehovah's Witnesses believe that children are allowed to have blood in an emergency.

16. A patient with anemia has difficulty with activities because of tissue hypoxia. Which task can be delegated to the UAP? *(1484)*
    1. Ask the patient how far he is able to ambulate and evaluate his abilities.
    2. Apply oxygen per nasal cannula if the patient reports shortness of breath.
    3. Explain the patient's limitations to visitors and encourage short visits.
    4. Assist the patient with self-care activities such as hygiene and toileting.

17. The nurse is caring for a trauma patient who must be observed for signs and symptoms of occult bleeding and injury. Which sign/symptom is an **early** manifestation of hypovolemic shock? *(1484)*
    1. Orthostatic blood pressure
    2. Decreased red blood cell count
    3. Restlessness
    4. Decreased urine output

18. The patient had major abdominal surgery yesterday. He reported abdominal pain, and the nurse gave him an opioid pain medication as directed; 2 hours later, he reports that the pain is worse. What should the nurse do **first**? *(1485)*
    1. Check the medication administration record for other pain or adjunctive medications.
    2. Explain to the patient that pain medication can only be given as prescribed every 4-6 hours.
    3. Reassess the abdomen and ask the patient to describe the pain to the best of his ability.
    4. Call the health care provider and obtain an order for laboratory studies or x-ray studies.

19. The nurse is caring for a postoperative patient who is demonstrating early symptoms of hypovolemic shock. The nurse is awaiting a return call from the health care provider. Which task can be delegated to the UAP? *(1485)*
    1. Take and report the blood pressure, pulse, and respirations every 15 minutes.
    2. Reinforce the dressings for saturation of blood or drainage.
    3. Apply oxygen and monitor the pulse oximetry readings every 5 minutes.
    4. Place the patient in a supine position and monitor respiratory effort.

20. The health care provider has recommended that the patient with sickle cell disease have a splenectomy. Which medication is likely to be discontinued for several days prior to the surgery? *(1488)*
    1. Folic acid supplement
    2. Hydroxyurea
    3. Blood thinner
    4. Antibiotic

21. The nurse is caring for a patient experiencing an initial sickle cell crisis. What is the **primary** sign/symptom that the nurse should expect during the crisis? *(1491)*
    1. Jaundice
    2. Fever
    3. Fatigue
    4. Pain

22. What health promotion points should be emphasized for patients who have sickle cell disease? **Select all that apply.** *(1492)*
    1. Avoid high altitudes
    2. Drink large amounts of iced fluids
    3. Stay current with vaccinations
    4. Maintain very cold room temperatures
    5. Stop smoking and alcohol consumption
    6. Maintain vigorous exercise routine

23. The patient is diagnosed with primary polycythemia. Which assessments are the **most** important? *(1493)*
    1. Palpating for abdominal distention and checking bowel movements
    2. Checking for pain, warmth, swelling, redness, and pulses in arms or legs
    3. Monitoring temperature and watching for other signs of infection
    4. Frequently assessing for fatigue and activity intolerance

24. The laboratory calls to inform the nurse that the patient has a white cell count of 1000/mm³ with a differential neutrophil count of less than 200/mm³. Which action is the **most** important for the nurse to initiate while waiting for the health care provider to respond to the phone message? *(1495)*
    1. Review current medication list.
    2. Start neutropenic precautions.
    3. Check for signs/symptoms of infection.
    4. Teach the importance of hand hygiene.

25. A 6-year-old child is hospitalized for treatment of acute lymphocytic leukemia. Which activity would the nurse suggest to the child and parents? *(1495, 1496)*
    1. Drawing pictures that accompany storytelling
    2. Playing with and petting the pet therapy dog
    3. Walking in the garden courtyard
    4. Attending a party in the pediatric play area

26. The nurse is examining the patient and notices several areas of ecchymoses and petechiae. Which question(s) will the nurse ask to follow up on this observation? **Select all that apply.** *(1498)*
    1. "What do you think is causing these bruises?"
    2. "Do you notice any bleeding when you brush your teeth?"
    3. "Have you had frequent nosebleeds?"
    4. "Are your stools a black or very dark red color?"
    5. "Are you using a hydrocortisone cream on these areas?"
    6. "How much dietary fiber do you consume per day?"

27. The patient has a very low platelet count. Which instruction will the nurse give to the UAP about the care of this patient? *(1498)*
    1. Always wear a mask to prevent spreading respiratory droplets.
    2. Handle the patient very gently to avoid bruising and injury.
    3. Encourage the patient to take fluids to prevent dehydration.
    4. Assist the patient with hygiene to prevent undue fatigue.

28. An adolescent with hemophilia A wants to participate in a high school sports activity. In consultation with the health care provider, which sport would be the **best**? *(1502)*
    1. Football
    2. Soccer
    3. Wrestling
    4. Golf

29. The home health nurse reads in the record that the patient has a medical diagnosis of Hodgkin's disease stage 1. Which sign/symptom would the nurse expect to see? *(1508)*
    1. Abnormal single lymph node
    2. Night sweats
    3. Weight loss
    4. Alcohol-induced pain

30. Based on the nurse's knowledge of non-Hodgkin's disease, what does the nurse consider when planning care for the patient who has recently started treatment? **Select all that apply.** *(1510)*
    1. Pain is likely to be localized in the spine and increases with movement.
    2. Disease is likely to be widespread and most body systems are affected.
    3. Patient could have side effects from chemotherapy.
    4. Patient and/or family may need support because prognosis is poor.
    5. Total assistance for activities of daily living is likely to be needed.

CRITICAL THINKING ACTIVITIES

Activity 1

31. A 63-year-old patient reports that her "heart is racing." She also has nausea, sore tongue, and difficulty swallowing. Upon oral examination, her tongue is smooth and erythematous. *(1486)*

    a. What medical diagnosis would the nurse anticipate? _____

    b. What treatment options are available for this patient? _____

    _____

    c. After completing 2 months of treatment, the patient states she is feeling well and now plans to discontinue the treatments. How should the nurse respond to the patient?

    _____

    _____

Activity 2

32. A 32-year-old female patient has fatigue, dizziness, and pallor. Her history includes childbirth 3 months ago, a subgastrectomy 3 years ago, and hernia repair 18 months ago. Her Hgb level is 10 g/dL. *(1489-1491)*

    a. Based on the nurse's knowledge, what is the anticipated medical diagnosis? _____

    _____

    b. What risk factors does this patient have that support development of this disorder? _____

    _____

    _____

    c. Identify other signs and symptoms that may accompany this disorder. _____

    _____

    _____

    d. Discuss six considerations for the administration of iron. _____

    _____

    _____

    _____

    _____

Activity 3

33. The nurse is caring for an older adult patient who reports bone pain that increases with movement. The medical diagnosis is multiple myeloma.

a. Discuss the benefits of ambulation and fluid for this patient. *(1488)*_____

_____

b. What can the nurse do to encourage the patient to walk if he says that moving increases the pain? *(1488)*

_____

_____

Activity 4

34. You are caring for a patient who is having massive hemorrhage from a wound on the thigh. The patient is in a room that is well-equipped with supplies to provide emergency care and resuscitation. There are other health care personnel on the unit. The health care provider has just ordered oxygen at 2 L/nasal cannula, 15-minute vital signs, start a peripheral IV and give a bolus of 2 L of normal saline, lower the head of the bed, apply direct pressure to the wound site then apply a pressure bandage, transfuse 1 unit of packed red blood cells, laboratory testing for platelet count and complete blood count, 1 unit of fresh frozen plasma "hold" for laboratory results, and transfer to the intensive care unit. The goals of care are 1) to stop blood loss, 2) treat for shock, and 3) restore lost volume. Discuss how you will prioritize and accomplish these orders. *(1484, 1485)*

a. List questions that you can ask yourself as you are formulating a plan to accomplish these orders.

_____

_____

_____

_____

b. Prioritize the health care provider's orders. _____

_____

_____

_____

_____

Care of the Patient With a Cardiovascular or a Peripheral Vascular Disorder

TRACING A DROP OF BLOOD

1. Directions: Trace a drop of blood around the pulmonary circulatory system. Start at the superior or inferior vena cava and identify the names of the blood vessels, the chambers of the heart, and the valves of the heart. End with the drop of blood at the aorta. *(1521)*

    Superior or inferior vena cava →

    _____ → _____ →

    _____ → _____ →

    _____ → _____ →

    _____ → _____ →

    _____ → _____ →

    _____ → Aorta

FIGURE LABELING

2. Directions: Label each of the coronary vessels that supply blood to the heart. *(1520)*

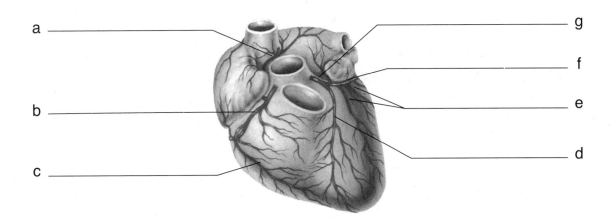

TABLE ACTIVITY

3. Directions: Complete the table with the description of what the nurse feels when palpating pulses according to the scale of: 0 to +4. *(1564)*

Scale	Description of Pulse
0	
+1	
+2	
+3	
+4	

SHORT ANSWER

Directions: Using your own words, answer each question in the space provided.

4. Directions: Identify the impulse pattern of the electrical conduction system of the heart. Start at the SA node. *(1519)*

   SA node →

   _____ → _____ →

   _____ → _____

5. List at least five nonpharmacologic therapies for hypertension. *(1568, 1569)* _____

   _____

   _____

   _____

   _____

6. What are the classic five Ps for assessing arterial occlusion? *(1570)* _____

   _____

   _____

MULTIPLE CHOICE
Directions: Select the best answer(s) for each of the following questions.

7. The health care provider instructs the nurse to immediately report laboratory results to confirm the diagnosis of myocardial infarction. Which laboratory result should the nurse seek out **first**? *(1524)*
   1. Creatine phosphokinase
   2. Creatine kinase
   3. Troponin T
   4. Troponin I

8. The home health nurse is reviewing the patient's laboratory results and sees that the overall serum cholesterol level is 230 mg/dL. Based on the laboratory results, which patient education topic is the nurse **most** likely to review with the patient? *(1527)*
   1. Importance of ambulation and mobility
   2. Coping and stress reduction techniques
   3. Dietary sources of fat and weight reduction
   4. Methods to increase medication compliance

9. Under what circumstances would the nurse expect to observe sinus tachycardia if the patient were on a cardiac monitor? *(1529)*
   1. Patient has an untreated high fever.
   2. Patient demonstrates obstructive sleep apnea.
   3. Patient faints during a bowel movement.
   4. Health care provider performs carotid massage.

10. Which physical assessment would the nurse perform to assist the health care provider in identifying atrial fibrillation? *(1530)*
    1. Take a manual blood pressure on both arms.
    2. Compare bilateral peripheral pulses.
    3. Count the apical pulse for a full minute.
    4. Obtain help and check for a pulse deficit.

11. The health care provider tells that nurse the patient has occasional premature ventricular contractions (PVC). Based on this information, what would the nurse expect to observe when assessing the patient? *(1531)*
    1. Shallow, rapid respiration with PVCs
    2. Chest pain when the PVCs are occurring
    3. Irregular rate and rhythm when palpating pulse
    4. Blood pressure lower than 120/80 mm Hg

12. What are the signs/symptoms of cardiac arrest? **Select all that apply.** *(1534)*
    1. Pupil constriction
    2. Absence of carotid pulse
    3. Gasping respirations followed by apnea
    4. Lethargic and difficult to arouse
    5. Abrupt loss of consciousness
    6. Pallor and cyanosis

13. The health care provider is reviewing the 12-lead electrocardiogram and tells the nurse that the patient has a STEMI MI. Based on this information, what is the **priority** intervention? *(1543)*
    1. Administer beta-adrenergic blocker as prescribed.
    2. Transfer to the intensive care unit.
    3. Prepare patient for thrombolytic therapy.
    4. Administer oxygen at 2 L/minute.

14. The nurse hears in report that the patient with heart failure has 4+ pitting edema in the lower extremities. Based on this information, what is the **priority** assessment that the nurse will perform? *(1518)*
    1. Check for edema in the sacrum.
    2. Weigh the patient.
    3. Observe respiratory effort.
    4. Observe for jugular vein distention.

15. The patient has pulmonary edema and is prescribed furosemide. Which laboratory result is the **most** important for the nurse to monitor? *(1551)*
    1. Complete blood count
    2. Electrolytes
    3. Coagulation studies
    4. Serum lipids

16. Which patient is the **most** likely candidate to meet the criteria for a cardiac transplant? *(1562)*
    1. Has type 1 diabetes with end-organ damage
    2. Has heart disease stabilized by medication
    3. Has a history of mental illness
    4. Has inoperable coronary artery disease

17. The nurse is caring for a patient who is on anticoagulant therapy. Which laboratory values are the **most** important to monitor? *(1579)*
    1. Prothrombin time, International Normalized Ratio, and partial thromboplastin time
    2. Blood glucose, potassium, sodium, calcium, and magnesium
    3. Enzyme creatine kinase, creatine phosphokinase, and myoglobin
    4. B-type natriuretic peptide and troponins 1 and 2

18. Laboratory results show a low hemoglobin for a patient diagnosed with myocardial infarction. What is the **first** intervention that the nurse would perform to address this laboratory result? *(1524)*
    1. Obtain an order for an intramuscular iron supplement.
    2. Help the patient to order an iron-rich meal tray.
    3. Obtain an order for type and cross for blood transfusion.
    4. Check to see that oxygen is delivered as prescribed.

19. The nurse is planning care for several patients who are scheduled to have diagnostic testing for cardiac disorders. Which patient will require postprocedural checks for peripheral pulses, color, and sensation of the extremity every 15 minutes for 1 hour? *(1521)*
    1. Needs cardiac catheterization to diagnose extent of atherosclerotic heart disease
    2. Is scheduled for electrocardiogram to identify specific cardiac dysrhythmias
    3. Requires chemically induced stress electrocardiogram for poor exercise tolerance
    4. Must have positron emission tomography because of coronary artery disease

20. The nurse is discussing modifiable risk factors for cardiovascular disease with a 23-year-old patient who is currently asymptomatic. What does the nurse recommend? *(1528)*
    1. Find out if any first-degree relatives had cardiovascular problems before the age of 50.
    2. Stop smoking or consider greatly reducing the number of cigarettes smoked per day.
    3. Ask the health care provider for a cholesterol-lowering drug such as simvastatin.
    4. Monitor weight and calorie intake to maintain a body mass index of 30.

21. During a discharge teaching session, the young patient voices concern about her risk for heart disease because she has diabetes mellitus. Which self-care measures would the nurse teach the patient? **Select all that apply.** *(1528)*
    1. Keep the blood glucose level under control.
    2. Monitor blood pressure at home: goal less than 120/80 mm Hg.
    3. Eat a low-fat diet rich in fruits and vegetables.
    4. Exercise 3-5 times a week for at least 30 minutes.
    5. Take low-dose aspirin once a day.

22. Which psychosocial behaviors are **more** likely to be associated with increased cardiovascular symptoms? *(1528)*
    1. Frequently in a hurry and generally impatient
    2. Easygoing and usually enjoys life
    3. Neat, organized, and pays attention to detail
    4. Pessimistic and generally expresses negativity

23. The patient's cardiac monitor shows a regular rhythm with a rate of 65 beats/min, P waves precede each QRS complex, QRS complexes are symmetrical and regularly spaced, and a normal T wave shows repolarization. What is the nurse's interpretation of the monitor display? *(1528)*
    1. Vital signs should be immediately assessed.
    2. The monitor indicates a normal sinus rhythm.
    3. The monitor is showing a benign dysrhythmia.
    4. The patient should be assessed for chest pain.

24. The patient experiences dizziness and lightheadedness while trying to pass a bowel movement. An immediate pulse check shows 45 beats/min that rapidly recovers to a regular rate of 70. What is the **most** probable cause of this episode of sinus bradycardia? *(1529)*
    1. Digitalis toxicity
    2. Endocrine disturbance
    3. Intracranial tumor
    4. Vagal stimulation

25. For which dysrhythmia would a pacemaker **most** likely be necessary? *(1531)*
    1. Sinus tachycardia
    2. Premature ventricular contractions
    3. Third-degree heart block
    4. Atrial fibrillation

26. The patient who had a myocardial infarction 2 weeks ago is now having frequent episodes of ventricular tachycardia. For this patient, what is the clinical significance of this dysrhythmia? *(1531)*
    1. Warning sign for ventricular fibrillation
    2. Expected finding at this stage
    3. Reaction to a beta-adrenergic blocker
    4. Treatment is given only for symptoms

27. The patient is on the cardiac monitor undergoing a diagnostic procedure. Suddenly, the health care provider says, "The patient is having ventricular fibrillation." Which piece of equipment is the **most** vital? *(1532)*
    1. Temporary pacemaker
    2. Defibrillator
    3. Bag-valve-mask
    4. Crash cart

28. A patient is being discharged after receiving a permanent pacemaker. What is the **best** rationale to give to the patient about refraining from sports such as tennis, swimming, golf, and weight-lifting for the first 6-8 weeks? *(1535)*
    1. "First, you have to be able to climb at least two flights of stairs."
    2. "Active sports will interfere with the pacemaker's fixed mode."
    3. "These sports are too strenuous and rapidly increase the heart rate."
    4. "The arm on the pacemaker side should not be lifted over the head."

29. The patient had a percutaneous transluminal coronary angioplasty with stent placement. What type of medication is the patient **most** likely to be prescribed for at least 3 months? *(1539)*
    1. Digitalis preparation
    2. Diuretic
    3. Opioid pain medication
    4. Anticoagulant

30. Which instruction would the nurse give to the patient for self-administration of nitrate medications? *(1541)*
    1. Refrigerate the oral tablets and nitroglycerin patches until use.
    2. Apply patches in the morning and remove them at bedtime.
    3. A burning sensation on the tongue indicates an allergic reaction.
    4. Pain relief should occur after a minimum of two doses.

31. For a patient with myocardial infarction, what symptom is the **most** important? *(1542)*
    1. Diaphoresis
    2. Palpitations
    3. Pain
    4. Shortness of breath

32. A 63-year-old patient presents with fever, increased pulse, epistaxis, and joint involvement. Heart murmurs are auscultated. The patient has a history of inadequately treated childhood group A β-hemolytic streptococci pharyngitis. These findings and history are consistent with which medical diagnosis? *(1556)*
    1. Cardiomyopathy
    2. Angina
    3. Left-sided heart failure
    4. Rheumatic heart disease

33. A neighbor tells the nurse that he has indigestion that has lasted 60 minutes. He tried "taking nitroglycerin, but that didn't help." What should the nurse do **first**? *(1541)*
    1. Tell the neighbor to take an aspirin and then drive to the emergency department.
    2. Stay with the neighbor, assist him to remain calm, and call 911.
    3. Assess the neighbor's use of nitroglycerin and assess for other symptoms.
    4. Phone the neighbor's health care provider and ask for recommendations.

34. The health care provider is considering tissue plasminogen activator (TPA) for a patient who is having an acute myocardial infarction. The wife suddenly rushes to the nurse and says, "We forgot to tell you something." Which disclosure is a contraindication for TPA? *(1543)*
    1. "My husband is a Jehovah's Witness."
    2. "My husband recently had a head injury."
    3. "He forgot to take his insulin this morning."
    4. "He had a small heart attack last year."

35. The nurse is caring for a patient who is 40 hours post–myocardial infarction. Which instruction should be given to the unlicensed assistive personnel (UAP)? *(1545)*
    1. Assist the patient to ambulate in the hall three times.
    2. Check to see if the patient is too tired to get up.
    3. Encourage the patient to independently get out of bed.
    4. Help the patient get to the commode chair.

36. What is the **best** method to help a patient comply with dietary restrictions associated with atherosclerotic heart disease? *(1569)*
    1. Tell him to avoid all foods that are high in fats.
    2. Remind him that total fat intake is 35%-40% of total caloric intake.
    3. Tell him to eat 10-15 grams of soluble fiber every day.
    4. Teach him how to read the nutritional labels on food products.

37. The nurse is caring for a patient who has right ventricular heart failure. After therapy, the nurse sees that the patient has lost 5 pounds of weight. Assuming that all the weight represents fluid loss, how much fluid has the patient lost? _____ L *(1548)*

38. The patient with a history of heart failure tells the home health nurse, "Every night I sleep in this recliner chair. I feel better if I sleep with my head up." What will the nurse assess **first**? *(1546)*
    1. Check for dependent edema in the lower extremities.
    2. Look at accessibility to the bedroom and bathroom.
    3. Assess ability to independently move and ambulate.
    4. Ask about compliance with low-sodium, low-fat diet.

39. The nurse is assessing a patient who had an embolectomy in the right lower extremity. Which assessment finding is cause for **greatest** concern? *(1573)*
    1. Sudden absence of pulse in the affected extremity
    2. Capillary refill in extremity is greater than 2 seconds
    3. Affected extremity is erythematous and edematous
    4. Patient reports a tingling sensation in extremity

40. The patient arrives in the emergency department with severe dyspnea, agitation, cyanosis, audible wheezes, and a cough with blood-tinged sputum. What is the **priority** nursing action? *(1554)*
    1. Obtain a blood sample for arterial blood gases.
    2. Administer oxygen.
    3. Auscultate lung sounds.
    4. Establish a peripheral IV.

41. The nurse is caring for a patient with valvular heart disease. Which task could be assigned to the UAP? *(1557)*
    1. Identify activities of daily living that cause fatigue.
    2. Check meal trays for high-sodium foods.
    3. Weigh the patient at the same time every day.
    4. Explain the plan for rest periods.

42. Which disorder of the cardiovascular system places the patient at **highest** risk for the potentially life-threatening condition of cardiac tamponade? *(1559)*
    1. Pericarditis
    2. Valvular heart disease
    3. Buerger's disease
    4. Endocarditis

43. Which sign/symptom indicates to the nurse that a patient with endocarditis is experiencing a serious and common complication of the disease? *(1559)*
    1. Fever and chills
    2. Joint pains and aches
    3. Sudden shortness of breath
    4. Petechiae on neck and chest

44. The nurse sees an older woman sitting in the waiting room and she is crying, "My granddaughter was just diagnosed with infective endocarditis." Which therapy is the nurse **most** likely to explain to the grandmother? *(1561)*
    1. Prosthetic valve replacement
    2. Intensive antibiotic therapy
    3. Complete bedrest
    4. Anticoagulation therapy

45. Which patient should be counseled about the risk of cardiomyopathy related to lifestyle choices? *(1561)*
    1. High-risk sexual behavior
    2. Poor intake of dietary fiber
    3. Use of "crack" cocaine
    4. Social consumption of alcohol

46. The patient had a recent cardiac transplant. Which intervention is required for posttransplant care? *(1562)*
    1. Immunosuppressive therapy
    2. Pericardiocentesis
    3. Percutaneous transluminal angioplasty
    4. Contact isolation

47. A younger patient has had several blood pressure readings that are consistently staying around 130/80 mm Hg. What treatments and/or advice should be given to this patient? *(1566)*
    1. Diuretics and low-sodium diet
    2. Beta-adrenergic blockers and weight loss
    3. Angiotensin II receptor blockers and low-fat diet
    4. Lifestyle change and routine health appointments

48. The nurse is caring for a patient who has peripheral arterial disease with burning pain in the right leg that occurs at rest. Which intervention will the nurse use? *(1572)*
    1. Elevate the leg on a pillow.
    2. Use a covered ice compress.
    3. Place the leg in a dependent position.
    4. Encourage aerobic exercise for circulation.

49. A patient receives a prescription for anticoagulant medication for treatment of arterial emboli. What dietary information should the nurse give? *(1573)*
    1. Do not increase intake of dark-green vegetables because of vitamin K.
    2. Take extra dairy products to ensure calcium intake and vitamin D.
    3. Eat fruits such as citrus and bananas that provide potassium.
    4. Avoid eating saturated fats by limiting use of butter, oils, and red meats.

50. The nurse is monitoring a patient who is waiting for diagnostic testing to determine if he has an aortic aneurysm. The patient suddenly reports severe chest pain. He becomes pale, weak, and confused. His pulse is 130 beats/min and blood pressure is 85/50 mm Hg. What should the nurse do **first**? *(1575)*
    1. Call the health care provider.
    2. Put the patient in a supine position.
    3. Assess pain and give opioid medication.
    4. Establish a patent peripheral IV.

51. The nurse is caring for a postsurgical patient. Which intervention is the **most** important in preventing venous thrombosis in the legs? *(1580)*
    1. Applying elastic compression stockings
    2. Elevating the lower extremities
    3. Ensuring early ambulation and mobility
    4. Measuring the calf circumference daily

CRITICAL THINKING ACTIVITIES

Activity 1

52. A 56-year-old man with a history of angina arrives in the emergency department seeking care. He reports crushing chest pain that radiates down his left shoulder and arm. "The pain is more severe and has lasted longer than a typical angina episode." *(1541-1545)*

    a. What data should the nurse collect? _____

    _____

    _____

    _____

    b. What does the nurse anticipate this patient's medical diagnosis will be? _____

    _____

    c. What are the goals of the medical management of this patient? _____

    _____

    d. Identify at least six nursing interventions for this patient's care._____

    _____

    _____

    _____

    _____

    _____

    _____

Activity 2

53. A 43-year-old Native American woman presents with "heaviness in her chest." She reports that it radiates down her left inner arm. Her medical history includes childbirth, pancreatitis, and hypertension. The medical diagnosis of angina is made. *(1536, 1537)*

   a.   What risk factors for heart disease does the patient have? _____

   _____

   _____

   b.   What medications are used to treat angina? _____

   _____

   _____

Activity 3

54. A home health nurse is caring for a 73-year-old man who has heart failure. He has been hospitalized twice for exacerbations, but is currently stable and able to live independently in his own home.

   a.   What changes related to aging would the nurse expect to find for this patient's cardiac system? *(1526)*

   _____

   _____

   b.   What are common signs and symptoms of heart failure? *(1549)* _____

   _____

   _____

   c.   Identify medication classes that are used in the medical management of heart failure. *(1550-1551)*

   _____

   _____

   d.   Discuss patient teaching points for heart failure. *(1554)* _____

   _____

   _____

Activity 4

55. The nurse is working in an ambulatory walk-in clinic in an urban area. Many of the patients are homeless and the clinic staff sees many patients who have venous stasis ulcers.

   a.   What is the pathophysiology of stasis ulcers and why are the homeless at risk for this disorder? *(1581)*

   _____

   b.   Describe how the nurse would use PATCHES to assess venous disorders. *(1564)* _____

   _____

   _____

   _____

   c.   Identify the signs and symptoms of venous stasis ulcers. *(1581)* _____

   _____

   _____

d. Review the treatment options available for venous stasis ulcers and suggest how the nurse can assist homeless patients to obtain care. *(1581)*

_____

_____

_____

Activity 5

56. Check the cupboards of an older relative or patient (or your own cupboards) and read nutritional labels on packages. Determine if a typical day's use of the products on the shelf would meet the nutritional restrictions for someone on a cardioprotective diet. (Don't forget to check condiments, if they are likely to be included in daily use.) Record your findings and the recommendations that you would make about the choice of food products. *(1547)*

_____

_____

_____

_____

_____

_____

_____

_____

_____

Care of the Patient With a Respiratory Disorder

MATCHING

Medication Used for Respiratory Disorders

Directions: Match the medication used for a respiratory disorder on the left to the associated characteristic (action, side effect, or nursing implication) on the right. Indicate your answers in the spaces provided. (1615-1617)

Medication	Actions, Side Effects, or Nursing Implications
_____ 1. Acetylcysteine	a. Vasoconstrictor used for nasal congestion
_____ 2. Salmeterol	b. Beta$_1$- and beta$_2$-receptor agonist; could cause tachycardia, palpitations, angina, chest pain, myocardial infarction, dysrhythmias, hypertension, restlessness, agitation, anxiety
_____ 3. Prednisone	
_____ 4. Epinephrine	
_____ 5. Albuterol	c. Bronchodilator; can cause anxiety, restlessness, insomnia, headache, seizures, tachycardia, dysrhythmias
_____ 6. Isoniazid	d. Mucolytic agent; also used as antidote in acetaminophen overdose
_____ 7. Oxymetazoline	
_____ 8. Theophylline	e. Used in prevention of exercise-induced asthma
_____ 9. Rifampin	f. Antiinflammatory agent; do not discontinue medication abruptly; dosage must be tapered slowly
_____ 10. Zafirlukast	g. "Rescue therapy;" short-acting inhaled beta$_2$-agonist
	h. Antitubercular agent; monitor liver function tests
	i. For long-term treatment of asthma
	j. Antitubercular agent; long-term therapy

TABLE ACTIVITY

11. Directions: Complete the table by filling in the normal values for an arterial blood gas. *(1597)*

pH:	
Pa$_{CO_2}$:	
Pa$_{O_2}$:	
HCO$_3^-$:	
Sa$_{O_2}$:	

MULTIPLE CHOICE

Directions: Select the best answer(s) for each of the following questions.

12. The inner linings of the pharynx and the eustachian tube are continuous. In children, this normal anatomical structure contributes to what common disorder? *(1600)*
    1. Asthma
    2. Epistaxis
    3. Laryngitis
    4. Ear infections

13. If the epiglottis fails to perform its intended function, how would this affect the patient? *(1589)*
    1. Increased risk for aspiration
    2. Increased incidence of throat infections
    3. Decreased respiratory drive
    4. Decreased forced expiratory volume

14. The nurse is assessing a newborn who was brought to the clinic for the initial well-baby physical. The newborn demonstrates a respiratory rate of 50 breaths/min. How does the nurse interpret this data? *(1592)*
    1. Newborn's respiratory rate suggests a hypermetabolic state, such as fever.
    2. Newborn must be immediately taken to resuscitation area for respiratory distress.
    3. Newborn's respiratory rate is within the expected range for developmental age.
    4. Newborn's respiratory rate is borderline high and should be closely monitored.

15. The patient has increased intracranial pressure and the nurse knows that the medulla oblongata and pons of the brain have a role in respiration. If increased intracranial pressure is uncontrolled and excessive, what is the potential adverse effect on respiratory function? *(1592)*
    1. Respiratory infection
    2. Respiratory arrest
    3. Respiratory edema
    4. Respiratory acidosis

16. The nurse is assessing a child who is "having an asthma attack." Which assessment finding is cause for **greatest** concern? *(1593)*
    1. Audible wheezing on expiration
    2. Subjective sensation of chest tightness
    3. Increased pulse and respiratory rate
    4. Substernal and clavicular retractions

17. A neighbor tells the nurse that he is "pretty healthy and doesn't take any medications" but seems to have nosebleeds that are occurring more frequently. What does the nurse suggest **first**? *(1599)*
    1. "To stop bleeding, hold pressure on the lower nose for 10-15 minutes."
    2. "Let's check your blood pressure for the next several mornings."
    3. "Make an appointment to have your clotting times checked."
    4. "Have your health care provider examine your nasal septum."

18. What is an **early** sign of cancer of the larynx? *(1603)*
    1. Pain radiating to the ear
    2. Difficulty swallowing
    3. Feeling of a lump in the throat
    4. Progressive or persistent hoarseness

19. Which persons should be advised to get pneumococcal vaccination? **Select all that apply.** *(1619)*
    1. 18-month-old child with no known health problems
    2. 25-year-old nurse with no known health problems
    3. 80-year-old with chronic conditions who lives in a nursing home
    4. 35-year-old with diabetes mellitus that is well-controlled with insulin
    5. 40-year-old in good general health, who travels outside the United States
    6. 19-year-old who smokes two packs of cigarettes per day

20. The nurse is caring for a patient who sustained rib fractures during a car accident. The patient reports sudden sharp chest pain over the fracture area, with difficulty breathing. Which assessment finding supports the nurse's suspicion of pneumothorax? *(1627)*
    1. Bilateral wheeze during inspiration and expiration
    2. Decreased breath sounds over the affected area
    3. Coarse crackles heard in early inspiration
    4. Dry creaking and grating when breath is held

21. The patient had a permanent tracheostomy several months ago. At this point, what is the **priority** concern? *(1605)*
    1. Breathing independently and safely.
    2. Secreting adequate amounts of mucus.
    3. Being unable to produce normal speech.
    4. Swallowing without choking or gagging.

22. A patient with a chronic lung disorder comes to the clinic and tells the nurse, "I feel like I am getting sick again." What questions would the nurse ask? **Select all that apply.** *(1592)*
    1. "How's your breathing? Can you describe it?"
    2. "Are you coughing? Can you describe the cough?"
    3. "When did you first notice the worsening of symptoms?"
    4. "What were your last arterial blood gas results?"
    5. "Do you use oxygen at home? If so, does it help?"
    6. "Have you noticed a change in your ability to do routine activities?"

23. The patient arrives at the emergency department and displays significant respiratory distress. Which objective finding is generally regarded as a **late** sign of respiratory distress? *(1593)*
    1. Shows increased respiratory rate
    2. Has adventitious breath sounds
    3. Assumes orthopneic position
    4. Demonstrates flaring of nostrils

24. A patient was brought to the emergency department because he was involved in a motor vehicle accident. The patient shows mild respiratory distress and expansion of the right side of the chest is decreased compared to the left. The history and data are indicative of which disorder? *(1627)*
    1. Pleural effusion
    2. Pneumothorax
    3. Empyema
    4. Pulmonary edema

25. Which patient has the **greatest** need for a helical computed tomography scan? *(1594)*
    1. A disoriented older patient who may have a pulmonary embolus
    2. A toddler who might have swallowed a metallic foreign body
    3. A patient who requires a sample of lymph node tissue for biopsy
    4. A patient who was exposed to tuberculosis several decades ago

26. The nurse is caring for a patient who had a bronchoscopy. Which task can be delegated to the unlicensed assistive personnel (UAP)? *(1595)*
    1. Give clear fluids after checking for the gag reflex.
    2. Assist the patient to a semi-Fowler's position.
    3. Report signs of laryngeal edema such as stridor.
    4. Check sputum for signs of hemorrhage.

27. The patient needs a thoracentesis for therapeutic removal of fluid. Which position should the nurse help the patient to assume for the procedure? *(1596)*
    1. Seated on the bed; head and arms resting on a pillow placed on an overbed table
    2. Placed in a supine position with the anterior lateral chest draped for ready access
    3. Positioned in a recumbent prone position with head resting on forearms and hands
    4. Situated in a side-lying position on affected side and uncovered to the waist

28. The nurse hears in handover report that 1600 mL of fluid was removed during the therapeutic thoracentesis procedure. What is the **most** important intervention that the nurse will plan to do? *(1623)*
    1. Perform routine postprocedure assessments.
    2. Increase the fluid intake to compensate for the loss.
    3. Watch for signs and symptoms of pulmonary edema.
    4. Follow up to get the results of the fluid specimen.

29. When an arterial blood gas is obtained from a patient who is taking warfarin, what special consideration is needed? *(1597)*
    1. The dietary therapy associated with the drug is likely to alter the results.
    2. The drug increases fragility of the vessels, so the specimen is hard to obtain.
    3. The drug alters the amount of oxygen that hemoglobin can carry.
    4. The clotting time is prolonged; pressure is held for 20 minutes on the puncture site.

30. The nursing student uses an automatic blood pressure cuff to take vital signs. To be efficient, the student simultaneously attaches the pulse oximeter to the patient's same hand. The pulse oximeter reading is below 90%. What should the student do **first**? *(1598)*
    1. Report the findings to the nurse or instructor.
    2. Redo the pulse oximeter reading on the other hand.
    3. Assess the patient for shortness of breath.
    4. Document the finding in the patient's record.

31. A patient was treated for epistaxis with nasal packing saturated with 1:1000 epinephrine. During the postprocedure assessment, the nurse notices that the patient swallows frequently. Which question should the nurse ask? *(1599)*
    1. "Does your throat feel swollen or painful?"
    2. "Would you like some cool fluids to drink?"
    3. "Is blood running down the back of your throat?"
    4. "Are you tasting epinephrine in your throat?"

32. What is likely to be included in the discharge instructions for a patient who was treated for epistaxis? **Select all that apply.** *(1599)*
    1. Use a vaporizer.
    2. Use saline nose drops.
    3. Apply nasal lubricants.
    4. Take aspirin for pain as needed.
    5. Vigorously blow to remove clots.
    6. Avoid inserting foreign objects into nose.

33. What is the nurse's role in allergy testing? *(1601)*
    1. Uses a lancet to prick the skin with different allergens
    2. Evaluates the response to different allergens
    3. Advises the patient about allergens to avoid
    4. Determines schedule for retesting questionable allergens

34. The nurse is eating in a restaurant. At a nearby table, several men are talking, laughing, drinking alcohol, and eating steak. Suddenly, the nurse hears, "Hey! Are you all right?" Which behavior signals a need to intervene for choking? *(1603)*
    1. Vigorous coughing
    2. Running from the room
    3. Hand over throat
    4. Waving hands frantically

35. A patient is diagnosed with viral laryngitis. Which discharge instruction is the **most** important to relieve the inflammation and edema of the vocal cords? *(1608)*
    1. Use a mild analgesic such as acetaminophen for pain.
    2. Complete the full course of antibiotics.
    3. Rest the voice; communicate with gestures or by writing.
    4. Suck on throat lozenges to promote comfort.

36. The nurse is performing a rapid strep screen. What is the rationale for obtaining two throat swabs? *(1608)*
    1. The first swab is likely to be contaminated, so a backup swab is needed.
    2. If the rapid strep test is negative, the second swab is sent for culture.
    3. The second swab is given to the patient, in case the rapid strep is positive.
    4. The first and second swabs are grown in different types of culture media.

37. A patient comes to the clinic and reports decreased appetite, generalized malaise, and a decreased sense of smell. Gentle palpation over the sinus area elicits pain. Which piece of equipment should the nurse obtain so the health care provider can do some diagnostic testing during the physical examination? *(1609)*
    1. Tongue blade
    2. Percussion hammer
    3. Penlight
    4. Cotton-tipped applicator

38. A patient is diagnosed with acute bronchitis. Although the patient is instructed to increase fluids to 3000-4000 mL per day, which fluid is specifically not recommended because of the respiratory condition? *(1610)*
    1. Coffee
    2. Soda
    3. Orange juice
    4. Milk

39. What is the **primary** problem for the health care team in identifying potentially life-threatening respiratory disorders such as Legionnaires' disease, severe acute respiratory syndrome, and anthrax? *(1611, 1612)*
    1. They are agents used in global germ warfare.
    2. The percentage of morbidity and mortality is high.
    3. They require isolation because transmission is airborne.
    4. At first, symptoms are similar to other respiratory disorders.

40. What is the **major** problem for patients who are being treated for tuberculosis? *(1618)*
    1. All the patient's contacts must be identified and treated.
    2. Infection control measures are complex and expensive.
    3. Many have rapid disease progression with mortality rates up to 89%.
    4. Drug therapy lasts 6-9 months and about 50% of patients are noncompliant.

41. A patient recently diagnosed with peripherally located lung cancer reports he is experiencing severe chest pain. Based on the nurse's knowledge of the pathophysiology of this pain, which therapy does the nurse anticipate? *(1592, 1628)*
    1. Bronchodilators
    2. Thoracentesis
    3. Mechanical ventilation
    4. Corticosteroids

42. The patient is diagnosed with pleurisy. During auscultation of the lungs, what is the nurse **most** likely to hear? *(1593)*
    1. Interrupted crackling or bubbling sounds more common on inspiration
    2. Deep, loud, low, coarse sound (like a snore) during inspiration or expiration
    3. Dry, creaking, grating, with a machinelike quality loudest over anterior chest
    4. High-pitched, musical, whistlelike sound during inspiration or expiration

43. A patient being treated for atelectasis has been prescribed acetylcysteine. What is the purpose of this medication? *(1615)*
    1. Reduce the risk of infection
    2. Dilate the bronchioles
    3. Enhance the cough reflex
    4. Reduce viscosity of secretions

44. For a patient with a chest tube, which task could be delegated to the UAP? *(1624)*
    1. Assist to ambulate with water-seal below the level of the chest.
    2. Check to make sure that all connections are secure and intact.
    3. Observe for and report hypoventilation or increased dyspnea.
    4. Assess quantity and quality of drainage in the collection chamber.

45. The nurse is reviewing the admission orders for a patient who was stabilized in the emergency department and then admitted for a diagnosis of pulmonary edema. Which order is the nurse **most** likely to question? *(1630)*
    1. Oxygen 2 L per nasal cannula
    2. Notify provider with all blood gas results
    3. IV normal saline at 250 mL per hour
    4. Place on telemetry monitor

46. A patient is admitted for venous thrombosis in the left leg. He is in good spirits during the AM assessment, but later in day he reports feeling mildly short of breath with a sense of impending doom. What should the nurse do **first**? *(1632)*
    1. Obtain an order for an arterial blood gas.
    2. Check the vital signs and pulse oximeter reading.
    3. Assess the left leg for warmth, redness, or swelling.
    4. Alert the RN about possible pulmonary embolus.

47. Which patient has the **highest** mortality risk related to acute respiratory distress syndrome? *(1633)*
    1. Was diagnosed and treated for sepsis 5 days ago
    2. Had direct trauma to chest during a fight 10 days ago
    3. Has a history of chronic obstructive pulmonary disease
    4. Has been treated for asthma since early childhood

48. Which instruction would the nurse give to the UAP about assisting the patient who has emphysema to accomplish activities of daily living (ADLs)? *(1638)*
    1. Divide hygienic care into short sessions with 90 minutes of rest between.
    2. Defer the hygienic care until the patient has better activity tolerance.
    3. Assess the patient's response to ambulating and shorten walks accordingly.
    4. Perform range-of-motion exercises, unless the patient declines them.

49. For a patient with chronic bronchitis, what is the physiologic cause of polycythemia? *(1639)*
    1. Medication side effect
    2. Dehydration and fluid shifting
    3. Nutritional deficiency
    4. Compensation for chronic hypoxemia

50. For a patient with newly diagnosed asthma, what is the **best** rationale for assessing the home environment? *(1640)*
    1. Identify any activity intolerance related to the design of the home.
    2. Assess the safety of the environment related to the use of home oxygen.
    3. Identify stimulants or allergens that are triggering the asthma attacks.
    4. Evaluate the need for a home health aide to accomplish ADLs.

51. The home health nurse reads in the patient's record that he has smoked for the past 30 years and was recently diagnosed with emphysema. Which assessment finding does the nurse expect as the **primary** manifestation? *(1636)*
    1. Dyspnea on exertion
    2. Copious thick sputum
    3. Barrel-chest appearance
    4. Bulbous, shiny fingernails

CRITICAL THINKING ACTIVITIES

Activity 1

52. A 34-year-old man comes to the clinic for fatigue and headaches in the morning. The nurse's assessment reveals he is 5'9" and weighs 293 pounds. His blood pressure is 155/92 mm Hg. His health history reveals elevated blood pressure, hernia repair, appendectomy, and recent injuries suffered from a motor vehicle accident after falling asleep while driving. During the interview, his wife states he should never be tired because he snores so loudly at night that she is the one who is kept awake. *(1601, 1602)*

    a. Based on the nurse's knowledge, what medical diagnosis is anticipated? _____

    _____

    b. What risk factors and elements of the patient's personal history support this diagnosis? _____

    _____

    _____

    _____

    c. Discuss the medical management of this condition. _____

    _____

    _____

    _____

    _____

Activity 2

53. A 72-year-old man is transferred from the nursing home to the hospital with a diagnosis of viral pneumonia. *(1620, 1621)*

    a. What signs and symptoms are associated with this type of pneumonia? _____

    _____

    _____

    b. What diagnostic tests can the nurse expect to be completed for this patient? _____

    _____

    _____

    c. What types of medications may be prescribed for this patient? _____

    _____

    _____

d. Identify nursing assessments that should be performed for this patient._____
_____
_____

Activity 3

54. a. Discuss factors that may influence medication compliance for tuberculosis patients. *(1614, 1618)*
_____
_____
_____
_____

b. Suggest interventions to increase compliance. *(1618)* _____
_____
_____
_____
_____
_____
_____
_____

Activity 4

55. The nurse hears in report that the patient has a closed chest drainage system. *(1616)*

a. What nursing assessments should be performed for this patient? _____
_____
_____

b. How should the tubing and the chest drainage system be positioned? _____
_____
_____

c. How does the nurse interpret the absence of tidaling (air bubbling) in the water seal chamber?
_____
_____

d. What does constant bubbling in the water seal chamber indicate? _____
_____
_____

Care of the Patient With a Urinary Disorder

SHORT ANSWER

Directions: Using your own words, answer each question in the space provided.

1. What are the three major functions of the nephron? *(1649)*

    a. _____

    b. _____

    c. _____

2. Summarize the three phases of urine formation. *(1650)*

    a. _____

    b. _____

    c. _____

3. Identify at least three life span considerations for older adults related to the urinary system. *(1652)*

    _____

    _____

    _____

4. What are the major functions of the kidneys? *(1651)* _____

    _____

    _____

    _____

    _____

    _____

    _____

TABLE ACTIVITY

Directions: Complete the table below by supplying the normal range for urinalysis results and identify at least one factor that could influence the results. The first constituent is completed for you. (1653)

5. Urinalysis

Constituent	Normal Range	Influencing Factors
Color	Pale yellow to amber	Diabetes insipidus, biliary obstruction, medications, diet
Turbidity		
Odor		
pH		
Specific gravity		
Glucose		
Protein		
Bilirubin		
Hemoglobin		
Ketones		
Red blood cells		
White blood cells		
Casts		
Bacteria		

FIGURE LABELING

6. Directions: Identify the ileal conduit, stoma, and anastomosis on the figure below. *(1693)*

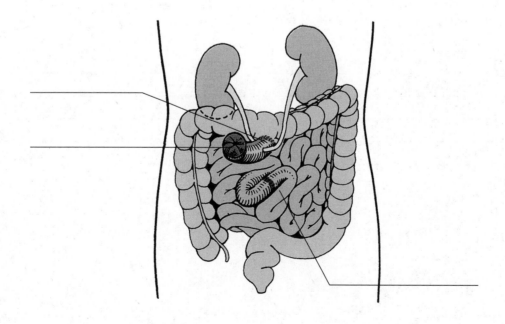

MULTIPLE CHOICE

Directions: Select the best answer(s) for each of the following questions.

7. The nurse is reviewing laboratory results for a young healthy patient who has no known health problems. The blood urea nitrogen (BUN) level is 26 mg/dL. What question is the nurse **most** likely to ask to clarify this laboratory result? *(1654)*
   1. "Have you had an exposure to a sexually transmitted infection?"
   2. "Did you eat or drink anything before you had the blood drawn?"
   3. "Do you have a family history of diabetes or liver problems?"
   4. "Are you having any problems with starting the urine stream?"

8. The nurse hears in report that the patient is in the diuretic phase of acute renal failure. What assessment findings does the nurse expect? *(1685)*
   1. BUN is over 50 mg/dL, serum creatinine is greater than 5 mg/dL, urine output is less than 30 mL/hour.
   2. BUN and serum creatinine levels begin to normalize and urinary output is 1 to 2 L/24 hours.
   3. Glomerular filtration rate rises and kidneys are at normal or near-normal function.
   4. BUN and serum creatinine levels rise and urinary output is less than 400 mL/24 hours.

9. The nurse is caring for several patients who need diagnostic testing for problems associated with the urinary system. Which patient is **most** likely to need insertion of an indwelling urinary catheter prior to having the procedure? *(1655)*
   1. Patient needs an intravenous pyelogram for possible hydronephrosis.
   2. Patient needs renal venography for possible dysfunction of venous drainage.
   3. Patient needs a renal ultrasonography for possible congenital anomaly.
   4. Patient needs a voiding cystourethrogram for possible abnormal urethra.

10. The nurse is caring for a patient who returned to the unit after a cystoscopy for diagnosis of a disorder of the urinary bladder. Which post-procedure assessment would be considered a normal finding? *(1655)*
    1. Increased output and low specific gravity
    2. Urinary retention and bladder distention
    3. Blood-tinged urine at the first void
    4. Mild flank pain and low-grade fever

11. Which staff member should not be assigned to care for a patient who has returned from a renal scan that used a radionuclide tracer substance? *(1656)*
    1. Unlicensed assistive personnel (UAP) who is in the first trimester of pregnancy
    2. LPN/LVN who is taking medication for a urinary tract infection
    3. RN who is immunosuppressed secondary to a splenectomy
    4. UAP who has allergies to iodine, seafood, and latex

12. Which patient is **most** likely to benefit from patient education pamphlets about urodynamic studies and rectal electromyography? *(1656)*
    1. Patient has renal cancer, staging yet to be determined.
    2. Patient has risk for polycystic kidney disease.
    3. Patient has urinary incontinence related to neurologic disorder.
    4. Patient has signs/symptoms of chronic glomerulonephritis.

13. The nurse is caring a patient who is prescribed furosemide for acute renal failure. What nursing interventions are related to the medication and acute renal failure? **Select all that apply.** *(1657)*
    1. Keep accurate intake and output (I&O) records.
    2. Assess BUN and serum electrolytes.
    3. Teach the patient to avoid overuse of salt.
    4. Monitor for flank and abdominal pain.
    5. Record and monitor daily morning weights.

14. Which breakfast tray is the **best** example of foods that adhere to the acid-ash diet? *(1659)*
    1. Blueberry pancakes with maple syrup and tea
    2. Coffee, orange juice, and granola with raisins
    3. Whole-grain toast, boiled egg, and prunes
    4. Low-fat milk, banana, and peanut butter toast

15. What instructions would the nurse give to the UAP about the care of a patient who has an indwelling catheter and urinary collection bag? **Select all that apply.** *(1660)*
    1. Never rest the collecting bag on the floor.
    2. Cleanse the perineum from front to back with mild soap and warm water, then pat dry.
    3. Inspect the catheter entry site for blood, exudate, or other signs of infection.
    4. Avoid kinks or compression of the drainage tubing.
    5. Assist the patient to ambulate; hold drainage bag below the catheter insertion site.

16. A patient is prescribed sulfamethoxazole-trimethoprim. What is the **most** important point to stress in teaching the patient about this medication? *(1666)*
    1. Expect an increase in urination and try to take the medication in the morning.
    2. Complete the full course of medication even if feeling better after a day or two.
    3. The medication makes the urine a bright orange color, but this is harmless.
    4. Drink at least 2000 mL of water every day to prevent crystal precipitation.

17. For patients with diabetes mellitus or starvation states, urinalysis will show the abnormal presences of ketones. What is the underlying pathophysiology for this abnormality? *(1651)*
    1. Fatty acids are rapidly catabolized.
    2. Glucose is converted to ketones.
    3. Insulin levels are excessive.
    4. Glucose is transformed into fat.

18. Which patient condition is **most** likely to result in casts in the urine specimen? *(1683)*
    1. Type 1 diabetes mellitus
    2. Stress incontinence
    3. Acute pyelonephritis
    4. Ureter structure trauma

19. The nurse sees that the urine specific gravity results are 1.000 g/mL. Which patient condition is **most** likely to result in this abnormal finding? *(1653)*
    1. Diabetic ketoacidosis
    2. Hyperemesis gravidarum
    3. Diabetes insipidus
    4. Febrile with poor skin turgor

20. Identify the renal disorders associated with an abnormal elevation in serum creatinine. **Select all that apply.** *(1654)*
    1. Stress incontinence
    2. Glomerulonephritis
    3. Pyelonephritis
    4. Acute tubular necrosis
    5. Acute renal failure

21. A 49-year-old man's prostate-specific antigen (PSA) result is 9.5 ng/mL. Which condition(s) could be associated with this result? **Select all that apply.** *(1654)*
    1. Had a recent prostate biopsy
    2. Could be related to prostate cancer
    3. Suggests urinary tract infection
    4. Indicative of prostatitis
    5. Within normal limits for age

22. The nurse is planning care for several patients who will have diagnostic testing for urinary disorders. Which procedure is going to require the **most** time for postprocedural care? *(1655)*
    1. Kidney-ureter-bladder radiography
    2. Intravenous pyelogram
    3. Renal angiography
    4. Renal ultrasonography

23. During a urodynamic study, a patient is given bethanechol, a cholinergic drug. What is the expected effect of the medication? *(1656)*
    1. Relaxes the patient
    2. Reduces urine production
    3. Stimulates the atonic bladder
    4. Increases the uptake of dye

24. What instructions would the nurse give to the UAP for assisting a patient for the first 24 hours after a renal biopsy? *(1656)*
    1. Assist the patient to ambulate to the bathroom.
    2. Ask the patient about dizziness before ambulating.
    3. Withhold all foods and fluids for 24 hours.
    4. Remind the patient about bedrest for 24 hours.

25. The nurse is reviewing medication prescriptions for a patient with advanced end-stage renal disease. The nurse would question the use of which type of medication? *(1658)*
    1. Antiemetic
    2. Antipruritic
    3. Vitamin supplement
    4. Osmotic diuretic

26. The nurse is caring for several older male patients who have problems with urinary disorders. Which patient is the **best** candidate for an external condom? *(1660)*
    1. Has Alzheimer's disease and recently pulled out an indwelling catheter
    2. Has urge incontinence and functional incontinence related to a hip fracture
    3. Has a urinary tract infection and is currently taking antibiotics
    4. Has an enlarged prostate and occasionally has trouble starting the stream

27. What is an **early** sign of bladder cancer? *(1676)*
    1. Change in voiding pattern
    2. Dusky yellow-tan or gray skin color
    3. Painless, intermittent hematuria
    4. Difficult starting the stream of urine

28. The nurse sees that the patient who is being discharged is prescribed spironolactone. Which laboratory result will the nurse verify before the patient goes home? *(1657)*
    1. Urinalysis
    2. Potassium level
    3. White cell count
    4. Blood urea nitrogen

29. A patient with benign prostatic hyperplasia (BPH) tells the nurse that he uses over-the-counter (OTC) medications. Which medication is likely to create additional problems related to the BPH? *(1662)*
    1. Acetaminophen
    2. Diphenhydramine
    3. Vitamin K supplement
    4. Iron supplement

30. Which patient is **most** likely to benefit from learning about Kegel exercises? *(1663)*
    1. Experiences loss of urine during sneezing and lifting
    2. Has urinary retention secondary to chronic infection
    3. Has urge incontinence due to advanced Parkinson's disease
    4. Has a spastic bladder due to upper motor neuron lesion

31. The nurse and UAP are aware that no tension should be placed on urinary catheters; however, the nurse should reinforce this principle for which patient? *(1682)*
    1. Has a suprapubic catheter for long-term management
    2. Has a three-way catheter for continuous bladder irrigation
    3. Has an indwelling catheter after reconstruction of urethra
    4. Has a catheter and urometer for hourly measurements

32. For patients with nephrotic syndrome, which signs/symptoms is the nurse **most** likely to observe? *(1682)*
    1. Periorbital edema, pitting edema in legs, and crackles in lungs
    2. Sore throat or skin infection with fever and malaise
    3. Burning with urination, low back pain, hematuria, and fatigue
    4. Dysuria, weak stream, and increasing pain with bladder distention

33. The patient with acute glomerulonephritis is placed on bedrest. Which vital sign is of **primary** interest as an indicator of the success of the therapy? *(1684)*
    1. Temperature
    2. Pulse rate
    3. Respiratory rate
    4. Blood pressure

34. What is an indicator of chronic glomerulonephritis? *(1684)*
    1. Residual urine
    2. Albumin in the urine
    3. Ketones in the urine
    4. Prostate-specific antigen

35. A student nurse is assessing the function of an arteriovenous fistula after a dialysis treatment. When would the supervising nurse intervene? *(1689)*
    1. Flushes with saline using strict aseptic technique.
    2. Palpates a thrill and auscultates for a bruit.
    3. Assesses the distal pulses and checks for sensation.
    4. Asks the patient about pain or discomfort at the site.

CRITICAL THINKING ACTIVITIES

Activity 1

36. A 42-year-old patient has a history of frequent urinary tract infections and is admitted to the unit with a diagnosis of pyelonephritis. *(1669, 1670)*

    a. What signs and symptoms would the nurse anticipate the patient to demonstrate? _____

    _____

    _____

    b. Discuss the diagnostic tests that may be used in the treatment of the patient and the probable results.

    _____

    _____

Activity 2

37. A patient comes to the emergency department for severe flank pain, nausea, and vomiting. The patient reports that the pain starts in the flank area and radiates to the groin and inner thigh. A urinalysis reveals the presence of hematuria. *(1672, 1673)*

    a. What medical diagnosis does the nurse anticipate? _____

    _____

    b. Discuss the conservative and invasive techniques that may be used in the management of this condition.

    _____

    _____

    c. After successful treatment, the nurse is preparing the patient for discharge. Discuss long-term preventive management options. Include diet and medications.

    _____

    _____

Activity 3

38. A 53-year-old man was in a motor vehicle accident 4 days ago. He sustained serious trauma with hypovolemia that was treated in the emergency department. He has been diagnosed with acute renal failure and is currently in the oliguric phase. *(1685, 1686)*

    a. What potential clinical manifestations should the nurse be aware of when completing the nursing assessment?

    _____

    _____

    b. Discuss the three phases of acute renal failure. _____

    _____

    _____

    _____

    c. The patient's wife asks if she can bring him a hamburger and fries from a local fast-food restaurant. How will the nurse respond?

    _____

    _____

Activity 4

39. A 22-year-old woman seeks care at the health care provider's office complaining of burning with urination, perineal pain, and blood-tinged urine. She is diagnosed with a urinary tract infection. *(1658, 1667)*

    a. Why are women more prone to urinary tract infections compared to men? _____

    _____

    b. What other signs and symptoms may be present? _____

    _____

    _____

    c. What medical treatments can be anticipated in the management of this patient? _____

    _____

    _____

    d. What self-care measures should the nurse suggest to the patient to prevent urinary tract infections?

    _____

    _____

    _____

chapter

Care of the Patient With an Endocrine Disorder

51

MATCHING

Directions: Match the hormone produced by the gland to the action on the target organ. Indicate your answer in the space provided.

Hormone (Endocrine Gland)

_____ 1. oxytocin (posterior pituitary) *(1699)*

_____ 2. antidiuretic (posterior pituitary) *(1699)*

_____ 3. thyroxine (thyroid) *(1701)*

_____ 4. calcitonin (thyroid) *(1701)*

_____ 5. parathormone (parathyroid) *(1701)*

_____ 6. mineralocorticoids (adrenal cortex) *(1701)*

_____ 7. glucocorticoids (adrenal cortex) *(1701)*

_____ 8. epinephrine (adrenal medulla) *(1702)*

_____ 9. norepinephrine (adrenal medulla) *(1702)*

_____ 10. insulin (pancreas) *(1702)*

_____ 11. glucagon (pancreas) *(1702)*

_____ 12. melatonin (pineal) *(1702)*

Action on Target Organ

a. Causes the kidneys to conserve water by decreasing the amount of urine produced

b. Promotes the release of milk and stimulates uterine contractions during labor

c. Decreases blood calcium levels by causing calcium to be stored in the bones

d. Growth and development; metabolism

e. Involved in glucose metabolism; provides extra reserve energy in times of stress; exhibits antiinflammatory properties

f. Causes the heart rate and blood pressure to increase

g. Increases the concentration of calcium in the blood and regulates phosphorus in the blood

h. Water and electrolyte balance; indirectly manages blood pressure

i. Secreted in response to decreased levels of glucose in the blood

j. Inhibits reproductive activities by inhibiting the gonadotropic hormones

k. Combines with epinephrine to produce "fight-or-flight" response

l. Secreted in response to increased levels of glucose in the blood

FIGURE LABELING

13. Directions: Label the figure below by indicating the position of the glands of the body. *(1699)*

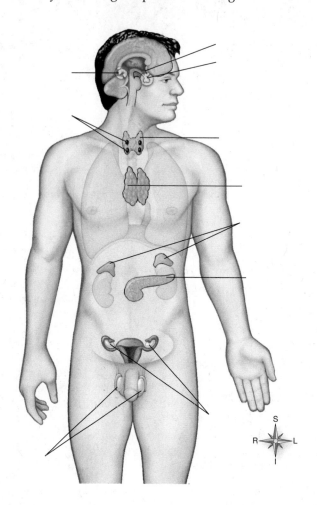

TABLE ACTIVITY

14. Directions: Complete the table below with the correct information about different types of insulin. *(1730)*

Type of Insulin	Injection Time (Before Meal)	Risk Time for Hypoglycemic Reaction	Onset of Action	Duration
Lispro (Humalog)				
Regular Humulin R Novolin R ReliOn R				
NPH/Regular Mix 70/30 Humulin Mix 70/30				
Glargine (Lantus)				

MULTIPLE CHOICE

Directions: Select the best answer(s) for each of the following questions.

15. Which electrolyte disorder is **most** likely to trigger early symptoms of syndrome of inappropriate antidiuretic hormone (SIADH)? *(1708)*
    1. Hypokalemia
    2. Hyponatremia
    3. Hypercalcemia
    4. Hyperglycemia

16. What instructions are given to the unlicensed assistive personnel (UAP) about the care of a patient with hypothyroidism? **Select all that apply.** *(1713)*
    1. Report frequency of bowel movements; straining; or small, hard stools.
    2. Allow extra time for physical care so the patient doesn't feel rushed.
    3. Make sure the patient does not become chilled during bathing.
    4. Observe patient's activity cycle and perform interventions accordingly.
    5. Encourage patient to select fruits, vegetables, and whole grains from menu.

17. A 53-year-old patient has just been informed that he has type 2 diabetes. Which patient education pamphlet is the nurse **most** likely to prepare for this patient? *(1728)*
    1. "A Step-by-Step Approach to Self-Administration of Insulin"
    2. "Side Effects of Common Oral Hypoglycemic Medications"
    3. "How to Manage Your Diabetes during Stress or Illness"
    4. "Using Exercise and Diet Modification for Weight Loss"

18. Which endocrine disorder is associated with the long-term complications of retinopathy; nephropathy; amputation of lower extremity; and cardiovascular conditions such as heart disease, hypertension, and stroke? *(1724)*
    1. Hyperparathyroidism
    2. Diabetes insipidus
    3. Cushing's syndrome
    4. Diabetes mellitus

19. Which patient always needs to have an emergency kit with 100 mg of IM hydrocortisone, syringes, and instructions for use? *(1722)*
    1. Patient has pheochromocytoma and is not a good candidate for the necessary surgery.
    2. Patient has Addison's disease and is having stress related to death of a family member.
    3. Patient has type 1 diabetes and is prone to episodes of sudden-onset hypoglycemia.
    4. Patient has hyperthyroidism and is having trouble tolerating the antithyroid drugs.

20. In the care of a patient with diabetic ketoacidosis, the nurse is **most** likely to contact the health care provider for clarification of which prescription? *(1729)*
    1. IV normal saline at 1000 L/hr until urinary output is at least 30 mL/hr
    2. Perform fingerstick for blood glucose level every hour
    3. Insert urinary catheter with urometer; monitor I&O every hour
    4. 100 units NPH insulin in 500 mL normal saline; titrate to blood glucose

21. What are **early** signs/symptoms of hypothyroidism? **Select all that apply.** *(1713)*
    1. Weight gain
    2. Difficulty concentrating
    3. Constipation
    4. Infertility
    5. Depression
    6. Mood swings

22. The nurse is talking to a 31-year-old woman who was recently diagnosed with acromegaly. The woman says, "My career is over. I'll become so hideous, I'm sure that I'll get fired." What is the **most** therapeutic response? *(1703)*
    1. "You have talents and abilities; surely those qualities will be considered."
    2. "Why don't you wait and cross that bridge when you come to it?"
    3. "You are thinking about how your life and career might change."
    4. "Let's talk about what you could do to enhance your appearance."

23. The school nurse is taking height and weight measurements for all children at the beginning of the school year. Measurement for one of the students shows a deviation over two percentile levels from the median. What should the nurse do? *(1705)*
    1. Call the parents and ask about the child's birth weight and growth patterns.
    2. Contact the parents and suggest they take the child to the health care provider.
    3. Recheck the child's height and weight once a month for the next several months.
    4. Track the child's growth over time and compare findings to siblings and classmates.

24. Which nursing interventions should be employed for a patient with diabetes insipidus? **Select all that apply.** *(1707)*
    1. Assessment of skin turgor
    2. Daily weight measurement
    3. Fluid restriction
    4. Monitor I&O
    5. Frequent ambulation

25. Which patient has the **greatest** risk for developing SIADH? *(1708)*
    1. Has malignant cancer
    2. Has dormant tuberculosis
    3. Suffered head trauma
    4. Received opioid medication

26. The nurse is caring for a patient who is diagnosed with SIADH. Which assessment finding indicates that the disorder has progressed to neurologic involvement? *(1708)*
    1. An increased urge to drink fluids
    2. A decrease in serum sodium
    3. Progression to shock symptoms
    4. A change in mental status

27. For the patient with SIADH, the health care provider orders fluid restriction. Which finding **best** indicates that the therapy is working? *(1708)*
    1. Patient reports that he feels better.
    2. Vital signs are at patient's baseline.
    3. Serum sodium is gradually increased.
    4. Diuretics are gradually discontinued.

28. The nurse is caring for a patient who had a thyroidectomy. Which routine postoperative intervention would the nurse clarify with the health care provider? *(1711)*
    1. Inspect dressing for bleeding and drainage.
    2. Give clear liquids; progress to soft diet.
    3. Encourage coughing and deep-breathing.
    4. Observe surgical site for signs of infection.

29. The health care provider tells the nurse that the patient needs diagnostic testing for possible hyperthyroidism. What symptoms is the patient **most** likely to exhibit? *(1709)*
    1. Weight loss, increased appetite, and nervousness
    2. Intolerance to cold, constipation, and lethargy
    3. Skeletal pain, pain on weight-bearing, and paranoia
    4. Polyphagia, polydipsia, and polyuria

30. The nurse is reviewing the patient's medication prescriptions and sees that the patient takes levothyroxine. Which laboratory result will indicate efficacy of therapy? *(1704)*
    1. Blood glucose less than 250 mg/dL
    2. Normalization of urine specific gravity
    3. Gradual improvement of serum sodium level
    4. Normalization of thyroid-stimulating hormone level

31. The nurse is caring for a patient who had a thyroidectomy 6 hours ago. The patient exhibits thyroid crisis and receives treatment. Which outcome statement indicates that the goals of therapy were met? *(1712)*
    1. Patient's sodium level is normalized, and fluid intake equals urinary output.
    2. Patient's low blood glucose returns to 60 mg/dL and mental status is at baseline.
    3. Patient displays euthyroid, blood pressure and temperature are at baseline.
    4. Patient's cortisol level returns to baseline, hypotension is resolved.

32. The health care provider tells the nurse that the patient has a firm, fixed, small, rounded, painless nodule that was palpated on the thyroid gland. The nurse prepares to support the patient when the provider informs about the need for diagnostic testing for which disorder? *(1715)*
    1. Myxedema
    2. Colloid goiter
    3. Thyroid cancer
    4. Cretinism

33. The nurse is caring for a patient who has a pathologic fracture secondary to hyperparathyroidism. Which food needs to be taken off the patient's breakfast tray? *(1717)*
    1. Glass of whole milk
    2. White toast with jam
    3. Sugared cereal flakes
    4. Fried egg with bacon

34. Why is furosemide (diuretic) prescribed for a patient with hyperparathyroidism? *(1717)*
    1. Preserve existing kidney function
    2. Decrease fluid retention and edema
    3. Encourage the elimination of serum calcium
    4. Decrease blood pressure

35. The LPN is assisting an RN with a patient who needs emergency administration of calcium gluconate for hypoparathyroid tetany. The RN is preparing the medication. What task should the LPN/LVN perform under the supervision of the RN? *(1717)*
    1. Assess the patient for medication allergies.
    2. Place the patient on electrocardiographic monitoring.
    3. Assess the patency of the intravenous access.
    4. Verify the prescription for calcium gluconate.

36. For patients who have hypoparathyroidism, why is it important for the nurse to encourage foods such as soy milk, white rice, jam, honey, lemon-lime soda, cucumbers, lettuce, peppers, tomatoes, and non-organ meats? *(1718)*
    1. These foods supply extra calcium, which is needed to treat hypocalcemia.
    2. These foods are low in phosphorus, and serum phosphorus is elevated.
    3. These foods supply vitamin D, which improves the absorption of calcium.
    4. These foods are low in fat and will not be metabolized into ketones.

37. Urine excreted by a patient with diabetes insipidus will exhibit which characteristics? *(1706)*
    1. Dilute, with a specific gravity of 1.005–1.030
    2. Dilute, with a specific gravity of 1.001–1.005
    3. Concentrated, with a specific gravity of 1.005–1.030
    4. Concentrated, with a specific gravity of 1.001–1.005

38. What is the pathophysiology of simple goiter? *(1714)*
    1. The growth is harmless, like a fluid-filled cyst that can be drained.
    2. There is fluid retention in the face and neck because of a blockage.
    3. The gland usually enlarges because of lack of iodine in the diet.
    4. The surrounding tissue becomes inflamed and swollen because of infection.

39. Cortisol is responsible for what bodily function? *(1701)*
    1. Regulates sodium levels
    2. Regulates potassium levels
    3. Provides energy during stress
    4. Responds to decreased glucose levels

40. What type of insulin administration is indicated in the management of hyperglycemia related to diabetic ketoacidosis? *(1729)*
    1. Glargine insulin given subcutaneously
    2. Humulin N insulin given subcutaneously
    3. NPH 70/30 given intravenously
    4. Regular insulin given intravenously

41. A patient is diagnosed with corticosteroid-induced Cushing's syndrome. Which statement by the patient indicates a need for additional teaching? *(1720)*
    1. "I would like to try a dose reduction."
    2. "I am going to stop taking the medication."
    3. "I prefer trying a gradual discontinuation."
    4. "I am changing to the alternate-day regimen."

42. The patient with Cushing's syndrome has high risk for skin breakdown. What instructions will the nurse give to the UAP to prevent skin impairment? *(1720)*
    1. Handle very gently to prevent bruising and ecchymosis.
    2. Assess for signs of erythema, edema, or infection.
    3. Frequently wash the skin to prevent irritation.
    4. Assist females to remove extra hair with a safety razor.

43. The nurse is caring for a patient who is admitted with Addison's disease. During the AM assessment, the nurse notes very high temperature and orthostatic hypotension. Laboratory results show hyponatremia and hyperkalemia. How does the nurse interpret these findings? *(1721)*
    1. These are expected findings for this disorder; continue routine assessment.
    2. The frequency of assessment should be increased; reassess status every 1-2 hours.
    3. These are signs of impending addisonian crisis; notify the health care provider.
    4. These should be documented as abnormal findings; compare data for trends.

44. The principal manifestation of pheochromocytoma is severe hypertension. What other symptoms are likely to accompany the excessive secretion of catecholamines (i.e., epinephrine and norepinephrine)? *(1722)*
    1. Lethargy, constipation, and depression
    2. Tachycardia, diaphoresis, and anxiety
    3. Kussmaul's respiration, hypotension, and drowsiness
    4. Excessive thirst, increased urine output, and lethargy

45. Which diagnostic test is the **best** for monitoring long-term compliance for patients with diabetes mellitus? *(1726)*
    1. Fasting blood glucose (FBG)
    2. Postprandial (after a meal) blood glucose (PPBG)
    3. Patient self-monitoring of blood glucose (SMBG)
    4. Glycosylated hemoglobin (HbA$_{1c}$)

46. Which patient needs to test the urine for ketones as part of self-care management? *(1727)*
    1. Gestational diabetic who has started insulin
    2. Type 2 diabetic who is preparing to exercise
    3. Type 1 diabetic who has a febrile infection
    4. An older diabetic who cannot perform SMBG

47. The pharmacy delivers a bag of insulin to be delivered as a piggyback infusion. The label says that 100 units of regular insulin is mixed in 500 mL of normal saline. How many mL would be required to deliver 3 units per hour? _____ mL/hr *(1738)*

48. A nurse hears in shift report that a diabetic patient has had nothing by mouth (NPO) since midnight for a surgical procedure that should happen this morning. On assessment, the patient is irritable and his skin is cool and clammy. His blood glucose is 45 mg/dL. What should the nurse do **first**? *(1737)*
    1. Give the patient some juice and a peanut butter sandwich.
    2. Administer 50% glucose per emergency protocol.
    3. Call the operating room and cancel the procedure.
    4. Call the health care provider and inform about findings.

CRITICAL THINKING ACTIVITIES

Activity 1

49. A 19-year-old woman seeks care because of excessive thirst, hunger, and fatigue. She reports she has not been able to sleep all night for the past few weeks because of needing to go to the bathroom.

    a. Based on the nurse's knowledge, what medical diagnosis is anticipated? *(1725)* _____

    b. What other clinical manifestations may occur in this patient? *(1725, 1726)* _____

    _____

    _____

    _____

    c. Describe what the nurse will teach the patient about administering insulin. *(1733)* _____

    _____

    _____

    _____

    _____

d. Upon realizing this condition is not curable, the patient asks what acute and long-term complications are associated with diabetes. How will the nurse respond to this inquiry? *(1724, 1735)*

_____

_____

_____

_____

Activity 2

50. The parents of a 6-year-old boy report to the health care provider with concerns about their son's height. They report that he is the smallest child in the school. The parents are of normal stature. Assessment reveals that the child is indeed significantly small for his age. *(1705, 1706)*

a. What diagnostic tests can be anticipated? _____

_____

_____

b. What other clinical manifestations may be exhibited by a child with dwarfism? _____

_____

_____

c. Another question voiced by the parents is the future implications for their child. How will the nurse respond?

_____

_____

_____

d. What medical treatment will be prescribed for this patient? _____

_____

_____

Activity 3

51. Discuss considerations for older adults related to endocrine disorders. *(1735)* _____

_____

_____

_____

_____

Activity 4

52. Why should patients with endocrine disorders be advised to wear medical alert jewelry? *(1707, 1731)*

_____

_____

_____

_____

Care of the Patient With a Reproductive Disorder

FIGURE LABELING

1   Directions: Label the parts of the female reproductive system. *(1749)*

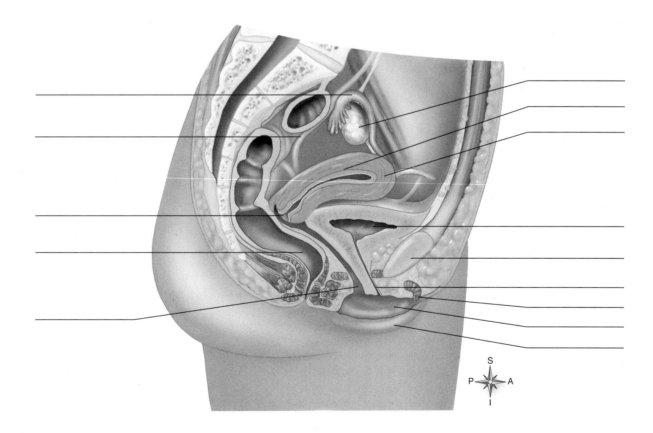

MATCHING

Directions: Match the birth control method with the description. Indicate your answers in the spaces provided. (1808)

Method	**Description**
____ 2. combination pill	a. Take two within 72 hours of coitus; repeat if vomiting occurs; take second dose 12 hours later
____ 3. morning-after pill	b. Consists of a thin flexible rod, which is inserted subdermally
____ 4. progestin-only pill	c. Rubber thimble-shaped shield covering cervix, held in place by suction
____ 5. medroxyprogesterone	d. Device inserted into uterus; flexible object made of plastic or copper wire
____ 6. Implanon	e. No pill-free days
____ 7. diaphragm	f. Double-ring system fitted into vagina up to 8 hours before intercourse
____ 8. cervical cap	g. Contains both estrogen and progesterone
____ 9. male condom	h. Only drug given by injection every 3 months
____ 10. female condom	i. Dome-shaped latex cap with flexible metal ring
____ 11. intrauterine device	j. Thin rubber sheath fitting over erect penis
____ 12. rhythm method	k. Bilateral surgical ligation and resection of ductus deferens
____ 13. tubal sterilization	l. Crushing, ligating, clipping, or plugging of fallopian tubes
____ 14. hysterectomy	m. Requires periodic abstinence during fertile portion of menstrual cycle
____ 15. vasectomy	n. Surgical removal of uterus; 100% effective

SHORT ANSWER

Directions: Using your own words, answer each question in the space provided.

16. Identify three functions of the organs of the male reproductive system. *(1747)*

    a. _____

    b. _____

    c. _____

17. What are three questions that the nurse would use to take a brief sexual history assessment? *(1753)*

    a. _____

    b. _____

    c. _____

18. What are the most common disturbances related to menstruation? *(1759)*

    a. _____

    b. _____

    c. _____

    d. _____

    e. _____

19. What are four main factors that contribute to sexually transmitted infections being among the world's most common communicable diseases? *(1801)*

    a. _____

    b. _____

    c. _____

    d. _____

FIGURE LABELING

20. Directions: Label the lymph nodes of the axilla. *(1787)*

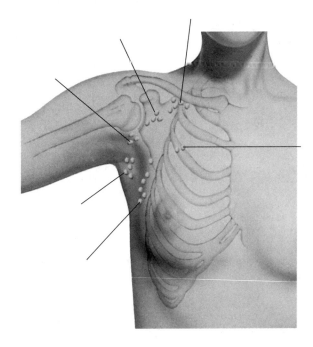

TABLE ACTIVITY

21. Directions: Using the 5 Ps, complete the table below with questions that the nurse would ask to assess risk factors for sexually transmitted infections. *(1801)*

Assessment of Risk Factors for Sexually Transmitted Infections Using the 5 Ps

5 Ps	Questions to Ask
Past STIs	
Partners	
Practices	
Prevention	
Pregnancy	

MULTIPLE CHOICE

Directions: Select the best answer(s) for each of the following questions.

22. The school nurse is reviewing the health records of children. Which parents should be contacted to follow up with the health care provider about their daughter's reproductive health? *(1759)*
    1. Girl was 9 years old when menarche started.
    2. Girl was 15 years old when menarche started.
    3. Girl is 11 years old and there is no breast development.
    4. Girl is 16 years old and menarche has not started.

23. Which person is the **best** example of fulfilling a gender role? *(1752)*
    1. Young woman pursues an intimate same-sex relationship.
    2. A 3-year old boy plays with a toy truck that's just like daddy's.
    3. Middle-aged man enjoys wearing his wife's clothes.
    4. Young woman investigates sex change procedures.

24. Which woman should be advised to have an annual clinical breast examination and mammogram? *(1787)*
    1. 18-year-old woman who has two children
    2. 65-year-old woman who is obese
    3. 40-year-old woman with average risk
    4. 35-year-old woman with average risk

25. Which illnesses can result in actual inability to function sexually? **Select all that apply.** *(1754)*
    1. Diabetes mellitus
    2. End-stage renal disease
    3. Primary syphilis
    4. Hypertension
    5. Spinal cord injuries

26. Which woman needs to be advised to have an annual Pap smear? *(1755)*
    1. A 17-year-old who has been sexually active since age 14
    2. A 19-year-old who has never been sexually active
    3. A 31-year-old who had three normal consecutive Pap smears
    4. A 25-year-old who had a hysterectomy for traumatic injury

27. A 23-year-old woman reports not having a period for several months. The health care provider tells the nurse that the patient needs diagnostic procedures/tests. Which procedures/tests does the nurse anticipate will be **first**? *(1760)*
    1. Serum hormone studies such as estradiol or prolactin
    2. Ultrasound and computed tomography scan
    3. Genetic testing and family history review for cancers
    4. Pregnancy test and pelvic examination

28. In caring for men who have had diagnostic testing of the reproductive system, the nurse would provide the comfort measures of scrotal support and an ice application for which diagnostic test? *(1758)*
    1. Semen analysis
    2. Prostatic smear
    3. Testicular biopsy
    4. Prostate-specific antigen

29. Following a cystoscopy, which finding would be considered normal? *(1758)*
    1. Elevated temperature
    2. Decreased urinary output
    3. Pink-tinged urine
    4. Low back pain

30. For which condition is the nurse **most** likely to use a heat application as a comfort measure? *(1761)*
    1. Amenorrhea
    2. Dysmenorrhea
    3. Menorrhagia
    4. Metrorrhagia

31. The nurse is interviewing a patient who reports that her menstrual periods seem heavier than usual. Which question(s) would the nurse ask? **Select all that apply.** *(1763)*
    1. "How many days have you had menstrual flow?"
    2. "How many days would your period typically last?"
    3. "How many pads or tampons are you saturating per day?"
    4. "How frequently would you normally change a pad/tampon?"
    5. "Do you take aspirin or other anticoagulant medications?"
    6. "Have you recently started a rigorous exercise program?"

32. The nurse is planning patient education for several patients. Which patient is **most** likely to need instructions on how to keep a journal for two or three menstrual cycles, which includes symptoms and activities that relate to the menses? *(1764, 1765)*
    1. 24-year-old woman reports irritability, fatigue, and depression with headache, backache, and breast tenderness
    2. 57-year-old woman reports feelings of being unwanted, fear of aging, hot flashes, and dyspareunia
    3. 18-year-old woman reports colicky pain prior to menses that radiates to perineum and back
    4. 34-year-old woman reports feeling angry, frustrated, and saddened because of inability to conceive

33. Which disorder is **most** likely to be treated with an antidepressant medication? *(1764)*
    1. Premenstrual syndrome
    2. Premenstrual dysphoric disorder
    3. Pelvic inflammatory disease
    4. Polycystic ovary syndrome

34. A 56-year-old woman reports that she went through menopause 3 years ago but has started to menstruate again and she wonders if she should start using birth control. What should the nurse say? *(1764)*
    1. "Resuming birth control is a good idea if you don't want to get pregnant."
    2. "Pregnancy is probably not likely since you went through menopause 3 years ago."
    3. "Vaginal bleeding after menopause is not expected. See your gynecologist."
    4. "Does your current flow look like it did before you went through menopause?"

35. What is the physiologic rationale that supports use of calcium and vitamin D supplements for postmenopausal women? *(1766)*
    1. These supplements are an alternative to hormone replacement therapy to relieve hot flashes.
    2. Decreased bone density occurs with menopause; calcium and vitamin D support bone health.
    3. Calcium and vitamin D mimic estrogen and progesterone in their structure and function in the body.
    4. Postmenopausal women are more likely to decrease active exercises that contribute to bone health.

36. For most menopausal women, which symptom/condition could be relieved by using a water-soluble lubricant? *(1767)*
    1. Pruritus
    2. Dysmenorrhea
    3. Dyspareunia
    4. Procidentia

37. The woman is undergoing a tubal insufflation test. Which outcome suggests that the fallopian tubes are blocked? *(1758)*
    1. No pain or other symptoms are experienced during the test.
    2. The patient experiences shoulder pain during the test.
    3. A high-pitched bubbling is auscultated over the abdomen.
    4. A radiographic film shows free gas under the diaphragm.

38. A 57-year-old male patient confides in the nurse that he doesn't feel as productive or sexually powerful as he used to. What should the nurse say **first**? *(1767)*
    1. "I understand how you feel; aging makes us feel like time is slipping away."
    2. "You'll be okay. Look at all the things you have accomplished so far."
    3. "What factors are contributing to the changes that you see in yourself?"
    4. "Let's talk about ways that you can cope with your loss of sexual power."

39. The nurse is reviewing the medication lists for several patients. Which combination of medications must be immediately brought to the attention of the provider? *(1768)*
    1. Sildenafil citrate and nitroglycerin tablets
    2. Vitamin B_6 supplement and ibuprofen
    3. Cefoxitin and steroids
    4. Danazol and vitamin E supplement

40. The nurse places the patient with pelvic inflammatory disease in Fowler's position. What is the rationale for using this position for this patient? *(1772)*
    1. Facilitate respiratory effort
    2. Prevent aspiration
    3. Facilitate vaginal drainage
    4. Decrease strain on the abdomen

41. What is an **early** manifestation of toxic shock syndrome? *(1773)*
    1. Decreased urine output
    2. Flulike symptoms
    3. Desquamation of palms
    4. Hypotension

42. What advice does the nurse give about tampon use to prevent toxic shock syndrome? *(1774)*
    1. Use an applicator to insert super-absorbent tampons.
    2. Wash hands thoroughly after inserting a tampon.
    3. Tampons should be changed every 8 hours.
    4. Alternate the use of tampons with use of pads.

43. The nurse hears in report that the patient has a vesicovaginal fistula. What assessment finding does the nurse expect? *(1775)*
    1. Trickling of urine from the vagina
    2. Expulsion of feces and flatus from the vagina
    3. Patient report of "something coming down"
    4. Vaginal flow similar to regular menses

44. Radiation has been scheduled for a patient diagnosed with breast cancer. When developing the plan of care, when should the nurse anticipate radiation will take place? *(1790)*
    1. Radiation will begin within 72 hours after surgery.
    2. Radiation will begin within 1 week after surgery.
    3. Radiation will begin 2-3 weeks after surgery.
    4. Radiation will begin 4-6 weeks after surgery.

45. What is an advantage of brachytherapy over traditional radiation therapy for early stage breast cancer ? *(1790)*
    1. Is more cost-effective
    2. Will take less time to complete
    3. Is associated with fewer side effects
    4. Uses a lower dosage of radiation

46. Anemia is a side effect associated with chemotherapy. Which medication may be prescribed to manage this complication? *(1790)*
    1. Epoetin alfa
    2. Prochlorperazine
    3. Granisetron
    4. Ondansetron

47. Tamoxifen has been prescribed for a patient diagnosed with breast cancer. Which characteristics are associated with tamoxifen? **Select all that apply.** *(1791)*
    1. Inhibits the growth-stimulating effects of estrogen
    2. Hormonal agent of choice for postmenopausal women
    3. Used to manage recurrent breast cancer
    4. Used to prevent breast cancer in high-risk individuals
    5. Used for women desiring continued fertility

48. An autologous bone marrow transplant is planned for a patient with breast cancer. Which action will the nurse perform? *(1791)*
    1. Maintain radiation safety while caring for the patient before the transplant.
    2. Prepare the patient to donate bone marrow, from which stem cells will be harvested.
    3. Administer chemotherapy after the stem cell transplant is completed.
    4. Reinforce explanation of plasmapheresis that is performed on the donor stem cells.

49. A 22-year-old woman who has a history of cervical dysplasia is scheduled for a conization procedure to remove a small eroded area on her cervix. What nursing care is appropriate for this procedure? *(1755)*
    1. Assess for allergies to seafood or iodine.
    2. Monitor for bleeding after the procedure.
    3. Encourage fluids prior to the procedure.
    4. Remind to refrain from using deodorants.

50. Which medications are used in the treatment of dysmenorrhea? **Select all that apply.** *(1761)*
    1. Oral contraceptives
    2. Ibuprofen
    3. Fluconazole
    4. Calcium
    5. Naproxen sodium

51. Endometrial cancer usually affects postmenopausal women. What is generally the **first** sign? *(1781)*
    1. Vague abdominal discomfort
    2. Offensive vaginal exudate
    3. Flulike symptoms
    4. Abnormal uterine bleeding

52. Which piece of equipment is the nurse **most** likely to obtain to assist the health care provider in differentiating hydrocele from a cancerous testicular mass? *(1798)*
    1. Doppler
    2. Flashlight
    3. Hemoccult card
    4. Culture swab

53. What is the treatment of choice for primary syphilis? *(1803)*
    1. Penicillin
    2. Acyclovir
    3. Valacyclovir
    4. Tetracycline

54. The health care provider tells the nurse that the male patient has gonorrhea. What signs/symptoms would the nurse expect to observe? *(1804)*
    1. Painful, erythematous, vesicular eruptions on or in the genitalia or rectum
    2. Painless erosion or papule with superficial ulceration and a scooped-out appearance
    3. Scanty white or clear exudate, burning around meatus, urinary frequency, and mild dysuria
    4. Urethritis, dysuria, frequent urination, pruritus, and purulent penile discharge

55. A patient and partner each received a prescription for a 7-day course of oral metronidazole for the treatment of trichomoniasis. In addition to sexual abstinence during treatment and completion of all prescribed antibiotics, what instructions will the nurse give about the medication? *(1762)*
    1. Notify provider of weight gain of 5 lb or more per week.
    2. Avoid drinking alcohol during therapy.
    3. Take medication with a full glass of water.
    4. Watch for and report edema in the extremities.

56. The nurse is chaperoning a group of adolescent girls on a camping trip. One of the girls goes to lie down in the tent, "because I'm on my period." On assessment, the girl has flulike symptoms, an elevated temperature, sore throat, diarrhea, headache, and a diffuse rash. Which question is the nurse **most** likely to ask? *(1773)*
    1. "Is there any chance you could be pregnant? If, so have you passed any clots or tissue?"
    2. "Are you sexually active? If so, have you been using barrier protection against disease?"
    3. "Are you wearing a tampon? If so, when was the last time you changed it?"
    4. "Is this a typical period for you? If so, how do you usually manage these symptoms?"

57. A patient who has a pessary reports foul-smelling discharge, vaginal irritation, and painful sexual intercourse. Which question should the nurse ask? *(1777)*
    1. "Have you been using vaginal douching?"
    2. "Are you having burning with urination?"
    3. "When was the pessary last cleaned?"
    4. "Do you use spermicidal for birth control?"

CRITICAL THINKING ACTIVITIES

Activity 1

58. A 20-year-old patient reports to the family planning clinic for painful, erythematous vesicles on her genitals. She is scared and voices many questions and concerns about her condition. *(1801, 1802)*

    a. Based on the nurse's knowledge, what is the anticipated medical diagnosis? _____

    _____
    _____
    _____
    _____

    b. What treatment options and interventions are available to the patient? _____

    _____
    _____
    _____

    c. What should be included in the patient education?_____

    _____
    _____
    _____
    _____

Activity 2

59. The nurse is preparing to discuss menstruation with a group of preteen girls. The nurse will include the following teaching points. *(1759)*

    a. At what age do girls typically begin menstruation? _____

    b. How long does a typical menstrual period last and approximately how much blood is lost during the average menstrual period?

        _____

        _____

    c. What will the nurse tell the girls about personal hygiene? _____

        _____

        _____

        _____

Activity 3

60. The nurse is originally from a very small farming town in the western United States, but after graduating, she decides to work in an urban clinic that serves an inner-city community in a very large city in the eastern part of the United States.

    a. What are the risk factors for the clinic population that are likely to contribute to reproductive disorders? *(1800)*

        _____

        _____

        _____

        _____

    b. What can the nurse do to prepare herself to help patients that may have gender identity beliefs or sexual practices that are different from her own? *(1752, 1753)*

        _____

        _____

        _____

        _____

Activity 4

61. Discuss the emotional impact for a couple who is undergoing diagnostic testing for infertility. *(1769, 1770)*

_____

_____

_____

_____

_____

_____

_____

_____

Care of the Patient With a Visual or Auditory Disorder

FIGURE LABELING

1. Directions: Label the anatomy of the eye. *(1817)*

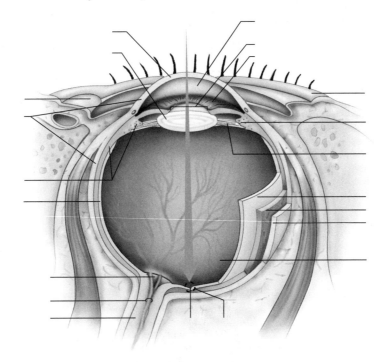

SHORT ANSWER

Directions: Using your own words, answer each question in the space provided.

2. What four basic processes are necessary to form an image? *(1818)*

    a. _____

    b. _____

    c. _____

    d. _____

3. Define the following types of blindness. *(1820)*

   a. Total blindness: _____

   b. Functional blindness: _____

   c. Legal blindness: _____

4. Briefly define the six types of hearing loss. *(1846)*

   a. _____

   b. _____

   c. _____

   d. _____

   e. _____

   f. _____

5. Identify the four taste sensations and the locations of the taste bud receptors. *(1858)*

   a. _____

   b. _____

   c. _____

   d. _____

FIGURE LABELING

6. Directions: Label the anatomy of the external, middle, and inner ear. *(1843)*

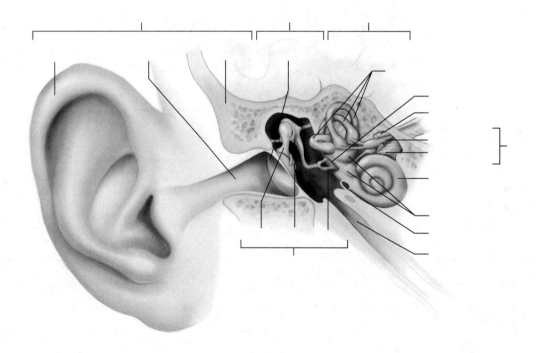

MULTIPLE CHOICE

Directions: select the best answer(s) for each of the following questions.

7. The patient is given a functional vision assessment (American Foundation for the Blind), and even with corrective lenses, the patient is unable to complete the distance task. For which task is the patient **most** likely to need assistance? *(1821)*
   1. Going up and down stairs
   2. Reading a label on a medication container
   3. Driving to a clinic appointment
   4. Preparing and cooking dinner

8. The patient shows loss and deterioration in the automated perimetry test. Which activity is the patient **most** likely to have difficulty with? *(1819)*
   1. Reading a newspaper or book
   2. Participating in a basketball game
   3. Looking at a laptop computer screen
   4. Going on a moonlight stroll down the street

9. Which diagnostic test requires an assessment of allergies to seafood or iodine? *(1819)*
   1. Snellen test
   2. Slit-lamp examination
   3. Fluorescein angiography
   4. Tonometry

10. The nurse is reviewing the medication prescriptions for several patients with disorders of the eye. The nurse would question the health care provider about the use of corticosteroids for which patient? *(1827)*
    1. Patient had cataract surgery
    2. Patient has dry eye with inflammation
    3. Patient had a corneal transplant
    4. Patient needs treatment for keratitis

11. The nurse hears in the shift report that the patient has diplopia. Which task will be the **most** difficult for the patient? *(1818)*
    1. Sitting upright in bed
    2. Reading an information brochure
    3. Listening to a radio broadcast
    4. Eating a sandwich with fries

12. The nurse is orienting the patient to the hospital environment. He is just learning to use a cane as an assistive device for partial blindness. Which interventions would the nurse use? **Select all that apply.** *(1821)*
    1. Walk silently beside the patient, so that he can hear environmental noises.
    2. Suggest that the cane be used to identify borders or objects in pathways.
    3. Walk behind the patient, so that the pathway is clear for him/her.
    4. Advise to walk slowly, especially since the environment is unfamiliar.
    5. Describe the general layout of the room and the adjacent hallway.

13. For which eye condition are patients **most** likely to try self-treatment with over-the-counter eyewear? *(1823)*
    1. Astigmatism
    2. Strabismus
    3. Myopia
    4. Hyperopia

14. A patient with myopia is thinking about having refractory surgery to correct the problem. What should the patient do prior to the surgery? *(1823)*
    1. Arrange to take at least 2 weeks off from work for recuperation.
    2. Stop wearing contact lenses for 1-2 weeks before surgical evaluation.
    3. Stop taking any medications for at least 2 days before the surgery.
    4. Use sterile hydrating eyedrops for at least 2 weeks prior to surgery.

15. The nurse's teenage son tells him that his contact lens fell out while he was hanging out in the park with his friends, so he used saliva to clean it off. Which question should the nurse ask? *(1824)*
    1. "Did you ask if anybody had contact lens solution or a lens case?"
    2. "You know you are not supposed to do that, don't you?"
    3. "So what are you planning to do if that happens again?"
    4. "Do you think glasses would be a better option for you?"

16. The nurse has a 10-year-old daughter who wants to invite two friends for a sleepover. Part of the entertainment for the night is to do "glamour makeovers." What should the nurse do? *(1840)*
    1. Tell the daughter that sharing eye makeup contributes to eye infections.
    2. Call the other parents and see if the friends currently have eye infections.
    3. Purchase three makeup kits from the drugstore and supervise the activity.
    4. Teach the children how to use a fresh cotton-tip applicator for application.

17. The home health nurse is supervising a parent who is demonstrating care for her child's conjunctivitis. The nurse would intervene if the mother performed which action? *(1826)*
    1. Used a clean washcloth to wipe away the secretions
    2. Applied a warm compress with a clean cloth for comfort
    3. Instilled the eyedrops in the lower conjunctival sac
    4. Taped an eyepad loosely over the affected eye

18. For a patient who is diagnosed with keratitis, which common symptom differentiates this disease from other inflammatory eye diseases? *(1826)*
    1. Elevated body temperature
    2. Severe eye pain
    3. Presence of halos or flashes
    4. Low white cell count

19. A patient has recently been diagnosed with keratoconjunctivitis sicca and a dry mouth. Which immune disorder is likely to be associated with this diagnosis and symptom? *(1827)*
    1. Sjögren's syndrome
    2. Acquired immunodeficiency syndrome
    3. Rheumatoid arthritis
    4. Type 1 diabetes mellitus

20. With Sjögren's syndrome, what would the nurse expect the patient to report? *(1827)*
    1. Seeing floaters in the field of vision
    2. Color blindness
    3. Feeling worse in the morning
    4. Sensation of grit in the eyes

21. What are the signs/symptoms of ectropion? **Select all that apply.** *(1828)*
    1. Tearing
    2. Redness of sclera
    3. Thick eye discharge
    4. Corneal dryness
    5. Outward turning of eyelid margin

22. What diagnostic test is used to confirm the presence of entropion? *(1828)*
    1. Amsler grid
    2. Snellen examination
    3. Ophthalmologic examination
    4. Pneumatic retinopexy

23. What type of visual distortion is associated with diabetic retinopathy? *(1832)*
    1. Tunnel vision that worsens in low lighting
    2. Loss of visual acuity accompanied by "floaters"
    3. Sudden onset of peripheral vision loss and eye discomfort
    4. Difficulty distinguishing colors

24. A 65-year-old patient reports visual deficits, including disturbances in color vision and visual clarity, and a darkened area in the center of vision. What medical diagnosis does the nurse anticipate will be made? *(1833)*
    1. Macular degeneration
    2. Glaucoma
    3. Herpetic keratitis
    4. Cataracts

25. Tonometry is used in the diagnosis of which condition? *(1836)*
    1. Corneal abrasions
    2. Blepharitis
    3. Glaucoma
    4. Retinal detachment

26. The patient has been diagnosed with a visual disorder. Contact lenses have been prescribed. Which statement indicates the need for further instruction? *(1824)*
    1. "Photophobia, dryness, burning, or tearing are expected symptoms."
    2. "I will use proper lens care solutions and a clean lens case."
    3. "I will need to be careful not to mix up my left and right lenses."
    4. "Washing and drying my hands before handling my lenses are essential."

27. Following cataract surgery, which activity is the ophthalmologist **most** likely to discourage? *(1830)*
    1. Going to the movies
    2. Lifting a grandchild
    3. Walking on a sunny day
    4. Sleeping with a spouse

28. Based on research, supplemental zinc, beta-carotene, vitamins C and E, and a diet rich in fruits and dark-green leafy vegetables would be recommended for which eye disorder? *(1832)*
    1. Age-related macular degeneration
    2. Senile cataracts
    3. Retinal detachment
    4. Glaucoma

29. A patient reports seeing flashing lights and floaters and a dark area in the outer peripheral vision. What is the **most** important question to ask for suspicion of retinal detachment? *(1834)*
    1. "Are you having severe pain in the affected eye?"
    2. "Is the darkened area getting progressively larger?"
    3. "Do you have type 1 diabetes mellitus?"
    4. "Do you have a family history of eye problems?"

30. What are the current recommendations for ophthalmologic examinations? **Select all that apply.** *(1838)*
    1. People between 40 and 64 years of age need examination every 2-4 years.
    2. People who wear contact lenses should have examinations every 6 months.
    3. African Americans in every age group should have more frequent examinations.
    4. People 65 years of age or older should be examined every 1-2 years.
    5. People with diabetes mellitus should have more frequent examinations.

31. The nurse's neighbor is trying to remove an eyelash from her eye. The nurse would intervene if the neighbor used which method? *(1840)*
    1. Flushed the eye gently with tap water
    2. Tried blinking and crying to stimulate tears
    3. Used a clean cotton-tipped swab to wipe the cornea
    4. Used a sterile pad to wipe the corner of the eye

32. The nurse is on a camping trip and one of the campers gets poked in the eye with a stick. The end of the stick is protruding from the eye. What should the nurse do **first**? *(1840)*
    1. Gently remove the stick and then flush the eye with water.
    2. Cover the injured eye with a paper cup and patch the uninjured eye.
    3. Have the camper sit quietly in the car and drive him to the hospital.
    4. Remain calm and control the bleeding with direct pressure.

33. What problem will the patient have if there is damage to the fine hair cell receptors in the organ of Corti? *(1844)*
    1. Difficulty with balance
    2. Overproduction of cerumen
    3. Loss of hearing
    4. Blurred distance vision

34. The nurse overhears a nursing student giving advice to a patient to "get a hearing aid." What is the **best** response that the nurse could give to the student and the patient? *(1846, 1847)*
    1. "Let's focus on nursing interventions that we can use today; for example, face each other and speak clearly."
    2. "The care, maintenance, and usage of a hearing aid can be complex, so we should first talk about those issues."
    3. "This is a good suggestion. We will make you an appointment with your health care provider."
    4. "The type of hearing loss must first be determined because the device won't work for all types of hearing loss."

35. Which patient is likely to be the **best** candidate for a hearing aid? *(1846)*
    1. Patient has congenital hearing loss secondary to oxygen deprivation at birth.
    2. Patient has conductive hearing loss due to stenosis of the external auditory canal.
    3. Patient has functional hearing loss after being trapped in a cave for several hours.
    4. Patient has central hearing loss secondary to a cerebrovascular accident (stroke).

36. The health care provider informs the nurse that the patient had an abnormal Romberg test. Which safety precaution will the nurse initiate? *(1846)*
    1. Make sure the room has adequate natural lighting.
    2. Do a physical demonstration of how to use the call light.
    3. Announce self to avoid suddenly startling the patient.
    4. Assist the patient to stand and get balance before walking.

37. The nurse's toddler received a prescription for antibiotics to treat acute otitis media. The antibiotics and acetaminophen where given as recommended, but the toddler is still crying with pain. What should the nurse try **first**? *(1849)*
    1. Have the toddler swallow cool fluids.
    2. Place a warm compress over the affected ear.
    3. Use distraction until the acetaminophen works.
    4. Call the provider and ask for a sedative prescription.

38. What is an **early** indicator of acute otitis media? *(1849)*
    1. Patient reports ear pain and is pulling on the pinna.
    2. Patient reports partial hearing loss.
    3. There is yellow discharge with a pungent odor.
    4. Patient reports sensation of blockage in ear canal.

39. During the night, which strategy for environmental control is **best** to help the patient with tinnitus? *(1855)*
    1. Have the patient lie very still.
    2. Play soft background music.
    3. Keep the room dark and quiet.
    4. Turn on the television.

40. The nurse is reviewing the patient's medication list and sees the patient takes meclizine. What instructions should be given to the unlicensed assistive personnel (UAP)? *(1857)*
    1. Face the patient directly when speaking to him.
    2. Assist the patient to ambulate because he gets dizzy.
    3. Keep the head of the bed elevated at least 30 degrees.
    4. Assist the patient to clean his eyes with a clean washcloth.

41. Which intervention applies to positioning the patient after a stapedectomy? *(1857)*
    1. Keep the operative side facing upward.
    2. Elevate the head of the bed to at least 90 degrees.
    3. Turn, cough, and deep-breathe every 2 hours.
    4. Use a neck brace for the first 2 hours.

42. If there is a disturbance in proprioception, which function will the patient have difficulty performing? *(1858)*
    1. Walking up the stairs
    2. Understanding informed consent
    3. Reading prescription labels
    4. Listening to the provider's instructions

CRITICAL THINKING ACTIVITIES

Activity 1

43. An 18-year-old patient has just returned from surgery for the enucleation of his right eye after injuries suffered in an accident. *(1841)*

    a. Discuss the nursing interventions that will be required over the next 24 hours. _____

    _____
    _____
    _____

    b. What findings are indicative of complications and warrant an immediate report to the health care provider?

    _____
    _____

    c. The patient expresses concerns about his appearance. How will the nurse address his concerns?

    _____
    _____

Activity 2

44. A 20-year-old patient reports worsening ear pain. After completing his history, it is determined he recently had an ear infection and he failed to take the full course of prescribed medications. His other signs and symptoms include fever, headache, malaise, and purulent exudate. *(1851, 1852)*

 a. What should the nurse anticipate the patient's medical diagnosis will be? _____

 _____

 b. How did this condition occur? _____

 _____

 _____

 c. Discuss the treatment and the prognosis for this condition. _____

 _____

 _____

 _____

 _____

 _____

 _____

Activity 3

45. The patient had vitrectomy surgery of the right eye. List the appropriate nursing interventions for this patient. *(1842)*

 _____

 _____

 _____

 _____

 _____

 _____

 _____

 _____

 _____

Activity 4

46. Refer to Box 53.2 and identify behaviors that you have noticed for someone who may be demonstrating hearing loss. Has that person admitted that he or she has hearing loss? *(1845)*

 _____

 _____

 _____

 _____

 _____

Activity 5

47. If you were to suddenly lose your vision or hearing, how would the loss affect your current lifestyle and future plans? *(1859)*

_____

_____

_____

_____

_____

_____

_____

_____

_____

_____

Care of the Patient With a Neurologic Disorder

FIGURE LABELING

1. Directions: Label the parts of the brain on the figure below. *(1866)*

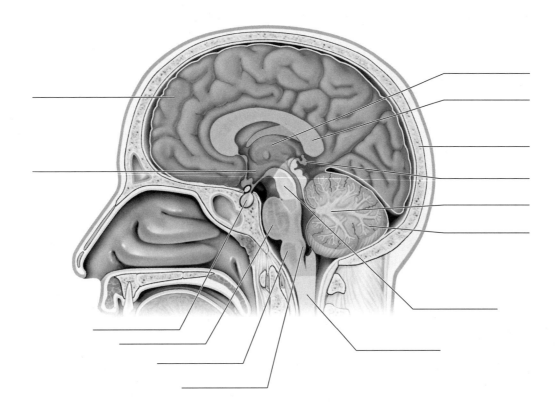

MATCHING

Directions: Match the cranial nerves to their functions. Indicate your answers in the spaces provided. (1868)

Cranial Nerve		Functions
_____	2. I—olfactory	a. Eye movements, extraocular muscles, pupillary control (pupillary constriction)
_____	3. II—optic	b. Hearing; sense of balance (equilibrium)
_____	4. III—oculomotor	c. Down and inward movement of eye
_____	5. IV—trochlear	d. Shoulder movements (trapezius muscle) and turning movements of head (sternocleidomastoid muscles)
_____	6. VI—abducens	e. Sense of smell
_____	7. VII—facial	f. Vision
_____	8. VIII—acoustic (vestibulocochlear)	g. Sense of taste on anterior two-thirds of tongue; contraction of muscles of facial expression
_____	9. IX—glossopharyngeal	h. Sensations of throat, taste, swallowing movements, gag reflex, taste on posterior one-third of tongue, secretion of saliva
_____	10. X—vagus	i. Lateral movement of eye
_____	11. XI—spinal accessory	j. Sensations of throat, larynx, and thoracic and abdominal organs; swallowing; voice production; slowing of heartbeat; acceleration of peristalsis
_____	12. XII—hypoglossal	k. Tongue movements

FIGURE LABELING

13. Directions: On the figures below, identify decorticate and decerebrate responses and the flexion and extension characteristics of the upper and lower extremities. *(1881)*

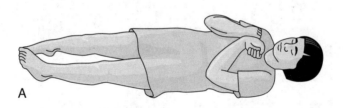

A

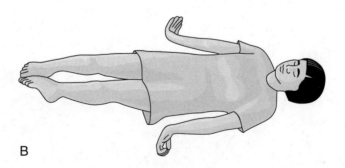

B

WORD SCRAMBLE

Levels of Consciousness

Directions: Unscramble the letters to reveal the correct spelling of terms related to level of consciousness and then match them to the correct definition or description. (1871)

Scrambled Term	Unscrambled Term	Definition or Characteristic
14. treal		
15. orientdisation		
16. porstu		
17. tosecomasemi		
18. esotamoc		

Description
a. Responds to verbal commands with moaning or groaning, if at all; seems unaware of surroundings
b. Is in impaired state of consciousness characterized by obtundation and stupor, from which a patient can be aroused only by energetic stimulation
c. Unable to respond to painful stimuli; cornea and pupillary reflexes are absent; cannot swallow or cough; is incontinent of urine and feces; electroencephalogram pattern demonstrates decreased or absent neuronal activity
d. Unable to follow simple commands; thinking slowed; inattentive; flat affect
e. Responds appropriately to auditory, tactile, and visual stimuli

MULTIPLE CHOICE
Directions: Select the best answer(s) for each of the following questions.

19. In Parkinson's disease, which neurotransmitter is decreased and therefore is a target of medication therapy? *(1893)*
    1. Acetylcholine
    2. Norepinephrine
    3. Dopamine
    4. Serotonin

20. In working with patients who have neurologic conditions that affect language function, which patient represents the **greatest** challenge to achieve communication? *(1873)*
    1. Patient has anomic aphasia that developed after removal of brain tumor.
    2. Patient has global aphasia due to progressive Alzheimer's disease.
    3. Patient has motor aphasia secondary to head injury.
    4. Patient has receptive aphasia residual to a stroke.

21. Which behavior(s) would be considered normal neurologic changes related to aging? **Select all that apply.** *(1870)*
    1. Drives slower to compensate for slowed reaction time
    2. Demonstrates slight tremor while holding teacup when tired
    3. Takes a foreign language class, but can't keep up with classmates
    4. Does needlework, but has more trouble with fine, small stitches
    5. Rearranges items on countertop, but action serves no purpose
    6. Frequently misplaces keys or eyeglasses, but can usually find them

22. The nurse is assessing the "fund of knowledge" component of the patient's awareness. Which question would the nurse use to assess this component? *(1871)*
    1. "What month is it? And what day of the week is it today?"
    2. "What did you have for dinner last night?"
    3. "If you had $3.00 and gave me half, what would you have?"
    4. "Who was the first president of the United States?"

23. The nurse is assessing a patient who had a serious head injury. During the assessment, the patient spontaneously opens his eyes; is oriented to person, place, and time; and can follow the nurse's commands. How would the nurse document his Glasgow coma score (GCS)? *(1871)*
    1. GCS within normal limits
    2. GCS insufficient
    3. GCS 3
    4. GCS 15

24. The nurse is using the FOUR Score coma scale to assess a patient who suffered a stroke. Which assessment is an integral part of this scale? *(1871)*
    1. Checking the blood pressure and pulse
    2. Checking orientation to person, place, and time
    3. Assessing the respiratory rate and pattern
    4. Evaluating the ability to make good judgments

25. The nurse hears in report that the patient has motor aphasia. Which intervention will the nurse plan to use when communicating with this patient? *(1872)*
    1. Talk slower, be patient, and enunciate very clearly.
    2. Face the patient so that he can watch the lips move.
    3. Obtain a set of picture cards and encourage gestures.
    4. Be kind and caring, but limit verbal communication.

26. The nurse is checking the gag reflex prior to giving liquids to a patient who had a bronchoscopy earlier in the day. Which cranial nerves is the nurse testing? *(1868)*
    1. Optic and oculomotor
    2. Abducens and trochlear
    3. Trigeminal and facial
    4. Glossopharyngeal and vagus

27. The nurse is caring for a patient who has unilateral neglect that includes the nondominant hand. For which task is the patient **most** likely to require assistance? *(1873)*
    1. Putting on her blouse
    2. Holding a drinking glass
    3. Using the remote control
    4. Writing a letter

28. The patient is scheduled to return from having a lumbar puncture. What instructions will the nurse give to the unlicensed assistive personnel (UAP) about the care of this patient? *(1874)*
    1. Help the patient ambulate in the halls.
    2. Keep the head of the bed at 30 degrees.
    3. Withhold fluids for several hours.
    4. Report any complaints of numbness or tingling.

29. The nurse is caring for a patient who had cerebral angiogram and the vascular system was accessed through the carotid artery. In the immediate postprocedure assessment, what is the **priority**? *(1876)*
    1. Watching for infection at the puncture site
    2. Assessing for reaction to contrast media
    3. Observing for respiratory difficulties
    4. Assessing for nausea and vomiting

30. A 35-year-old man who suffers from tension headaches requests opioid medications for the debilitating pain. Why is the health care provider unlikely to grant the patient's request? *(1878)*
    1. Opioids are avoided because of the risk of abuse.
    2. Tension headache pain does not warrant opioid use.
    3. Pain receptor sites will not respond to opioids.
    4. Tension headaches are controlled by reducing stress.

31. Which food may cause or worsen a migraine headache? *(1877)*
    1. Italian food
    2. Apples
    3. Dairy products
    4. Ripened cheese

32. In caring for a patient with a headache, which instruction will the nurse give to the UAP? *(1878)*
    1. Assist the patient to turn every 2 hours.
    2. Keep the room quiet and dark.
    3. Refresh warm compress as needed.
    4. Withhold fluids because of nausea.

33. The nurse is reviewing the medication list for a patient who is diabetic and sees that gabapentin is prescribed. Which pain assessment will the nurse make? *(1879)*
    1. Low back pain with movement
    2. Dull or throbbing headache
    3. Burning or tingling in lower legs
    4. Stiffness of joints in the morning

34. What is an **early** sign of increased intracranial pressure? *(1881)*
    1. Change in level of consciousness
    2. Decreased or abnormal respirations
    3. Increased systolic blood pressure
    4. Increased or widening pulse pressure

35. The night shift nurse has just finished giving report on four patients who have risk for increased intracranial pressure. The health care provider is aware of their status. Which patient will the oncoming nurse check **first**? *(1881)*
    1. Patient had a brief episode of Cheyne-Stokes respirations.
    2. Patient reported double vision and difficulty concentrating.
    3. Patient seemed restless and disoriented.
    4. Patient had a headache with nausea and vomiting.

36. The nurse is checking the pupils of a patient who sustained a serious head injury. Which pupil response is the **first** and most subtle clue of increased intracranial pressure? *(1881)*
    1. Pupil reacts, but is sluggish.
    2. Pupil is fixed and dilated.
    3. Pupil is dilated, but will slowly constrict.
    4. Pupil on affected side is larger.

37. Which patient is **best** demonstrating the use of intact sensory abilities to independently compensate for a sensory deficit? *(1886)*
    1. Patient with agnosia needs help for activities of daily living.
    2. Patient with loss of proprioception uses a walker.
    3. Patient with diabetic neuropathy inspects feet every day.
    4. Patient with hearing deficit speaks very loudly to others.

38. The nurse is planning patient education for several patients. Which patient is the **best** candidate for a teaching session on weight shifting? *(1884)*
    1. Patient with mild Alzheimer's has recently started wandering.
    2. Patient has Parkinson's and shows evidence of pill-rolling.
    3. Patient with paraplegia is transferring to a rehabilitation unit.
    4. Patient has unilateral neglect that is affecting the dominant side.

39. For a patient with hemiplegia, how does the staff use counterpositioning to protect the affected upper extremity? *(1884)*
    1. Positions the upper extremity with shoulder pulled inward and elbow extended
    2. Places the shoulder and upper arm in abduction with elbow flexed and wrist dorsiflexed
    3. Places the patient recumbent with arm beside body, elbow straight, and palmar surface upwards
    4. Elevates the elbow and forearm on a pillow above the level of the heart with wrist flexed

40. The home health nurse is reviewing the patient's medication list and sees that the patient takes phenytoin. Which question is the nurse **most** likely to ask? *(1889)*
    1. "When was the last time you had a seizure?"
    2. "Has the medication controlled your headaches?"
    3. "When did you first start taking medication for Parkinson's?"
    4. "Has the medication helped to reduce the spasms?"

41. Which measures should be implemented for a patient experiencing increased intracranial pressure? **Select all that apply.** *(1883)*
    1. Restrict fluid intake.
    2. Place head in flexed position.
    3. Avoid flexion of the hips.
    4. Administer enemas as needed.
    5. Administer oxygen.

42. The patient has residual hemiplegia following a stroke. Which instructions will the nurse give to the UAP? *(1884)*
    1. Assist the patient to ambulate to the bathroom.
    2. Put the affected arm through range of motion.
    3. Place in a prone position if the patient can tolerate it.
    4. Use pillows to keep the upper arm in adduction.

43. The nurse hears in report that the 33-year-old patient with multiple sclerosis (MS) is withdrawn, depressed, and emotionally labile. The nurse knows that emotional changes are part of the disease. What other aspect(s) of the disease are likely to be contributing to the patient's emotional state? **Select all that apply.** *(1891)*
    1. Exacerbations and remissions are continuous; deterioration progresses.
    2. The symptoms are vague, insidious, and widely distributed.
    3. No specific treatments exist, although many treatments have been tried.
    4. Multiple body systems are affected, and function is lost in every area.
    5. Earlier diagnosis and intervention could have stopped the deterioration.

44. A resident with Parkinson's disease lives at a long-term care facility. The patient has a flat facial expression, hand tremors, and bradykinesia. Which instruction will the nurse give to the UAP to address the bradykinesia? *(1893)*
    1. He has a shuffling gait and needs assistance to prevent bumping into objects.
    2. He has trouble bending to tie his shoes because of muscle soreness and aches.
    3. He has trouble using a fork and knife because of loss of fine motor control.
    4. He has resistance to motion, so he may seem stiff when you put on his shirt.

45. The health care provider tells that nurse that during hospitalization, the older patient is going to be on drug holiday from all medications that are normally prescribed for his Parkinson's disease. What is the **priority** problem related to the temporary cessation of the medications? *(1895)*
    1. Aspiration
    2. Constipation
    3. Tremors
    4. Postural hypotension

46. What is an **early** subjective symptom that the patient may report that would be characteristic of myasthenia gravis? *(1901)*
    1. Muscle weakness in the extremities
    2. Eyelid drooping and double vision
    3. Trouble swallowing
    4. Weak, nasal-sounding voice

47. What is the **priority** assessment for a patient with a severe exacerbation of myasthenia gravis? *(1903)*
    1. Assess for ocular signs/symptoms including ptosis and diplopia.
    2. Auscultate bowel sounds and assess bowel and bladder continence.
    3. Assess ability to ambulate, sustain a sitting position, and raise arms.
    4. Auscultate lungs, assess respiratory effort and ability to cough up secretions.

48. What is the single **most** important modifiable risk factor for stroke? *(1904)*
    1. Cigarette smoking
    2. Sedentary lifestyle
    3. Hypertension
    4. Obesity

49. The patient who had a stroke exhibits dysphagia. Which intervention will the nurse use? *(1909)*
    1. Mix solid and liquid foods together to facilitate swallowing.
    2. Assist the patient to drink water after every bite of food.
    3. Offer the patient a drinking straw or a covered plastic cup.
    4. Check mouth on the affected side for accumulation of food.

50. The patient comes to the clinic and is exhibiting stroke symptoms. The health care provider believes that the patient is a possible candidate for thrombolytic therapy. What are the **most** important actions for the clinic staff to perform? *(1907)*
    1. Rapid triage and transport to a stroke center
    2. Draw blood for coagulation tests and establish IV
    3. Obtain a CT or MRI to rule out hemorrhagic stroke
    4. Explain the risks and benefits of therapy to the patient

51. In caring for a patient with trigeminal neuralgia, what instructions would the nurse give to the UAP about assisting with hygiene and meals? *(1900)*
    1. Use gentle touch when assisting with shaving.
    2. Encourage the patient to drink cold liquids.
    3. Allow the patient to do his own care if he prefers.
    4. Offer to cut the patient's food into bite-sized pieces.

52. A patient who is diagnosed with Bell's palsy will need to know how to use which device? *(1911)*
    1. Eating utensil with a universal cuff
    2. Eyeshield to be applied at night
    3. Footboard for the end of the bed
    4. A volar wrist splint for extension

53. In caring for a patient who is diagnosed with Guillain-Barré syndrome, what is the **priority** assessment? *(1912)*
    1. Motion and sensation in the legs
    2. Respiratory depth and pattern
    3. Mental status and level of consciousness
    4. Loss of bowel and bladder control

54. The nurse is caring for a patient who is diagnosed with bacterial meningitis. For this patient, what is the rationale for keeping the room quiet and dark? *(1913)*
    1. Light and noise increase the subjective experience of pain.
    2. Patient needs extra rest and sleep to facilitate recovery.
    3. Any increased sensory stimulation may cause a seizure.
    4. Critically ill patients do better in quiet environments.

55. What is considered a prominent **early** sign of a brain tumor? *(1916)*
    1. Speech impairment
    2. Morning headache
    3. Change in personality
    4. Memory loss

56. A young man who sustained a serious head injury several years ago is a resident in a long-term care facility. After the injury, he demonstrated intermittent poor judgment and occasional physical aggression. Today, he is trying to leave the facility. What should the nurse do **first**? *(1918)*
    1. Speak calmly and redirect him to another activity.
    2. Obtain a prescription for an antianxiety medication.
    3. Allow him to wander around but keep an eye on him.
    4. Instruct a UAP to perform one-to-one observation.

57. The UAP tells the nurse that a patient with a spinal cord injury has a systolic blood pressure of 190/100 mm Hg. The nurse observes that the patient is diaphoretic, restless, and has "gooseflesh" and a headache. What should the nurse do **first**? *(1921)*
    1. Recheck the blood pressure.
    2. Check the bladder for distention.
    3. Check the rectum for impaction.
    4. Put the patient in a sitting position.

58. For patients with spinal cord injuries, which patient is **most** likely to achieve the rehabilitation potential of "Completely independent ambulation with short leg braces and canes; inability to stand for long periods." *(1920)*
    1. Patient has a level of injury at C8 sustained in a diving accident.
    2. Patient has a level of injury at T12 related to an occupational incident.
    3. Patient has a level of injury at L1 secondary to a gunshot wound.
    4. Patient has a level of injury at L4 sustained in a motorcycle accident.

CRITICAL THINKING ACTIVITIES

Activity 1

59. The school nurse is accompanying a group of children on a field trip. One of children suddenly reports feeling odd and then sits down on the ground. As the nurse eases her to a supine position, the child demonstrates tonic-clonic jerking movements of the body. The nurse notes secretions and drooling from the child's mouth and the lips are slightly cyanotic. The child is unable to respond to her name and her eyes are rolled back and upwards. *(1890)*

    a. Describe what the nurse should do. _____

    _____

    _____

    b. What information should the nurse record and report to the health care provider? _____

    _____

    _____

Activity 2

60. A 58-year-old man reports he experienced numbness in his right leg, a loss of sensation in his right arm, and an inability to speak; the entire event lasted only about 15 minutes. *(1905)*

    a. What condition/disorder has the patient experienced? _____

    b. Since the duration of this event was short, is it of any long-term significance? Why or why not?

    _____

    _____

    _____

    c. What is the most frequently prescribed antiplatelet agent for this condition? _____

    _____

Activity 3

61. a. It is likely that you know or will know someone who has Alzheimer's disease. What are the warning signs? *(1899)*

    _____

    _____

    _____

    _____

    b. Discuss the effect that Alzheimer's disease has on family and society. *(1900)*_____

    _____

    _____

    _____

    _____

    c. What can you teach your patients to do that will help prevent Alzheimer's disease? *(1899)* _____

    _____

    _____

    _____

    _____

Care of the Patient With an Immune Disorder

FIGURE LABELING

1. Directions. Label the figure below with the correct names of the organs of the immune system. *(1930)*

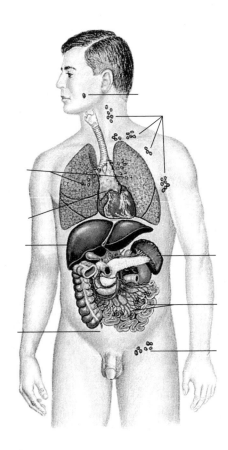

SHORT ANSWER
Directions: Using your own words, answer each question in the space provided.

2. What are the three main functions of the immune system? *(1928)*

   a. _____

   b. _____

   c. _____

3. What are the four Rs of the immune response? *(1932)*

   a. _____

   b. _____

   c. _____

   d. _____

4. Identify the five factors influencing hypersensitivity. *(1934)*

   a. _____

   b. _____

   c. _____

   d. _____

   e. _____

5. List 14 items in the health care environment that could contain latex. *(1938)* _____

   _____

   _____

MULTIPLE CHOICE
Directions: Select the best answer(s) for each of the following questions.

6. Which nursing action **best** supports the patient's innate immunity? *(1929)*
   1. Encourages the patient to complete full course of prescribed antibiotics
   2. Advises older patient to get an annual influenza vaccination
   3. Assists new mother who is learning to breastfeed her baby
   4. Assesses the skin of a patient who is at risk for a pressure injury

7. Which surgical procedure creates lifetime immunocompromise and vulnerability to infection? *(1940)*
   1. Thyroidectomy
   2. Splenectomy
   3. Appendectomy
   4. Cholecystectomy

8. One of the residents in a long-term care facility has uncharacteristic lethargy and disorientation. The nurse recognizes that these could be early signs of infection. What would the nurse do **first**? *(1933)*
   1. Obtain a prescription for white blood cell count.
   2. Obtain a urine specimen.
   3. Auscultate the breath sounds.
   4. Check the resident's temperature.

9. Which person needs to be advised to get the human papilloma virus vaccination? *(1933)*
   1. 21-year-old sexually active male who has never been previously vaccinated
   2. 3-month-old who needs a well-baby physical and routine vaccination
   3. 73-year-old with chronic health problems who lives in a long-term care facility
   4. 54-year-old who is undergoing renal dialysis and is on the transplant list

10. Based on the National Institute for Occupational Safety and Health (NIOSH) recommendations for preventing allergic reactions to latex in the workplace, what instructions would the nurse give to the unlicensed assistive personnel (UAP)? *(1938)*
    1. Avoid latex exposures and know the signs/symptoms of allergic response.
    2. Ask every patient about latex allergies before donning gloves.
    3. Do not use latex gloves unless there is visible evidence of blood and body fluid.
    4. Wash hands with a mild soap and dry thoroughly after removing latex gloves.

11. The home health patient thinks he has food allergies because he has diarrhea after eating certain foods. What would the nurse suggest **first**? *(1935)*
    1. See the health care provider for possible desensitization therapy.
    2. Keep a weekly food diary with a description of any untoward reactions.
    3. Eliminate soy, eggs, and strawberries because of chance for anaphylaxis.
    4. Eat a bland diet and add a new food every week to see if there is a reaction.

12. In caring for an older adult, what instructions would the nurse give to the UAP that address changes related to aging of the immune system. **Select all that apply.** *(1933)*
    1. Promptly assist with toileting to prevent urinary stasis.
    2. Increase fluids (unless contraindicated) to thin secretions.
    3. Apply a thin layer of lotion after bathing to prevent dry skin.
    4. Teach coughing and deep breathing as needed.
    5. Perform scrupulous hand hygiene and don clean gloves.
    6. Offer frequent oral hygiene because of decreased saliva production.

13. What is the theory behind progressively increasing the doses of the allergens during perennial immunotherapy? *(1933)*
    1. Inhibits the release of leukotrienes and reduces allergic symptoms
    2. Allows the individual to build up a tolerance without having symptoms
    3. Competes with histamine by attaching to the cell surface receptors
    4. Inhibits further release of chemical mediators from mast cells

14. If medications are administered in error to a patient who is hypersensitive, which route will produce the **most** rapid allergic reaction? *(1934)*
    1. Oral
    2. Transdermal
    3. Intravenous
    4. Topical

15. The nurse and a friend are ordering lunch. The friend takes 50 mg of diphenhydramine and then orders oysters, saying, "I'm allergic to oysters, but I just love them, so I take medication." What should the nurse say? *(1934)*
    1. "Do you have your cell phone, so we can call 911?"
    2. "Every time you eat oysters, the reaction will get worse."
    3. "You are an adult and you can make your own choices."
    4. "If I have to resuscitate you, I am not going to be happy."

16. The clinic nurse is trying to do an environmental assessment for an older patient who is having continuous allergic reactions, but the patient vaguely rambles on about pets, dust, a broken vacuum cleaner, and mold. What is the **best** intervention to use for this patient? *(1934)*
    1. Use simplified, focused yes-or-no questions.
    2. Make an environmental checklist for the patient.
    3. Obtain information from a close relative.
    4. Obtain an order for a home health nurse visit.

17. Within 15 minutes of initiating a blood transfusion, the patient reports shortness of breath, chills, and urticaria. After stopping the transfusion and notifying the health care provider, which laboratory test must be completed? *(1939)*
    1. Urinalysis
    2. Electrolytes
    3. Platelet count
    4. White blood cell count

18. What is the physiologic explanation for the suppressed humoral immune response in older adults? *(1940)*
    1. Degeneration of the spleen
    2. Decreased production of white blood cells
    3. Reduction in effectiveness of white blood cells
    4. Decreased immunoglobulin levels

19. During plasmapheresis, the plasma may be replaced with what? **Select all that apply.** *(1941)*
    1. Normal saline
    2. Lactated Ringer's solution
    3. Albumin
    4. 10% dextrose
    5. Fresh-frozen plasma
    6. Dextrose 5% and half normal saline

20. The nurse gives a patient his immunotherapy injection and immediately he demonstrates wheezes, impaired breathing, and hypotension. The nurse initiates the anaphylaxis protocol. What is the nurse's **first** action? *(1937)*
    1. Establish an IV to administer 1:10,000 epinephrine hydrochloride.
    2. Administer 1:1000 epinephrine hydrochloride subcutaneously.
    3. Prepare the equipment and assist the provider to intubate the patient.
    4. Administer a 50-mg oral dose of diphenhydramine.

21. What are examples of passive immunity? **Select all that apply.** *(1931)*
    1. Mother breastfeeds her baby
    2. Antivenom given after a snakebite
    3. Immunoglobulin administered postexposure
    4. Child gets hepatitis B vaccine
    5. Patient reports having measles during childhood

22. In caring for a patient who recently had an organ transplant, which instructions would the nurse give to the UAP to protect this immunosuppressed patient? *(1939)*
    1. The most dangerous period is 7-10 days after the transplant.
    2. Remind visitors to check at the nurses' station before entering.
    3. If you are pregnant, the patient's chemotherapy may harm the baby.
    4. If you have a cough or skin infection, don a mask and gown.

23. The nurse is caring for a patient who underwent plasmapheresis. What is the **most** important assessment to make after the procedure? *(1941)*
    1. Monitor intake and output.
    2. Check blood pressure.
    3. Assess mental status.
    4. Evaluate pain.

CRITICAL THINKING ACTIVITIES

Activity 1

24. A 22-year-old patient has just completed allergy testing. Her health care provider has prescribed a regimen of weekly allergy shots.

    a. What special precautions should be taken after the injection? *(1933)* _____

    _____

    _____

    b. What teaching should be provided for a patient who is receiving allergy shots at home? *(1936)*

    _____

    _____

    _____

    c. After administering the shots at home for more than a month, the patient calls and reports she has been ill and unable to take the medications for the past 2 weeks. How should the nurse advise the patient? *(1934)*

    _____

    _____

Activity 2

25. A 67-year-old patient voices concern about his health status. He reports he never used to "get sick," but now has been hospitalized three times in the last year with a variety of illnesses. *(1933)*

   a. Discuss how aging affects the immune system. _____

   _____

   _____

   _____

   b. For an older patient, what would the nurse recommend to decrease risk for infection? _____

   _____

   _____

   _____

Activity 3

26. Design actual questions that the nurse could use to take a detailed history about a rash to help the health care provider diagnose the patient's allergies. Include: (1) onset, nature, and progression of signs and symptoms; (2) aggravating and alleviating factors; (3) frequency and duration of signs and symptoms; and (4) environmental, household, and occupational factors. *(1934)*

   _____

   _____

   _____

   _____

   _____

   _____

   _____

Care of the Patient With HIV/AIDS

chapter

56

SHORT ANSWER

Directions: Using your own words, answer each question in the space provided.

1. List at least four common opportunistic diseases associated with HIV. *(1959)*_____

   _____

   _____

   _____

   _____

2. List at least four barriers to adherence with HIV treatment recommendations. *(1964)*_____

   _____

   _____

   _____

   _____

3. List three questions that the nurse should ask when talking to new patients to evaluate risk assessment specific to HIV and sexually transmitted infections, as well as blood-borne diseases. *(1967)*

   _____

   _____

   _____

MULTIPLE CHOICE

Directions: Select the best answer(s) for each of the following questions.

4. HIV is transmitted from human to human through infected body fluids. Which body fluids are considered vehicles of transmission? **Select all that apply.** *(1975)*
   1. Blood
   2. Semen
   3. Cervicovaginal secretions
   4. Rectal secretions
   5. Urine
   6. Saliva

5. The nurse is teaching a patient living with HIV and her family about transmission of HIV. Which actions can the family and patient feel reassured are safe? **Select all that apply.** *(1947)*
   1. Hugging
   2. Shaking hands
   3. Breastfeeding the baby
   4. Sharing a computer keyboard
   5. Sharing food and utensils
   6. Petting and playing with the family dog

6. The nurse is on a committee to plan a series of educational programs for prevention of HIV. For the first program, the committee decides to focus on the most common mode of transmission and the people at greatest risk. Which group will be the **first** target audience? *(1947)*
   1. Receptive partners of men who have sex with men
   2. Heterosexual women who have sex with infected partners
   3. People who inject illicit drugs and share needles with others
   4. Health care workers who have occupational exposure

7. Which behavior combined with viral load status creates the **highest** risk for contracting HIV? *(1947)*
   1. Infected partner in mid-stage HIV performs insertive oral intercourse.
   2. Uninfected partner receives anal intercourse from infected partner in primary stage.
   3. Infected partner in mid-stage receives vaginal intercourse from uninfected partner.
   4. Uninfected partner performs insertive oral intercourse on infected partner in late stage.

8. What factors increase the risk of HIV for intravenous drug users? **Select all that apply.** *(1976)*
   1. Poor nutritional status and poor hygiene
   2. Exchanges sexual activity for drugs
   3. Impaired judgment due to illicit drug use
   4. Less likely to use condoms during sex
   5. Has ready access to sterile equipment
   6. Shares cookers and other paraphernalia

9. Which health care worker has sustained the **greatest** risk for HIV after being exposed to body fluids from patients who are HIV-positive? *(1977)*
   1. Deep puncture with a hollow-bore needle filled with blood from a patient's vein
   2. Splashed in the face with saliva and mucus during oral suctioning and hygiene
   3. Glove tears while cleaning the perianal area of a patient who has postpartum bleeding
   4. Patient vomits copious amounts of bloody fluid over the front of the worker's uniform

10. For a health care worker who must take post-exposure antiviral therapy, which signs/symptoms suggest that the worker is developing the **most** likely adverse effect of the drug therapy? *(1949)*
    1. Fatigue, activity intolerance, and a low red blood cell count
    2. Decreased urine output and elevated blood urea nitrogen
    3. Jaundice, malaise, and abnormal liver function tests
    4. Chest pain, arrhythmias, and elevated troponin levels

11. Perinatal or vertical transmission has been reduced by initiating which combination of interventions? *(1949)*
    1. Breastfeeding, enhanced maternal nutrition, and voluntary HIV testing
    2. Bottle-feeding, antiretroviral therapy for HIV-infected mothers, and cesarean birth
    3. Early prenatal care, natural childbirth, and antiretroviral therapy for HIV-infected babies
    4. Inducing labor during mid-stage HIV, and giving zidovudine syrup to neonate at birth

12. For a CD_4^+ lymphocyte level of 200 cells/mm^3, which clinical manifestations are **most** likely to be observed? *(1944)*
    1. Generally asymptomatic
    2. Mild flulike symptoms
    3. Opportunistic infections
    4. Fatal respiratory complications

13. What differentiates typical progressors from long-term nonprogressors and rapid progressors? *(1945)*
    1. Their physiologic response to standard antiviral therapy
    2. The age of the patient (i.e., rapid progressors are usually older)
    3. The length of time between seroconversion and symptom onset
    4. The number and combination of risk factors at time of exposure

14. What is the **primary** concern for a patient who has acute retroviral syndrome? *(1954)*
    1. Focus of care is palliative and life expectancy is approximately 3 years.
    2. Risk for opportunistic infections is increased and infections are less responsive to medication.
    3. Fever, night sweats, chronic diarrhea, headaches, and fatigue affect activities of daily living.
    4. Viral load and risk of transmission are extremely high, but symptoms are minor and mild.

15. The patient is advised to be tested for viral load 4-6 months after exposure. What is the clinical significance of having a lower viral set point at this stage? *(1954)*
    1. Used to determine the risk for exposing partner to HIV
    2. Predicts minor transient respiratory or skin infections
    3. Helps to determine the type and timing of therapy
    4. Used as a predictor of long-term survival

16. A 32-year-old patient diagnosed with HIV reports she is looking into some alternative and complementary therapies to treat her disease. What is the **best** response? *(1960)*
    1. "You should only rely on prescribed medications."
    2. "Those therapies can be costly and ineffective."
    3. "What kind of therapies are you considering?"
    4. "Let me know how they work for you."

17. While caring for a known HIV-positive patient in the emergency department, the nurse notices the phlebotomist preparing to draw blood. Which nursing action is correct? *(1960)*
    1. Do nothing, because all patients should be treated with Standard Precautions.
    2. Pull the technician aside and inform him about the patient's HIV status.
    3. Flag the chart to let all health care professionals know the patient's status.
    4. Discreetly hand a second pair of gloves to the technician as a signal.

18. An HIV-positive patient voices concern about his recurring bouts of diarrhea because he is making every effort to follow the treatment plan. What factors contribute to the diarrhea? **Select all that apply.** *(1968)*
    1. Side effects of the medications
    2. Infections of the gastrointestinal tract
    3. Damage to the intestinal villi
    4. Malabsorption in the intestinal tract
    5. Insufficient personal hygiene

19. A 34-year-old patient has recently been diagnosed with HIV-associated cognitive motor complex. Which assessment will the home health nurse initiate? *(1971)*
    1. Presence of numbness or tingling in hands or feet
    2. Level of consciousness based on Glasgow coma scale
    3. Home safety assessment to identify obstacles in hallways
    4. Pain in the extremities when ambulating or bending

20. The nurse is talking to a 17-year-old sexually active adolescent who is reluctant to use condoms because "It just doesn't feel as good." Which barrier to prevention is the adolescent demonstrating? *(1974)*
    1. Denial of risk
    2. Fear of alienation
    3. Lack of access
    4. Anxiety about sex

21. Which sexual activity would be considered the **safest**? *(1975)*
    1. Mutual monogamy
    2. Mutual masturbation
    3. Vaginal sex with condom
    4. Serial monogamy

22. What is a common presenting condition for HIV-positive women? *(1955)*
    1. Shingles
    2. Syphilis
    3. Vaginal candidiasis
    4. Weakness in extremities

23. Which breakfast tray offers the **best** selection of foods for a patient who has oral thrush? *(1970)*
    1. Grapefruit, hash browns, and an egg
    2. Oatmeal, vanilla yogurt, and canned peaches
    3. Orange juice, whole-wheat toast and jam
    4. Breakfast burrito with egg, bacon, and salsa

24. Which instructions about hygiene would the nurse give to the unlicensed assistive personnel (UAP) in assisting the patient who is living with HIV? *(1962)*
    1. Avoid washing any skin lesions.
    2. Check for areas of dependent edema.
    3. Add oil to tub bath if rash is present.
    4. Use a soft toothbrush and nonabrasive toothpaste.

25. The home health nurse is visiting a patient who has end-stage HIV disease. The patient's partner is the primary caregiver and other members of the family are also available to help. What is the **most** important goal of palliative care for this patient and family? *(1964)*
    1. Make plans for long-term care or home health assistance.
    2. Ensure that family complies with medication therapy.
    3. Relieve suffering caused by pain or other symptoms.
    4. Assess for disenfranchised grief and use active listening.

CRITICAL THINKING ACTIVITIES

Activity 1

26. A nursing student has just been stuck by a needle while providing care for a patient whose lifestyle has placed him at high risk for HIV infection. After reporting to the clinic, she has questions. *(1977)*

   a. What course of action should be taken initially? _____

   _____

   _____

   _____

   b. What patient-based factors will affect her level of susceptibility? _____

   _____

   _____

   _____

   c. Upon hearing the recommendation for her to begin prophylactic drug therapy, she asks to wait a few days before beginning the medication regimen. What is the best advice?

   _____

   _____

   _____

   _____

   d. After a discussion of the need to begin the medications as soon as possible, she asks for an explanation concerning the pros and cons of taking the drugs.

   _____

   _____

   _____

   _____

   e. The student voices concerns about having contact with her husband and child. How will the nurse respond to her concerns?

   _____

   _____

   _____

   _____

Copyright © 2019, 2015, 2011, 2006, 2003, 1999, 1995, 1991 by Mosby, an imprint of Elsevier Inc. All rights reserved.

Activity 2

27. A commercial sex worker has used the clinic for treatment for sexually transmitted infections over the past 3 years, but has always declined testing for HIV. Recently, the worker started to come in for a variety of infections that never seemed to fully resolve. Several nurses and health care providers talked to this patient about HIV testing and the benefits of early detection, but the patient said she assumes a "don't know, don't tell" position and that she tries to get all of her customers to use condoms. Several months later, the worker is admitted to the hospital for treatment of opportunistic infection secondary to HIV disease. Discuss the legal and ethical dilemmas for the clinic staff. *(1977)*

_____

_____

_____

_____

_____

_____

_____

_____

_____

Activity 3

28. Think about your personal feelings and concerns about taking care of a patient with HIV or AIDS. If possible, interview a nurse (or a patient) who experienced the early days of the HIV epidemic. Compare your own personal feelings to those of people who experienced the early days of HIV disease. *(1943-1945, 2004)*

_____

_____

_____

_____

_____

_____

_____

_____

_____

_____

_____

Care of the Patient With Cancer

MATCHING

Directions: Match the terms to the correct definition. Indicate your answers in the spaces provided.

Terms		Definition
_____	1. benign *(1987)*	a. Malignant tumors
_____	2. carcinoma *(1988)*	b. Process by which tumor cells spread
_____	3. differentiated *(1987)*	c. Abnormal cell growth with a loss of normal role and function, and ability to spread to other body sites
_____	4. malignant *(1987)*	d. Malignant tumors of connective tissues
_____	5. metastasis *(1987)*	e. Uncontrolled or abnormal growth of cells
_____	6. neoplasm *(1987)*	f. Recognizable as being the same in size or shape as normal cells
_____	7. sarcoma *(1988)*	g. Not recurrent or progressive; nonmalignant

SHORT ANSWER

8. What are four quality-of-life factors that affect cancer patients and their families? *(2006)*

   a. _____

   b. _____

   c. _____

   d. _____

9. Name at least five common concerns voiced by cancer patients. *(2006)*

   a. _____

   b. _____

   c. _____

   d. _____

   e. _____

10. What are the leading primary cancer sites for men? *(1981)*

    a. _____

    b. _____

    c. _____

    d. _____

11. What are the leading primary cancer sites for women? *(1981)*

    a. _____

    b. _____

    c. _____

    d. _____

12. What are the eight warning signs of cancer? *(1986)*

    a. _____

    b. _____

    c. _____

    d. _____

    e. _____

    f. _____

    g. _____

    h. _____

FIGURE LABELING

13. Directions: On the figure below, identify the four types of biopsy depicted. *(1989)*

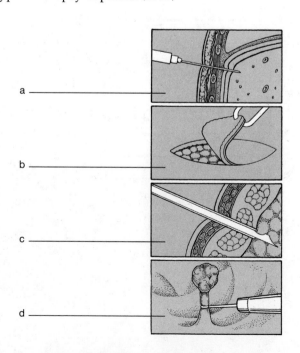

CLINICAL APPLICATION OF MATH

14. The American Cancer Society recommends adults engage in at least 150 minutes of moderate physical activity each week or 75 minutes of vigorous activity each week. *(1987)*
    a. Patient A desires to exercise five times a week doing moderate physical exercise. How many minutes per day will the patient have to spend for each session? _____ min
    b. Patient B desires to exercise six times a week doing moderate physical exercise. How many minutes per day will the patient have to spend for each session? _____ min
    c. Patient C desires to exercise three times a week doing vigorous physical exercise. How many minutes per day will the patient have to spend for each session? _____ min
    d. Patient D desires to exercise seven times a week doing vigorous physical exercise. How many minutes per day will the patient have to spend for each session? _____ min

15. The nurse knows that a 5% weight loss places the patient at risk for malnutrition and the health care provider should be notified. If the patient weighs 140 pounds, how many pounds would be considered a 5% loss? _____ pounds *(2005)*

16. The nutritionist tells the home health nurse that a 4.5 kg weight loss makes it difficult for the patient to maintain adequate nutritional status. The nurse closely monitors the patient's weight and nutritional intake. The patient weighed 123 lbs at the initial home health visit; today the patient weighs 118.5 lbs. How many kilograms has the patient lost? _____ kg *(2005)*

TABLE ACTIVITY

17. Directions: Fill in the normal values in the table below. *(1999)*

	Male	**Female**
Erythrocytes (RBCs)	million/mm³	million/mm³
Hemoglobin	g/dL	g/dL
Hematocrit	%	%

MULTIPLE CHOICE
Directions: Select the best answer(s) for each of the following questions.

18. Which person has the **greatest** risk for developing cancer? *(1983)*
    1. Older white male who started smoking at age 14
    2. Middle-age obese white female with sedentary lifestyle
    3. Young African American woman who is a vegetarian
    4. Older Asian American male who drinks socially

19. Based on the incidence of cancer and the mortality rate, which group has the **greatest** need for improvements in cancer prevention, detection, and treatment outcomes? *(1983)*
    1. Hispanic American females
    2. White American males
    3. Asian Americans
    4. African Americans

20. Which lunch tray contains the **best** selection of foods to reduce cancer risk? *(1983)*
    1. Three-bean salad with cheddar cheese and saltine crackers
    2. Cottage cheese with tomatoes and melon ball salad
    3. Bacon, lettuce, and tomato on wheat toast with potato chips
    4. Grilled fish with white rice and pickled vegetables

21. What is the clinical significance for persons who have the *BRCA1* and *BRCA2* genes? *(1984)*
    1. Increased incidence of lung cancer
    2. Increased incidence of leukemia
    3. Increased incidence of colon cancer
    4. Increased incidence of breast cancer

22. The nurse is volunteering at a local health fair and is talking with people about cancer prevention and screening recommendations. Which person should be referred for cancer risk assessment and genetic counseling? *(1984)*
    1. Admits to a long history of smoking tobacco and marijuana
    2. History of multiple primary cancers in one family member
    3. Has an occupational history of exposure to heavy metals
    4. Has a recent change in bowel movements with occasional bleeding

23. What is a clinical manifestation of testicular cancer? *(1985)*
    1. Erectile dysfunction
    2. Weak flow of urine
    3. An enlargement in either testicle
    4. Smooth consistency of testicles

24. Which person is the **most** likely candidate for low-dose helical CT for lung cancer screening? *(1986)*
    1. 35-year-old male who never smoked, but is anxious because his father died of lung cancer
    2. 55-year-old male quit smoking 5 years ago and is in fairly good health with a 30 pack-year history
    3. 25-year-old female has smoked for 10 years and is unable to accomplish smoking cessation
    4. 69-year-old female smoked for several years during her early twenties, but is currently healthy

25. What instructions should be given to boys and men about self-examination of the testes? **Select all that apply.** *(1985)*
    1. Should be done once a month.
    2. Feel for lumps or thickening.
    3. Check after a warm bath or shower.
    4. Self-examination should begin at puberty.
    5. Men older than 50 should stop self-examination.

26. Which dietary recommendation to decrease risk for cancer comes from the National Cancer Institute? *(1983)*
    1. Eat four to five servings of lean protein each day.
    2. Eat at least two servings of yellow cheese each day.
    3. Add several types of beans to your diet every week.
    4. Eat at least five servings of fruit and vegetables each day.

27. The patient states that she knows vitamin C is an important nutrient in the prevention of cancer, but she really dislikes citrus fruits. What is the **best** alternative source that the nurse could suggest? *(1983)*
    1. Taking a vitamin C supplement
    2. Trying citrus juice in place of fruit
    3. Eating strawberries or tomatoes
    4. Eating carrots or cauliflower

28. The nurse is talking to a 23-year-old woman about breast self-examination (BSE). What does the nurse tell the patient about timing and frequency of doing BSE? *(1984)*
    1. Perform the examination monthly on the first day of your menses.
    2. Perform the examination on the first day of every month.
    3. Perform the examination if you notice a discharge from the nipple.
    4. Perform the examination 2-3 days after your period ends.

29. A prostate-specific antigen (PSA) test is usually recommended at age 50. Beginning at age 40, members of which ethnic group need to be advised to get the test? *(1991)*
    1. Asian American
    2. African American
    3. Native American
    4. Hispanic American

30. According to clinical staging classification, which stage indicates the **most** extensive cancer with the poorest prognosis? *(1988)*
    1. Stage 0
    2. Stage I
    3. Stage III
    4. Stage IV

31. According to the TNM classification system, which set of parameters suggests the **best** prognosis? *(1988)*
    1. $T_0; N_0; M_0$
    2. $T_x; N_x; M_x$
    3. $T_{is}; N_1; M_1$
    4. $T_4; N_4; M_4$

32. The patient is having a radioisotope bone scan. He has had the radioactive material injected into his arm and the nurse encourages him to drink water for the next several hours. What is the purpose of encouraging fluids? *(1990)*
    1. Radioisotope that is not picked up by the bone will be flushed through the kidneys.
    2. The radioactive material could be harmful to the kidneys if not diluted and voided.
    3. The fluid enhances the contrast media and facilitates visualization of tumor areas.
    4. Extra fluid thins secretions and improves the visualization of the lung fields.

33. The health care provider is considering magnetic resonance imaging (MRI) for a patient who might have a spinal tumor. Prior to the MRI, the nurse would notify the provider if the patient disclosed which information? *(1990)*
    1. History of depression
    2. Family history of breast cancer
    3. History of hip fracture
    4. History of deep vein thrombosis

34. The health care provider informs the nurse that the patient may have metastasis to the bone. The provider requests that the nurse notify her immediately with the relevant results. Which test will the nurse be watching for? *(1990)*
    1. Serum calcitonin
    2. Alkaline phosphatase
    3. Carcinoembryonic antigen
    4. CA-125

35. The patient has a positive guaiac test, but he tells the nurse that he may have not followed the dietary instructions correctly. Which food substance is **most** likely to cause a false positive? *(1993)*
    1. A rare steak
    2. A double fudge sundae
    3. French fries with catsup
    4. Caffeinated soda

36. The nurse is present when the health care provider tells the patient that a combination of surgery, radiation, and chemotherapy are needed to treat his cancer. Afterwards, the patient angrily says, "I'm not going to spend my last days getting poked by that doctor. I'm leaving the hospital!" What should the nurse say? *(1994)*
    1. "I respect your decision, but is there anything I can do to help?"
    2. "Don't be hasty, you have just had bad news; wait for a while."
    3. "Please don't leave. The doctor is just trying to help you."
    4. "You are upset; that's understandable. Let me call your doctor."

37. The unlicensed assistive personnel (UAP) is assigned to assist with hygiene for a patient who is currently undergoing external radiation over a large portion of the trunk. What instructions will the nurse give? *(1995)*
    1. Gently clean the skin with a mild soap and flush with warm water.
    2. Do not put lotion, cream, or body powder over the marked areas.
    3. Help the patient take a shower, but use tepid water and a soft cloth.
    4. Shower according to usual procedure, but don't scrub the skin.

38. In caring for the patient who is being treated with internal radiation, what is the **most** important part of the nursing process for the nurse to prevent self-exposure? *(1996)*
    1. Assessment
    2. Planning
    3. Implementation
    4. Evaluation

39. The UAP is assigned to assist a patient who is being treated with radioactive material in the vagina. What instructions should the nurse give? *(1996)*
    1. Spend a maximum of 10 minutes to help with a bed bath from the waist up.
    2. Assist the patient with perineal care because vaginal discharge is likely.
    3. Help the patient ambulate to the shower if she is feeling well enough to walk.
    4. Turn the patient every 2 hours and remind her to do range-of-motion for her arms.

40. The patient is placed on neutropenic precautions for a neutrophil count of fewer than $1000/mm^3$. Which prescription would the nurse question? *(1997)*
    1. Take vital signs every 4 hours.
    2. Report temperature greater than 100.4° F (38° C).
    3. Catheterize for urine specimen.
    4. Administer filgrastim.

41. Which intervention is the nurse **most** likely to use for a patient who has "chemo brain"? *(1997)*
    1. Frequently orient the patient to person, place, and time.
    2. Perform the Glasgow coma scale at least once per shift.
    3. Help patient to establish routine and avoid multi-tasking.
    4. Instruct UAP to assist with most activities of daily living.

42. The patient has stomatitis secondary to chemotherapy. Which intervention will the nurse use? *(1998)*
    1. Suggest that the patient suck hard candy or chew gum.
    2. Help the patient rinse with mouthwash every 2-4 hours.
    3. Use a sponge-tipped applicator to perform frequent mouth care.
    4. Suggest drinking warm soup, tea, or other hot liquids.

43. The patient is receiving epoetin alfa. Which laboratory finding indicates that the therapy is helping? *(1999)*
    1. Normalization of the white cell count
    2. Improvement of the red cell count
    3. Increase in the platelet count
    4. Normalization of the electrolytes

44. Which observation would be consistent with a platelet count of fewer than 20,000/mm³? *(1999)*
    1. Extreme fatigue
    2. Decreased urine output
    3. High fever
    4. Bleeding gums

45. While caring for a 23-year-old patient undergoing chemotherapy, the patient voices concerns about her hair loss. What information would the nurse give to the patient? *(1999)*
    1. The loss of her hair will not be permanent.
    2. Hair loss will only affect facial areas.
    3. The hair just stops growing temporarily.
    4. When the hair grows back, it will be thicker.

46. During meal planning for a cancer patient, the patient reports that things have a "strange" taste, which is affecting her appetite. Which responses accurately pertain to her concern? **Select all that apply.** *(2005)*
    1. This is a common occurrence and will get better after the treatment ends.
    2. Taste alteration is a permanent consequence associated with treatment.
    3. Onion and ham may help to improve the taste of vegetables.
    4. Lemon juice is successfully used to mask strange taste sensations.
    5. Eat anything that seems appealing, just try to maintain the caloric intake.

47. Which factors are shown to have an impact on how a patient will cope with a diagnosis of cancer? **Select all that apply.** *(2006)*
    1. Age at the time of the diagnosis
    2. Availability of significant others
    3. Presence of symptoms
    4. Socioeconomic status
    5. Gender
    6. Ability to express feelings

48. The nurse is reviewing the patient's medication list and sees that the patient is taking ondansetron. What additional intervention will the nurse plan to use? *(2000)*
    1. Minimize food odors or noxious smells.
    2. Help the patient dangle before walking.
    3. Check the pulse before giving the drug.
    4. Place a sign on the door to limit visitors.

49. What is an **early** sign/symptom of tumor lysis syndrome? *(2001)*
    1. Anuria
    2. Muscle weakness
    3. Paresthesias
    4. Tetany

50. What is the **most** effective regimen to manage the patient's cancer pain? *(2004)*
    1. Patient-controlled analgesia
    2. Bolus dose for breakthrough pain
    3. Round-the-clock, fixed dose
    4. As needed, based on assessment

CRITICAL THINKING ACTIVITIES

Activity 1

51. During a routine checkup, a 40-year-old man voices questions about his potential for developing colon cancer. He relates his concerns about the recent death of his maternal grandfather from colon cancer.

    a. Discuss how a family history of colon cancer affects the recommendations for screening examinations for this patient. *(1984)*

    _____

    _____

    _____

    _____

b.   What preventive behaviors should be included in discussions with this patient? *(1987)* _____

_____

_____

_____

_____

Activity 2

52. A 32-year-old patient is being treated with unsealed internal radiation for thyroid cancer. Identify precautions to reduce radiation exposure to staff members who care for this patient. *(1996)*

_____

_____

_____

_____

_____

_____

_____

Professional Roles and Leadership

SHORT ANSWER

Directions: Using your own words, answer each question in the space provided.

1. What are the key components of a cover letter? *(2010, 2011)* _____

   _____

   _____

2. What are the advantages of membership in professional organizations? *(2016, 2017)* _____

   _____

   _____

3. For the NCLEX-PN® examination, identify the following. *(2019, 2020)*

   a. Minimum number of questions: _____

   b. Maximum number of questions: _____

   c. Maximum time allowed:_____

   d. Goal of computerized adaptive testing : _____

   e. Average time to receive results:_____

   f. Approval for candidate to take the test given by:_____

   g. Examples of alternate-item format questions:_____

4. List possible job settings for an LPN/LVN. *(2022)* _____

   _____

   _____

   _____

   _____

MULTIPLE CHOICE
Directions: Select the best answer(s) for each of the following questions.

5. A nurse is participating in a phone interview for a job at a pediatric walk-in clinic. Which question would be inappropriate for the interviewer to ask? *(2014)*
   1. "Have you ever been arrested for a criminal activity?"
   2. "Do you have hobbies or recreational activities that involve children?"
   3. "Do you think that pediatrics is part of your long-term career goals?"
   4. "Do you think that a person of your age could work with children?"

6. A newly graduated nurse is interviewing for her first job. Which question is the **most** important for the nurse to ask? *(2015)*
   1. "Is the employment contract verbal, implied, or written?"
   2. "What kind of internship or residency programs do you offer?"
   3. "How would I fit into the existing organizational chart?"
   4. "Would I have to take a competency test for medication or math?"

7. The LPN/LVN desires to have improved knowledge and skills in IV therapy. Which educational opportunity would be the **best** route for this nurse? *(2018)*
   1. Associate nursing degree
   2. In-service education
   3. Refresher course
   4. Certification

8. A smart, conscientious nursing student comes to see the nursing instructor immediately after taking the NCLEX-PN®. The student is distraught and tearful because "The questions were so hard. They seemed to get more difficult. At 85 questions, I got the message that the examination was over. I think I must have failed." What is the instructor's **best** response? *(2020)*
   1. "You seem really upset. Let's take a moment and talk about how you feel."
   2. "So, worst-case scenario, if you failed, what can do you to take the next steps?"
   3. "Difficult questions are selected by your performance; this reflects a high competence level."
   4. "Don't worry; generally having the system stop at 85 questions means that you have passed."

9. These nurses have recently relocated from another state and are working at a new job. Which nurse has the **greatest** need to clarify the nurse practice act before acting on the request? *(2018, 2021)*
   1. LPN/LVN gets a verbal order to insert a peripheral IV catheter; then push IV opioid medication.
   2. Supervising RN asks LPN/LVN to train and supervise new unlicensed assistive personnel (UAP).
   3. Patient requests that LPN/LVN explain the difference between power of attorney and living will.
   4. Another LPN/LVN asks if the nurse could switch a shift because of child care issues.

10. Under what circumstance would it be **most** appropriate for the nurse to contact the state board of nursing, if the nurse has already tried to go up the chain of command at the place of employment? *(2021)*
    1. LPN/LVN feels that competency testing was unfair because of culturally biased questions.
    2. Charge nurse shows favoritism to her friends when making out the patient assignments.
    3. Patient has threatened to name LPN/LVN in a lawsuit that involves physician malpractice.
    4. Supervising RN is making assignments that fall outside the LPN/LVN's scope of practice.

11. There has been an earthquake in the area, and disaster victims are being brought into the emergency department. In this situation, what type of leadership should the nurse manager use? *(2026)*
    1. Democratic
    2. Autocratic
    3. Situational
    4. Laissez-faire

12. The nursing student will be in a position to take the NCLEX-PN® within a few months. However, her fiancé is likely to be transferred to another state within the next year. What should the student do? *(2020)*
    1. Wait until the fiancé has moved and then apply to that state board of nursing to take NCLEX-PN®.
    2. Wait until after legally married to take the NCLEX-PN® so that the license will be issued under her married name.
    3. Apply to take the NCLEX-PN® in the current state of residency and investigate reciprocity or endorsement with other states.
    4. Apply to take the NCLEX-PN® in the current state of residency and then retake the NCLEX-PN® in the permanent state of residency.

13. A new nurse is unsure of the prescription that is written but believes that it is appropriate. What should the nurse do **first**? *(2029)*
    1. Transcribe it to the medication administration record.
    2. Report the problem to the nursing supervisor.
    3. Wait until the provider returns and ask for clarification.
    4. Ask a charge nurse or senior nurse to look at the prescription.

14. The patient had surgery in the morning, and during the evening requests medication for pain. The nurse administers a preoperative dose of an opioid medication. One hour later, the patient reports that the pain is unrelieved and the nurse realizes that she made an error. What should the nurse do **first**? *(2029, 2030)*
    1. Check the postoperative orders and give the correct dose.
    2. Inform the patient that additional medication cannot be given at this time.
    3. Report the error to the provider and ask for a one-time order for pain medication.
    4. Make out an incident report and document actions in the patient record.

15. The nurse is caring for several patients. Which tasks can be delegated to the UAP? **Select all that apply.** *(2027, 2028)*
    1. Taking the morning vital signs
    2. Changing the linens for isolation patients
    3. Restocking the medications and intravenous solutions
    4. Ambulating patients in the hallway
    5. Assessing skin condition while bathing
    6. Transcribing orders during the night shift

16. Which action could be considered negligence by the nurse and could potentially result in the loss of the nursing license? *(2021)*
    1. Fails to check patient allergies prior to administering medication, but patient suffers no harm
    2. Fails to report change of patient status to provider and later the patient has to be taken for emergency surgery
    3. Fails to give medication within the time limit established by the facility's policies and procedures
    4. Fails to come to work on time and so off-going nurse has to stay later to cover patient care

17. The nurse overhears another nurse, who is a friend, discussing patient information in the cafeteria. There are several visitors nearby and it appears that they are also overhearing the conversation. What should the nurse do **first**? *(2016)*
    1. Take the nurse aside and tell her that others are listening.
    2. Report the nurse to risk management.
    3. Walk over to the nurse and quickly change the subject.
    4. Write an incident report and submit it anonymously.

18. The nurse is assigned to be the chairman of a patient satisfaction committee. The committee will include nurses, UAP, and unit secretaries from other units in the hospital. Which style of leadership would be **most** useful? *(2027)*
    1. Autocratic
    2. Democratic
    3. Laissez-faire
    4. Situational

19. The nurse is working in a long-term care facility and instructs the UAP to assist several patients with morning hygiene and report back if anyone is having any problems. What delegation error has the nurse made? *(2027)*
    1. Has assigned the UAP too many patients
    2. Has given the UAP a task that is not within scope of practice
    3. Has given broad and generalized instructions to the UAP
    4. Has failed to give feedback on the UAP's performance

20. The new nurse is having difficulty with time management. She feels very frustrated and ends up staying late every day to complete her work. What should be the **first** step to improve time management? *(2027, 2028)*
    1. Ask for help if falling behind schedule.
    2. Stop socializing with colleagues.
    3. Reflect on how the time is being spent.
    4. Set goals every day and stick to them.

21. Which actions are considered part of the responsibilities of the nurse manager? **Select all that apply.** *(2026)*
    1. Submits staffing schedules for the unit
    2. Conducts regular staff meetings
    3. Role models nursing care for a group of assigned patients
    4. Recruits, interviews, and hires new employees
    5. Conducts routine staff evaluations
    6. Establishes necessary staff and interdisciplinary committees

CRITICAL THINKING ACTIVITIES

22. Identify a job or a practice setting that you would like to apply for. Describe what you will need to do to increase your chances of getting your first choice of position. *(2014)*

    _____

    _____

    _____

23. The nurse has just started a new job, but has never worked the night shift before. Identify self-care behaviors that the nurse could use for each of the following. *(2015)*

    a. Staying alert at work: _____

    _____

    b. Getting to sleep: _____

    _____

    c. Balancing life with work: _____

    _____

    d. While there are many disadvantages to working the night shift, the nurse is looking forward to the new job and decides to focus on some of the advantages. Identify several things that could be considered a benefit of being on this shift. (Hint: Interview several night-shift nurses to get a variety of opinions.)

    _____

    _____

    _____

24. a. Listen to several different nurses give change-of-shift report. Describe the strong points of the reports and describe parts of the reports that could have been improved. *(2030)*

    _____

    _____

    _____

    _____

    _____

b. Compare different styles of report that you have seen on clinical units (e.g., tape recordings, rounding on patients, etc.). If you have only seen one method, interview nurses and discuss with classmates or senior students. *(2030, 2031)*

_____

_____

_____

_____

Notes

Notes

Notes

Notes

Notes

Notes

Notes

Notes

Notes

Notes